Nursing Home Federal Requirements

Guidelines to Surveyors and Survey Protocols

Sixth Edition

New Topics in 2006 Edition

More than 25% of the federal guidelines have been modified in the past two years. In addition, the Survey protocols have been extensively modified to reflect the new QIS (quality indicators survey). In addition, we have added the following topics of direct relevance to the nursing home:

- Updated Definitions of Medicare and Medicaid
- Compliance Requirements With Title VI of the Civil Rights Act of 1964
- SNF/Hospice Requirements When SNF serves Hospice Patients
- SNF-Based Home Health Agencies
- Life Safety Code Requirements effective March 10, 2006
- Definitions of Certified Beds, Dually-Participating and Distinct Parts
- Changes in SNF Provider Status
- Surveyor Qualifications Standards
- Management of Complaints and Incidents

Using these guidelines and CMS forms

The following regulations, guidelines, procedures and probes are used by federal surveyors in certifying facilities for participation in Medicare and Medicaid, issuing deficiencies, requiring plans of correction, and imposing fines. The only official copy of these guidelines is the original copy retained by the U.S. government, hence this copy is not for official interpretations.

Quality assurance / Risk management

Facilities which implement these federal requirements will, by adopting these guidelines, have outstanding quality assurance and risk management programs in place! In short, these federal requirements, taken together, are a quality assurance program which Congress, the federal Centers for Medicare and Medicaid (CMS) and those others in authority over nursing facilities in the U.S. require that nursing facilities implement.

Updates are routinely posted on the CMS website.

Nursing Home Federal Requirements

Guidelines to Surveyors and Survey Protocols

2006

A user-friendly rendering of the
Centers for Medicare and Medicaid's (CMS)
nursing home inspection and requirement forms

6th Edition

James E. Allen, PhD, MSPH, CNHA
Associate Professor of Health Policy and Administration
University of North Carolina and Chapel Hill

Springer Publishing Company, LLC
11 West 42nd Street
New York, NY 10036-8002

Acquisitions Editor: Sheri W. Sussman
Managing Editor: Toni Ann Scaramuzzo
Production Editor: Megha Jain
Cover design by Mimi Flow
Composition: International Graphic Services

05 06 07 08 09 / 5 4 3 2 1

Library of Congress Cataloging-in-Publication Data

Allen, James E. (James Elmore), 1935-
Nursing home federal requirements : guidelines to surveyors and survey protocols / James E. Allen.— 6th ed.
  p. ; cm.
  Includes index.
  ISBN 0-8261-0267-0 1.
  Nursing homes—Law and legislation—United States. 2. Medicaid—Law and legislation.
3. Medicare—Law and legislation. [DNLM: 1. Nursing Homes—legislation & jurisprudence—United States. 2. Homes for the Aged—legislation & jurisprudence—United States.
3. Homes for the Aged—standards—United States—Legislation. 4. Medicaid—legislation &
jurisprudence. 5. Medicare—legislation & jurisprudence. WX 32 AA1 A42n 2006] I. Title.
KF3826.N8A3 2006 *2007*
344.7303'216—dc22   2006003754

Table of Contents by Subject

Medicare & Medicaid Final Requirements
&
Guidelines to Surveyors

§483.1   Basis and Scope

§483.5   Definitions

§483.10   Resident rights

(d) Free choice

(e) Privacy and confidentiality

(f) Grievances

(g) Examination of survey results

(h) Work

(i) Mail

(j) Access and visitation rights

(k) Telephone

(l) Personal property

(m) Married couples

(n)   Self-administration of drugs

(o)   Refusal of certain transfers

§483.12   Admission, transfer, and discharge rights

(a)   Transfer and discharge

(b)   Notice of bed-hold policy and readmission

(c)   Equal access to quality care

(d)   Admissions policy

§483.13   Resident behavior and facility practices

(a)   Restraints

(b)   Abuse

(c)   Staff treatment of residents

§483.15   Quality of life

(a)   Dignity

(b)   Self-determination and participation

(c)   Participation in resident and family groups

§483.20   Resident assessment

(c)   Accuracy of assessments

(d)   Comprehensive care plans

(e)   Discharge summary

(f)   Preadmission screening

§483.25   Quality of care

(a)   Activities of daily living

(b)   Vision and hearing

(k)   Special needs

(l)   Unnecessary drugs

(m)   Medication errors

§483.30   Nursing services

(a)   Sufficient staff

(b)   Registered nurse

(c)   Nursing facilities: waiver

(d)   SNFs: waiver

§483.35 Dietary services

§483.40   Physician services

(a)   Physician supervision

(b)   Physician visits

(c)   Frequency of physician visits

(d)   Availability of physicians for emergency care

(e)   Physician delegation of tasks in SNFs

(f)   Performance of physician tasks in NFs

§483.45   Specialized rehabilitative services

(a)   Provision of services

(b)   Qualifications

§483.55   Dental services

(a)   Skilled nursing facilities

(b)   Nursing facilities

§483.60   Pharmacy services

(a)   Procedures

(b)   Service consultation

(c)   Drug regimen review

(d)   Labeling of drugs
and biologicals

(d)   Resident rooms

(e)   Toilet facilities

(f)   Resident call systems

(g)   Dining and resident activities

(h)   Other environmental conditions

§483.75   Administration

(a)   Licensure

(b)   Compliance and

(c)   Relationship to
other HHS regulations

(d)   Governing body

(e)   Required training of
nursing aides

(f)   Proficiency of nurse aides

(g)   Staff qualifications

(h)   Use of outside resources

(i)   Medical director

(j)   Laboratory services

(k)   Radiology and other diagnostic services

(l)   Clinical records

(m)   Disaster and emergency preparedness

(n)   Transfer agreement

(o)   Quality assessment and assurance

(p)   Disclosure of ownership

Survey Protocol for Long-term Care Facilities

INDEX

(Rev. 9, 08-05-05)

New Topics in 2006 Edition

Appendix

CMS MANUAL SYSTEM

Department of Health & Human Services (DHHS)

Pub. 100-07 State Operations

Provider Certification

Centers for Medicare & Medicaid Services (CMS)

Transmittal 12

Date: OCTOBER 14, 2005

Table of Contents

(Rev.12, 10-14-05)

§483.13(c) Staff Treatment of Residents (F224 and F226)

§483.15 Quality of Life   Tags 240 – 258

§483.15(a) Dignity
§483.15(b) Self-Determination and Participation
§483.15(c) Participation in Resident and Family Groups
§483.15(d) Participation in Other Activities
§483.15(e) Accommodation of Needs
§483.15(f) Activities
§483.15(g) Social Services
§483.15(h) Environment

§483.20 Resident Assessment   Tags 271 – 285

§483.20(a) Admission Orders
§483.20(b) Comprehensive Assessments
§483.20(c) Quality Review Assessment
§483.20(d) Use
§483.20(e) Coordination
§483.20(f) Automated Data Processing Requirement
§483.20(g) Accuracy of Assessment
§483.20(h) Coordination
§483.20(i) Certification
§483.20(j) Penalty for Falsification
§483.20(k) Comprehensive Care Plans
§483.20(l) Discharge Summary
§483.20(m) Preadmission Screening for Mentally Ill Individuals and Individuals With Mental Retardation

§483.25 Quality of Care   Tags 309 – 354

§483.25(a) Activities of Daily Living
§483.25(b) Vision and hearing
§483.25(c) Pressure Sores
§483.25(d) Urinary Incontinence
§483.25(e) Range of motion
§483.25(f) Mental and Psychosocial Functioning
§483.25(g) Naso-Gastric Tubes
§483.25(h) Accidents
§483.25(i) Nutrition
§483.25(j) Hydration
§483.25(k) Special Needs
§483.25(l) Unnecessary Drugs
§483.25(m) Medication Errors

§483.65 Infection Control   Tags 441 – 445

§483.65(a) Infection Control Program
§483.65(b) Preventing Spread of Infection
§483.65(c) Linens

§483.70 Physical Environment   Tags 454 – 469

§483.70(a) Life Safety From Fire
§483.70(b) Emergency Power
§483.70(c) Space and equipment
§483.70(d) Resident Rooms
§483.70(e) Toilet Facilities
§483.70(f) Resident Call System
§483.70(g) Dining and Resident Activities
§483.70(h) Other Environmental Conditions

§483.75 Administration   Tags 490 – 522

§483.75(a) Licensure
§483.75(b) Compliance With Federal, State, and Local Laws and Professional Standards
§483.75(c) Relationship to Other HHS Regulations
§483.75(d) Governing Body
§483.75(e) Required Training of Nursing Aides
§483.75(f) Proficiency of Nurse Aides
§483.75(g) Staff Qualifications
§483.75(h) Use of Outside Resources
§483.75(i) Medical Director
§483.75(j) Laboratory Services
§483.75(k) Radiology and Other Diagnostic Services
§483.75(l) Clinical Records
§483.75(m) Disaster and Emergency Preparedness
§483.75(n) Transfer Agreement
§483.75(o) Quality Assessment and Assurance
§483.75(p) Disclosure of Ownership

§483.5 Definitions   Tag 150

§483.10 Resident Rights   Tags 151 – 177

§483.10(a) Exercise of Rights
§483.10(b) Notice of Rights and Services
§483.10(c) Protection of Resident Funds
§483.10(d) Free Choice
§483.10(e) Privacy and Confidentiality
§483.10(f) Grievances
§483.10(g) Examination of Survey Results
§483.10(h) Work
§483.10(i) Mail
§483.10(j) Access and Visitation Rights
§483.10(k) Telephone
§483.10(l) Personal Property
§483.10(m) Married Couples
§483.10(n) Self-Administration of Drugs
§483.10(o) Refusal of Certain Transfers

F150 Definition SNF, NF, resident rights overview

(Rev. 5, Issued: 11-19-04, Effective: 11-19-04, Implementation: 11-19-04)

§483.5 Definitions

(a) Facility defined. For purposes of this subpart "facility" means, a skilled nursing facility (SNF) or a nursing facility (NF) which meets the requirements of §§1819 or 1919(a), (b), (c), and (d) of the Social Security Act, the Act. "Facility" may include a distinct part of an institution specified in §440.40 of this chapter, but does not include an institution for the mentally retarded or persons with related conditions described in §440.150 of this chapter. For Medicare and Medicaid purposes (including eligibility, coverage, certification, and payment), the "facility" is always the entity which participates in the program, whether that entity is comprised of all of, or a distinct part of a larger institution. For Medicare, a SNF (see §1819(a)(1)), and for Medicaid, a NF (see §1919(a)(1)) may not be an institution for mental diseases as defined in §435.1009.

Interpretive Guidelines §483.5

The following are the statutory definitions at §§1819(a) and 1919(a) of the Act for a SNF and a NF:

"Skilled nursing facility" is defined as an institution (or a distinct part of an institution) which is primarily engaged in providing skilled nursing care and related services for residents who require medical or nursing care, or rehabilitation services for the rehabilitation of injured, disabled, or sick persons, and is not primarily for the care and treatment of mental diseases; has in effect a transfer agreement (meeting the requirements of §1861(1)) with one or more hospitals having agreements in effect under §1866; and meets the requirements for a SNF described in subsections (b), (c), and (d) of this section.

"Nursing facility" is defined as an institution (or a distinct part of an institution) which is primarily engaged in providing skilled nursing care and related services for residents who require medical or nursing care, rehabilitation services for the rehabilitation of injured, disabled, or sick persons, or on a regular basis, health-related care and services to individuals who because of their mental or physical condition require care and services (above the level of room and board) which can be made available to them only through institutional facilities, and is not primarily for the care and treatment of mental diseases; has in effect a transfer agreement (meeting the requirements of §1861(1)) with one or more hospitals having agreements in effect under §1866; and meets the requirements for a NF described in subsections (b), (c), and (d) of this section.

If a provider does not meet one of these definitions, it cannot be certified for participation in the Medicare and/or Medicaid programs.

NOTE: If the survey team finds substandard care in §§483.13, 483.15, or 483.25, follow the instructions for partial extended or extended surveys.

---

§483.10 Resident Rights

The resident has a right to a dignified existence, self-determination, and communication with and access to persons and services inside and outside the facility. A facility must protect and promote the rights of each resident, including each of the following rights:

Interpretive Guidelines §483.10

All residents in long-term care facilities have rights guaranteed to them under Federal and State law. Requirements concerning resident rights are specified in §§483.10, 483.12, 483.13, and 483.15. Section 483.10 is intended to lay the foundation for the remaining resident's rights requirements which cover more specific areas. These rights include the resident's right to:

- Exercise his or her rights (§483.10(a));
- Be informed about what rights and responsibilities he or she has (§483.10(b));
- If he or she wishes, have the facility manage his personal funds (§483.10(c));
- Choose a physician and treatment and participate in decisions and care planning (§483.10(d));

- Privacy and confidentiality (§483.10(e));
- Voice grievances and have the facility respond to those grievances (§483.10(f));
- Examine survey results (§483.10(g));
- Work or not work (§483.10(h));
- Privacy in sending and receiving mail (§483.10(i));
- Visit and be visited by others from outside the facility (§483.10(j));
- Use a telephone in privacy (§483.10(k));
- Retain and use personal possessions (§483.10(1)) to the maximum extent that space and safety permit;
- Share a room with a spouse, if that is mutually agreeable (§483.10(m));
- Self-administer medication, if the interdisciplinary care planning team determines it is safe (§483.10(n)); and
- Refuse a transfer from a distinct part, within the institution (§483.10(o)).

A facility must promote the exercise of rights for each resident, including any who face barriers (such as communication problems, hearing problems, and cognition limits) in the exercise of these rights. A resident, even though determined to be incompetent, should be able to assert these rights based on his or her degree of capability.

F151 Resident exercise of rights without reprisal

§483.10(a) Exercise of Rights

§483.10(a)(1) The resident has the right to exercise his or her rights as a resident of the facility and as a citizen or resident of the United States.

§483.10(a)(2) The resident has the right to be free of interference, coercion, discrimination, and reprisal from the facility in exercising his or her rights.

Interpretive Guidelines §483.10(a)(1)

Exercising rights means that residents have autonomy and choice, to the maximum extent possible, about how they wish to live their everyday lives and receive care, subject to the facility's rules, as long as those rules do not violate a regulatory requirement.

Intent §483.10(a)(2)

This regulation is intended to protect each resident in the exercise of his or her rights.

Interpretive Guidelines §483.10(a)(2)

The facility must not hamper, compel, treat differentially, or retaliate against a resident for exercising his/her rights. Facility behaviors designed to support and encourage resident participation in meeting care planning goals as documented in the resident assessment and care plan are not interference or coercion.

Examples of facility practices that may limit autonomy or choice in exercising rights include reducing the group activity time of a resident trying to organize a residents' group; requiring residents to seek prior approval to distribute information about the facility; discouraging a resident from hanging a religious ornament above his or her bed; singling out residents for prejudicial treatment such as isolating residents in activities; or purposefully assigning inexperienced aides to a resident with heavy care needs because the resident and/or his/her representative, exercised his/her rights.

Procedures §483.10(a)(2)

Pay close attention to resident or staff remarks and staff behavior that may represent deliberate actions to promote or to limit a resident's autonomy or choice, particularly in ways that affect independent functioning. Because reprisals may indicate abuse, if the team determines that a facility has violated this requirement through reprisals taken against residents, then further determine if the facility has an effective system to prevent the neglect and abuse of residents. (§483.13(c), F224-F225.)

F152 Resident rights exercised by surrogates

§483.10(a)(3) — In the case of a resident adjudged incompetent under the laws of a State by a court of competent jurisdiction, the rights of the resident are exercised by the person appointed under State law to act on the resident's behalf.

§483.10(a)(4) — In the case of a resident who has not been adjudged incompetent by the State court, any legal-surrogate designated in accordance with State law may exercise the resident's rights to the extent provided by State law.

Interpretive Guidelines §483.10(a)(3) and (4)

When reference is made to "resident" in the Guidelines, it also refers to any person who may, under State law, act on the resident's behalf when the resident is unable to act for himself or herself. That person is referred to as the resident's surrogate or representative. If the resident has been formally declared incompetent by a court, the surrogate or representative is whoever was appointed by the court — a guardian, conservator, or committee. The facility should verify that a surrogate or representative has the necessary authority. For example, a court-appointed conservator might have the power to make financial decisions, but not health care decisions.

A resident may wish to delegate decision-making to specific persons, or the resident and family may have agreed among themselves on a decision-making process. To the degree permitted by State law, and to the maximum extent practicable, the facility must respect the resident's wishes and follow that process.

The rights of the resident that may be exercised by the surrogate or representative include the right to make health care decisions. However, the facility may seek a health care decision (or any other decision or authorization) from a surrogate or representative only when the resident is unable to make the decision. If there is a question as to whether the resident is able to make a health care decision, staff should discuss the matter with the resident at a suitable time and judge how well the resident understands the information. In the case of a resident who has been formally declared incompetent by a court, lack of capacity is presumed. Notwithstanding the above, if such a resident can understand the situation and express a preference, the resident should be informed and his/her wishes respected to the degree practicable. Any violations with respect to the resident's exercise of rights should be cited under the applicable tag number.

The involvement of a surrogate or representative does not automatically relieve a facility of its duty to protect and promote the resident's interests. For example, a surrogate or representative does not have the right to insist that a treatment be performed that is not medically appropriate, and the right of a surrogate or representative to reject treatment may be subject to State law limits.

Procedures §483.10(a)(3) and (4)

Determine as appropriate if the rights of a resident who has been adjudged incompetent or who has a representative acting on his/her behalf to help exercise his/her rights are exercised by the legally appointed individual.

F153 Resident rights to all records

§483.10(b)(2) – The resident or his or her legal representative has the right—

(i) Upon an oral or written request, to access all records pertaining to himself or herself including current clinical records within 24 hours (excluding weekends and holidays); and

(ii) After receipt of his or her records for inspection, to purchase at a cost not to exceed the community standard photocopies of the records or any portions of them upon request and 2 working days advance notice to the facility.

Interpretive Guidelines §483.10(b)(2)

An oral request is sufficient to produce the current record for review.

In addition to clinical records, the term "records" includes all records pertaining to the resident, such as trust fund ledgers pertinent to the resident and contracts between the resident and the facility.

"Purchase" is defined as a charge to the resident for photocopying. If State statute has defined the "community standard" rate, facilities should follow that rate. In the absence of State statute, the "cost not to exceed the community standard" is that rate charged per copy by organizations such as the public library, the Post Office or a commercial copy center, which would be selected by a prudent buyer in addition to the cost of the clerical time needed to photocopy the records. Additional fees for locating the records or typing forms/envelopes may not be assessed.

F154 Resident rights to full total health status information

(Rev. 5, Issued: 11-19-04, Effective: 11-19-04, Implementation: 11-19-04)

§483.10(b)(3) — The resident has the right to be fully informed in language that he or she can understand of his or her total health status, including but not limited to, his or her medical condition;

Interpretive Guidelines §483.10(b)(3)

"Total health status" includes functional status, medical care, nursing care, nutritional status, rehabilitation and restorative potential, activities potential, cognitive status, oral health status, psychosocial status, and sensory and physical impairments. Information on health status must be presented in language that the resident can understand. This includes minimizing use of technical jargon in communicating with the resident, having the ability to communicate in a foreign language and the use of sign language or other aids, as necessary. (See §483.10(d)(3), F175, for the right of the resident to plan care and treatment.)

Procedures §483.10(b)(3)

Look, particularly during observations and record reviews, for on-going efforts on the part of facility staff to keep residents informed. Look for evidence that information is communicated in a manner that is understandable to residents and communicated at times it could be most useful to residents, such as when they are expressing concerns, or raising questions, as well as on an on-going basis.

§483.10(d)(2) — The resident has the right to be fully informed in advance about care and treatment and of any changes in that care or treatment that may affect the resident's well-being;

Interpretive Guidelines §483.10(d)(2)

"Informed in advance" means that the resident receives information necessary to make a health care decision, including information about his/her medical condition and changes in medical condition, about the benefits and reasonable risks of the treatment, and about reasonable available alternatives.

F155 Resident rights to advance directives, to refuse treatment and/or research

§483.10(b)(4) — The resident has the right to refuse treatment, to refuse to participate in experimental research, and to formulate an advance directive as specified in paragraph (8) of this section; and

Interpretive Guidelines §483.10(b)(4)

"Treatment" is defined as care provided for purposes of maintaining/restoring health, improving functional level, or relieving symptoms.

"Experimental research" is defined as development and testing of clinical treatments, such as an investigational drug or therapy, that involve treatment and/or control groups. For example, a clinical trial of an investigational drug would be experimental research.

"Advance directive" means a written instruction, such as a living will or durable power of attorney for health care, recognized under State law relating to the provision of health care when the individual is incapacitated.

As provided under State law, a resident who has the capacity to make a health care decision and who withholds consent to treatment or makes an explicit refusal of treatment either directly or through an advance directive, may not be treated against his/her wishes.

A facility may not transfer or discharge a resident for refusing treatment unless the criteria for transfer or discharge are met. (See §483.12(a)(1) and (2).)

If the resident is unable to make a health care decision, a decision by the resident's surrogate or representative to forego treatment may, subject to State law, be equally binding on the facility. The facility should determine exactly what the resident is refusing and why. To the extent the facility is able, it should address the resident's concern. For example, a resident requires physical therapy to learn to walk again after sustaining a fractured hip. The resident refuses therapy. The facility is expected to assess the reasons for this resident's refusal, clarify and educate the resident as to the consequences of refusal, offer alternative treatments, and continue to provide all other services.

If a resident's refusal of treatment brings about a significant change, the facility should reassess the resident and institute care planning changes. A resident's refusal of treatment does not absolve a facility from providing a resident with care that allows him/her to attain or maintain his/her highest practicable physical, mental, and psychosocial well-being in the context of making that refusal.

The resident has the right to refuse to participate in experimental research. A resident being considered for participation in experimental research must be fully informed of the nature of the experiment (e.g., medication, treatment) and understand the possible consequences of participating. The opportunity to refuse to participate in experimental research must occur prior to the start of the research. Aggregated resident statistics that do not identify individual residents may be used for studies without obtaining residents' permission.

Procedures §483.10(b)(4)

If the facility participates in any experimental research involving residents, does it have an Institutional Review Board or other committee that reviews and approves research protocols? In this regard, §483.75(c), Relationship to Other HHS Regulations applies (i.e., the facility must adhere to 45 CFR Part 46, Protection of Human Subjects of Research).

See §483.10(b)(8), F156 with respect to the advance directive requirement.

F156 Resident rights to information on medical care and insurance coverage

(Rev. 5, Issued: 11-19-04, Effective: 11-19-04, Implementation: 11-19-04)

§483.10(b)(1) — The facility must inform the resident both orally and in writing in a language that the resident understands of his or her rights and all rules and regulations governing resident conduct and responsibilities during the stay in the facility. The facility must also provide the resident with the notice (if any) of the State developed under §1919(e)(6) of the Act. Such notification must be made prior to or upon admission and during the resident's stay. Receipt of such information, and any amendments to it, must be acknowledged in writing;

Intent §483.10(b)(1)

This requirement is intended to assure that each resident knows his or her rights and responsibilities and that the facility communicates this information prior to or upon admission, as appropriate during the resident's stay, and when the facility's rules change.

Interpretive Guidelines §483.10(b)(1)

"In a language that the resident understands" is defined as communication of information concerning rights and responsibilities that is clear and understandable to each resident, to the extent possible considering impediments which may be created by the resident's health and mental status. If the resident's knowledge of English or the predominant language of the facility is inadequate for comprehension, a means to communicate the information concerning rights and responsibilities in a language familiar to the resident must be available and implemented. For foreign languages commonly encountered in the facility locale, the facility should have written translations of its statements of rights and responsibilities, and should make the services of an interpreter available. In the case of less commonly encountered foreign languages, however, a representative of the resident may sign that he or she has explained the statement of rights to the resident prior to his/her acknowledgement of receipt. For hearing impaired residents who communicate by signing, the facility is expected to provide an interpreter. Large print texts of the facility's statement of resident rights and responsibilities should also be available.

"Both orally and in writing" means if a resident can read and understand written materials without assistance, an oral summary, along with the written document, is acceptable.

Any time State or Federal laws relating to resident rights or facility rules change during the resident's stay in the facility, he/she must promptly be informed of these changes.

"All rules and regulations" relates to facility policies governing resident conduct. A facility cannot reasonably expect a resident to abide by rules he or she has never been told about. Whatever rules the facility has formalized, and by which it expects residents to abide, should be included in the statement of rights and responsibilities.

§483.10(b)(5) — The facility must—

(i) Inform each resident who is entitled to Medicaid benefits, in writing, at the time of admission to the nursing facility or, when the resident becomes eligible for Medicaid of—

(A) The items and services that are included in nursing facility services under the State plan and for which the resident may not be charged;

(B) Those other items and services that the facility offers and for which the resident may be charged, and the amount of charges for those services; and

(ii) Inform each resident when changes are made to the items and services specified in paragraphs (5)(i)(A) and (B) of this section.

§483.10(b)(6) — The facility must inform each resident before, or at the time of admission, and periodically during the resident's stay, of services available in the facility and of charges for those services, including any charges for services not covered under Medicare or by the facility's per diem rate.

Interpretive Guidelines §483.10(b)(5) and (6)

Residents should be told in advance when changes will occur in their bills. Providers must fully inform the resident of services and related changes.

"Periodically" means that whenever changes are being introduced that will affect the residents liability and whenever there are changes in services.

A Medicare beneficiary who requires services upon admission that are not covered under Medicare may be required to submit a deposit provided the notice provisions of §483.10(b)(6), if applicable, are met.

Procedures §483.10(b)(5) and (6)

See §483.10(c)(8) for those items and services that must be included in payment under skilled nursing and nursing facility benefits.

§483.10(b)(7) — The facility must furnish a written description of legal rights which includes—

(i) A description of the manner of protecting personal funds, under paragraph (c) of this section;

(ii) A description of the requirements and procedures for establishing eligibility for Medicaid, including the right to request an assessment under section 1924(c) which determines the extent of a couple's non-exempt resources at the time of institutionalization and attributes to the community spouse an equitable share of resources which cannot be considered available for payment toward the cost of the institutionalized spouse's medical care in his or her process of spending down to Medicaid eligibility levels;

(iii) A posting of names, addresses, and telephone numbers of all pertinent State client advocacy groups such as the State survey and certification agency, the State licensure office, the State ombudsman program, the protection and advocacy network, and the Medicaid fraud control unit; and

(iv) A statement that the resident may file a complaint with the State survey and certification agency concerning resident abuse, neglect, and misappropriation of resident property in the facility, and non-compliance with the advance directives requirements.

Interpretive Guidelines §483.10(b)(7)

"The protection and advocacy network" refers to the system established to protect and advocate the rights of individuals with developmental disabilities specified in the Developmental Disabilities Assistance and Bill of Rights Act, and the protection and advocacy system established under the Protection and Advocacy for Mentally Ill Individuals Act.

Procedures §483.10(b)(7)

At the Entrance Conference, request a copy of the written information that is provided to residents regarding their rights and review it to determine if it addresses the specified requirements. Additional requirements that address the implementation of these rights are cross-referenced below.

§483.10(b)(8) — The facility must comply with the requirements specified in subpart I of part 489 of this chapter relating to maintaining written policies and procedures regarding advance directives. These requirements include provisions to inform and provide written information to all adult residents concerning the right to accept or refuse medical or surgical treatment and, at the individual's option, formulate an advance directive. This includes a written description of the facility's policies to implement advance directives and applicable State law

Interpretive Guidelines §483.10(b)(8)

This provision applies to residents admitted on or after December 1, 1991. 42 CFR 489.102 specifies that at the time of admission of an adult resident, the facility must:

- Provide written information concerning his/her rights under State law (whether or not statutory or recognized by the courts of the State) to make decisions concerning medical care, including the right to accept or refuse medical or surgical treatment, and the right to formulate advance directives;
- Document in the resident's medical record whether or not the individual has executed an advance directive;
- Not condition the provision of care or discriminate against an individual based on whether or not the individual has executed an advance directive;
- Ensure compliance with requirements of State law regarding advance directives;
- Provide for educating staff regarding the facility's policies and procedures on advance directives; and
- Provide for community education regarding the right under State law (whether or not recognized by the courts of the State) to formulate an advance directive and the facility's written policies and procedures regarding the implementation of these rights, including any limitations the facility may have with respect to implementing this right on the basis of conscience.

The facility is not required to provide care that conflicts with an advance directive. In addition, the facility is not required to implement an advance directive if, as a matter of conscience, the provider cannot implement an advance directive and State law allows the provider to conscientiously object. (See §483.10(b)(4), F155.)

The sum total of the community education efforts must include a summary of the State law, the rights of residents to formulate advance directives, and the facility's implementation policies regarding advance directives. Video and audio tapes may be used in conducting the community education effort. Individual education programs do not have to address all the requirements if it would be inappropriate for a particular audience.

Procedures §483.10(b)(8)

During Resident Review, review the records of two selected sampled residents admitted on or after December 1, 1991, for facility compliance with advance directive notice requirements.

- Determine to what extent the facility educates its staff regarding advance directives.
- Determine to what extent the facility provides education for the community regarding one's rights under State law to formulate advance directives.

§483.10(b)(9) — The facility must inform each resident of the name, specialty, and way of contacting the physician responsible for his or her care.

Interpretive Guidelines §483.10(b)(9)

"Physician responsible for his or her care" is defined as the attending or primary physician or clinic, whichever is responsible for managing the resident's medical care, and excludes other physicians whom the resident may see from time to time. When a resident has selected an attending physician, it is appropriate for the facility to confirm that choice when complying with this requirement. When a resident has no attending physician, it is appropriate for the facility to assist residents to obtain one in consultation with the resident and subject to the resident's right to choose. (See §483.10(d)(1), F163.)

If a facility uses the services of a clinic or similar arrangement, it may be sufficient for residents to have the name and contact information for the primary physician and/or a central number for the clinic itself.

§483.10(b)(10) — The facility must prominently display in the facility written information, and provide to residents and applicants for admission oral and written information about how to apply for and use Medicare and Medicaid benefits, and how to receive refunds for previous payments covered by such benefits.

Interpretive Guidelines §483.10(b)(10)

To fulfill this requirement, the facility may use written materials issued by the State Medicaid agency and the Federal government relating to these benefits. Facilities may fulfill their obligation to orally inform residents or applicants for admission about how to apply for Medicaid or Medicare by assisting them in contacting the local Social Security Office or the local unit of the State Medicaid agency. Nursing facilities are not responsible for orally providing detailed information about Medicare and Medicaid eligibility rules.

"Refunds for previous payments" refers to refunds due as a result of Medicaid and Medicare payments when eligibility has been determined retroactively.

As part of determining Medicaid eligibility, at the time of admission, a married couple has the right to request and have the appropriate State agency assess the couple's resources.

F157 Notifications required upon change in resident's condition or resident's rights

§483.10(b)(11) — Notification of changes.

(i) A facility must immediately inform the resident; consult with the resident's physician; and if known, notify the resident's legal representative or an interested family member when there is—

(A) An accident involving the resident which results in injury and has the potential for requiring physician intervention;

(B) A significant change in the resident's physical, mental, or psychosocial status (i.e., a deterioration in health, mental, or psychosocial status in either life-threatening conditions or clinical complications);

(C) A need to alter treatment significantly (i.e., a need to discontinue an existing form of treatment due to adverse consequences, or to commence a new form of treatment); or

(D) A decision to transfer or discharge the resident from the facility as specified in §483.12(a).

(ii) The facility must also promptly notify the resident and, if known, the resident's legal representative or interested family member when there is—

(A) A change in room or roommate assignment as specified in §483.15(e)(2); or

(B) A change in resident rights under Federal or State law or regulations as specified in paragraph (b)(1) of this section.

(iii) The facility must record and periodically update the address and phone number of the resident's legal representative or interested family member.

Interpretive Guidelines §483.10(b)(11)

For purposes of §483.10(b)(11)(i)(B), life-threatening conditions are such things as a heart attack or stroke. Clinical complications are such things as development of a stage II pressure sore, onset or recurrent periods of delirium, recurrent urinary tract infection, or onset of depression. A need to alter treatment "significantly" means a need to stop a form of treatment because of adverse consequences (e.g., an adverse drug reaction), or commence a new form of treatment to deal with a problem (e.g., the use of any medical procedure, or therapy that has not been used on that resident before).

In the case of a competent individual, the facility must still contact the resident's physician and notify interested family members, if known. That is, a family that wishes to be informed would designate a member to receive calls. Even when a resident is mentally competent, such a designated family member should be notified of significant changes in the resident's health status because the resident may not be able to notify them personally, especially in the case of sudden illness or accident.

The requirements at §483.10(b)(1) require the facility to inform the resident of his/her rights upon admission and during the resident's stay. This includes the resident's right to privacy (§483.10(e), F164). If, after being informed of the right to privacy, a resident specifies that he/she wishes to exercise this right and not notify family members in the event of a significant change as specified at this requirement, the facility should respect this request, which would obviate the need to notify the resident's interested family member or legal representative, if known. If a resident specifies that he/she does not wish to exercise the right to privacy, then the facility is required to comply with the notice of change requirements.

In the case of a resident who is incapable of making decisions, the representative would make any decisions that have to be made, but the resident should still be told what is happening to him or her.

In the case of the death of a resident, the resident's physician is to be notified immediately in accordance with State law.

The failure to provide notice of room changes could result in an avoidable decline in physical, mental, or psychosocial well-being.

F158 Resident's right to manage his/her financial affairs

§483.10(c)(1) Protection of Resident Funds

The resident has the right to manage his or her financial affairs, and the facility may not require residents to deposit their personal funds with the facility.

F159 Facility requirements when managing resident funds

§483.10(c)(2) Management of Personal Funds

Upon written authorization of a resident, the facility must hold, safeguard, manage, and account for the personal funds of the resident deposited with the facility, as specified in paragraphs (c)(3)-(8) of this section.

§483.10(c)(3) Deposit of Funds

(i) Funds in excess of $50. The facility must deposit any residents' personal funds in excess of $50 in an interest bearing account (or accounts) that is separate from any of the facility's operating accounts, and that credits all interest earned on resident's funds to that account. (In pooled accounts, there must be a separate accounting for each resident's share.)

(ii) Funds less than $50. The facility must maintain a resident's personal funds that do not exceed $50 in a non-interest bearing account, interest-bearing account, or petty cash fund.

NOTE: The Social Security Amendments of 1994 amended §1819(c)(6)(B)(i) to raise the limit from $50.00 to $100.00 for the minimum amount of resident funds that facilities must entrust to an interest-bearing account. This increase applies only to Medicare SNF residents. While a facility may continue to follow a minimum of $50.00, the regulations do not require it.

Interpretive Guidelines §483.10(c)(1) through (3)

This requirement is intended to assure that residents who have authorized the facility in writing to manage any personal funds have ready and reasonable access to those funds. If residents choose to have the facility manage their funds, the facility may not refuse to handle these funds, but is not responsible for knowing about assets not on deposit with it.

Placement of residents' personal funds of less than $50.00 ($100.00 for Medicare residents) in an interest bearing account is permitted. Thus, a facility may place the total amount of a resident's funds, including funds of $50.00 ($100.00 for Medicare residents) or less, into an interest-bearing account. The law and regulations are intended to assure that residents have access to $50.00 ($100.00 for Medicare residents) in cash within a reasonable period of time, when requested. Requests for less than $50.00 ($100.00 for Medicare residents) should be honored within the same day. Requests for $50.00 ($100.00 for Medicare residents) or more should be honored within three banking days. Although the facility need not maintain $50.00 ($100.00 for Medicare residents) per resident on its premises, it is expected to maintain amounts of petty cash on hand that may be required by residents.

If pooled accounts are used, interest must be prorated per individual on the basis of actual earnings or end-of-quarter balance.

Residents should have access to petty cash on an ongoing basis and be able to arrange for access to larger funds.

"Hold, safeguard, manage and account for" means that the facility must act as fiduciary of the resident's funds and report at least quarterly on the status of these funds in a clear and understandable manner. Managing the resident's financial affairs includes money that an individual gives to the facility for the sake of providing a resident with a noncovered service (such as a permanent wave). It is expected that in these instances, the facility will provide a receipt to the gift giver and retain a copy.

"Interest-bearing" means a rate of return equal to or above the passbook savings rate at local banking institutions in the area.

Although the requirements are silent about oral requests by residents to have a facility hold personal funds, under the provisions regarding personal property (§483.10(l)), and misappropriation of property (§483.13(c)), residents may make oral requests that the facility temporarily place their funds in a safe place, without authorizing the facility to manage those funds. The facility has the responsibility to implement written procedures to prevent the misappropriation of these funds.

If you determine potential problems with funds through interviews, follow up using the following procedures as appropriate:

If the facility does not have written authorization to handle resident's funds, but is holding funds for more than a few days, determine if the facility is managing these funds without written authorization. There must be written authorization for the facility to be in compliance with this requirement.

To assure that facilities are not using oral requests by residents as a way to avoid obtaining written authorization to hold, manage, safeguard, and account for residents' funds, make sure that:

- There is a written declaration by the resident that the funds are being held for no more than a few days by the facility at the resident's request;
- These funds are not held for more than a few days; and
- The facility provides the resident a receipt for these funds and retains a copy for its records.

Review the administrative or business file and the bookkeeping accounts of residents selected for a comprehensive review who have authorized the facility to handle their personal funds.

- Are residents' funds over $50.00 ($100.00 for Medicare residents) or, at the facility's option, all resident funds, in an interest bearing account(s)?
- What procedure was followed when residents requested their funds?
- How long does it take for residents to receive: (a) petty cash allotments; (b) funds needing to be withdrawn from bank accounts?
- Were limits placed on amounts that could be withdrawn? If yes, was the reason based on resident care needs or facility convenience?
- Are funds records treated with privacy as required at F164?

NOTE: Banks may charge the resident a fee for handling their funds. Facilities may not charge residents for managing residents' funds because the services are covered by Medicare or Medicaid.

If problems are identified, review also §483.10(b)(7), Tag F156.

Monies due residents should be credited to their respective bank accounts within a few business days.

§483.10(c)(4) Accounting and Records

The facility must establish and maintain a system that assures a full and complete and separate accounting, according to generally accepted accounting principles, of each resident's personal funds entrusted to the facility on the resident's behalf.

(i) The system must preclude any commingling of resident funds with facility funds or with the funds of any person other than another resident.

(ii) The individual financial record must be available through quarterly statements and on request to the resident or his or her legal representative.

Interpretive Guidelines §483.10(c)(4)

This requirement constitutes the overall response of the facility to the resident's right to have the facility manage the resident's funds.

"Generally accepted accounting principles" means that the facility employs proper bookkeeping techniques, by which it can determine, upon request, the amount of individual resident funds and, in the case of an interest-bearing account, how much interest these funds have earned for each resident, as last reported by the banking institution to the facility.

Proper bookkeeping techniques would include an individual ledger card, ledger sheet, or equivalent established for each resident on which only those transactions involving his or her personal funds are recorded and maintained. The record should have information on when transactions occurred, what they were, as well as maintain the ongoing balance for every resident.

Anytime there is a transaction the resident should be given a receipt and the facility retains a copy.

Monies due residents should be credited to their respective bank accounts within a few business days.

"Quarterly statements" are to be provided in writing to the resident or the resident's representative within 30 days after the end of the quarter.

§483.10(c)(5) Notice of Certain Balances

The facility must notify each resident that receives Medicaid benefits—

(i) When the amount in the resident's account reaches $200 less than the SSI resource limit for one person, specified in section 1611(a)(3)(B) of the Act; and

(ii) That, if the amount in the account, in addition to the value of the resident's other nonexempt resources, reaches the SSI resource limit for one person, the resident may lose eligibility for Medicaid or SSI.

Interpretive Guidelines §483.10(c)(5)

The Social Security District Office can provide you with information concerning current SSI resource limits.

Procedures §483.10(c)(5)

If problems are identified for sampled residents who are Medicaid recipients, review financial records to determine if their accounts are within $200.00 of the SSI limit. If there are sampled residents in this situation, ask them or their representatives if they have received notice.

F160 Conveyance of resident's funds upon death within 30 days

483.10(c)(6) Conveyance upon Death

Upon the death of a resident with a personal fund deposited with the facility, the facility must convey within 30 days the resident's funds, and a final accounting of those funds, to the individual or probate jurisdiction administering the resident's estate.

Procedures §483.10(c)(6)

As part of closed records review, determine if within 30 days of death, the facility conveyed the deceased resident's personal funds and a final accounting to the individual or probate jurisdiction administering the individual's estate as provided by State law.

F161 Surety bond or equivalent to protect resident funds

483.10(c)(7) Assurance of Financial Security

The facility must purchase a surety bond, or otherwise provide assurance satisfactory to the Secretary, to assure the security of all personal funds of residents deposited with the facility.

Interpretive Guidelines §483.10(c)(7)

A surety bond is an agreement between the principal (the facility), the surety (the insurance company), and the obligee (depending on State law, either the resident or the State acting on behalf of the resident), wherein the facility and the insurance company agree to compensate the resident (or the State on behalf of the resident) for any loss of resident's funds that the facility holds, safeguards, manages, and accounts for.

The purpose of the surety bond is to guarantee that the facility will pay the resident (or the State on behalf of the resident) for losses occurring from any failure by the facility to hold, safeguard, manage, and account for the resident's funds, i.e., losses occurring as a result of acts or errors of negligence, incompetence, or dishonesty.

Unlike other types of insurance, the surety bond protects the obligee (the resident or the State), not the principal (the facility), from loss. The surety bond differs from a fidelity bond, which covers no acts or errors of negligence, incompetence, or dishonesty.

The surety bond is the commitment of the facility in an objective manner to meet the standard of conduct specified in §483.10(c)(2), that the facility will hold, safeguard, manage, and account for the funds residents have entrusted to the facility. The facility assumes the responsibility to compensate the obligee for the amount of the loss up to the entire amount of the surety bond.

Reasonable alternatives to a surety bond must:

- Designate the obligee (depending on State law, the resident individually or in aggregate, or the State on behalf of each resident) who can collect in case of a loss;
- Specify that the obligee may collect due to any failure by the facility, whether by commission, bankruptcy, or omission, to hold, safeguard, manage, and account for the resident's funds; and
- Be managed by a third party unrelated in any way to the facility or its management.

The facility cannot be named as a beneficiary.

Self-insurance is not an acceptable alternative to a surety bond. Likewise, funds deposited in bank accounts protected by the Federal Deposit Insurance Corporation, or similar entity, also are not acceptable alternatives.

Procedures §483.10(c)(7)

As part of Phase 2, if your team has any concerns about residents' funds, check the amount of the surety bond to make sure it is at least equal to the total amount of residents' funds, as of the most recent quarter.

If the State survey agency determines that individual circumstances associated with a facility's surety bond or its alternative are such that the survey agency cannot determine whether or not the facility is in compliance with the requirements at §483.10(c)(7), then it would be appropriate to make the referral to the State's fiscal department.

If a corporation has a surety bond that covers all of its facilities, there should be a separate review of the corporation's surety bond by the appropriate State agency, such as the State's fiscal department, to ensure that all the residents in the corporation's facilities within the State are covered against any losses due to acts or errors by the corporation or any of its facilities. The focus of the review should be to ensure that if the corporation were to go bankrupt or otherwise cease to operate, the funds of the residents in the corporation's facilities would be protected.

F162 Limitations on charges to personal funds: chargeable, non-chargeable items

§483.10(c)(8) Limitation on Charges to Personal Funds

The facility may not impose a charge against the personal funds of a resident for any item or services for which payment is made under Medicaid or Medicare (except for applicable deductible and coinsurance amounts).

The facility may charge the resident for requested services that are more expensive than or in excess of covered services in accordance with §489.32 of this chapter. (This does not affect the prohibition on facility charges for items and services for which Medicaid has paid. See §447.15, which limits participation in the Medicaid program to providers who accept, as payment in full, Medicaid payment plus any deductible, coinsurance, or copayment required by the plan to be paid by the individual.)

(i) Services included in Medicare or Medicaid payment. During the course of a covered Medicare or Medicaid stay, facilities may not charge a resident for the following categories of items and services:

(A) Nursing services as required at §483.30 of this subpart.

(B) Dietary services as required at §483.35 of this subpart.

(C) An activities program as required at §483.15(f) of this subpart.

(D) Room/bed maintenance services.

(E) Routine personal hygiene items and services as required to meet the needs of residents, including, but not limited to, hair hygiene supplies, comb, brush, bath soap, disinfecting soaps or specialized cleansing agents when indicated to treat special skin problems or to fight infection, razor, shaving cream, toothbrush, toothpaste, denture adhesive, denture cleaner, dental floss, moisturizing lotion, tissues, cotton balls, cotton swabs, deodorant, incontinence care and supplies, sanitary napkins and related supplies, towels, washcloths, hospital gowns, over the counter drugs, hair and nail hygiene services, bathing, and basic personal laundry.

(F) Medically-related social services as required at §483.15(g) of this subpart.

(ii) Items and services that may be charged to resident's funds. Listed below are general categories and examples of items and services that the facility may charge to resident's funds if they are requested by a resident, if the facility informs the resident that there will be a charge, and if payment is not made by Medicare or Medicaid:

(A) Telephone;

(B) Television/radio for personal use;

(C) Personal comfort items, including smoking materials, notions and novelties, and confections;

(D) Cosmetic and grooming items and services in excess of those for which payment is made under Medicaid or Medicare;

(E) Personal clothing;

(F) Personal reading matter;

(G) Gifts purchased on behalf of a resident;

(H) Flowers and plants; and

(I) Social events and entertainment offered outside the scope of the activities program, provided under §483.15(f) of this subpart.

(J) Noncovered special care services such as privately hired nurses or aides.

(K) Private room, except when therapeutically required (for example, isolation for infection control).

(L) Specially prepared or alternative food requested instead of the food generally prepared by the facility, as required by §483.35 of this subpart.

Intent §483.10(c)(8)

The intent of this requirement is to specify that facilities not charge residents for items and services for which payment is made under Medicare or Medicaid.

Interpretive Guidelines §483.10(c)(8)

The facility may charge the resident the difference for requested services that are more expensive than or in excess of covered services in accordance with §489.32 of this chapter. (This does not affect the prohibition on facility charges for items and services for which Medicaid has paid. See §447.15, which limits participation in the Medicaid program to providers who accept, as payment in full, Medicaid payment plus any deductible, coinsurance, or copayment required by the plan to be paid by the individual.) If a State plan does not cover an item or service, such as eyeglasses, the resident may purchase that item or service out of his/her funds. See §483.15(g), F250 for the facility's responsibility to assist the resident in obtaining those services.

Procedures §483.10(c)(8)

As appropriate during Phase 2 of the survey, review the written information given to Medicare/Medicaid eligible residents and family members on admission that notifies them of the items and services that are covered under Medicare or the State plan. Review a sample of residents' monthly statements to ensure that personal funds are not used to pay for covered services. If charges found on monthly statements indicate that residents may have paid for covered items or services, determine if these items or services are over and above what is paid by Medicare or Medicaid.

If, through observations or interviews of residents selected for comprehensive or focused review, the team determines that families or residents hire sitters, and/or that a large number of residents or families are paying for outside food, determine if these practices reflect inadequate staffing and/or food.

Interpretive Guidelines §483.10(c)(8)(i)(E)

Prescription drugs are part of the pharmaceutical services that facilities are required to provide. (See §483.25(l) and (m), and §483.60.) However, at times, a resident needs a medical service that is recognized by State law, but not covered by the State plan. Such a medical service includes a prescription drug that is not on the State's formulary or that exceeds the number of medications covered by Medicaid. It may also include prescription eyeglasses or dentures. If a resident needs a recognized medical service over what is allowed by the State plan, the resident has the right under the Medicaid statute to spend his/her income on that service. If the service is more than what Medicaid pays, the resident may deduct the actual cost of the service from the Medicaid share of the cost. The facility must assist the resident in exercising his or her right to the uncovered medical expense deduction and may not charge the resident for such services.

"Hair hygiene supplies" refers to comb, brush, shampoos, trims, and simple haircuts provided by facility staff as part of routine grooming care. Haircuts, permanent waves, hair coloring, and relaxing performed by barbers and beauticians not employed by a facility are chargeable.

"Nail hygiene services" refers to routine trimming, cleaning, filing, but not polishing of undamaged nails, and on an individual basis, care for ingrown or damaged nails.

"Basic personal laundry" does not include dry cleaning, mending, washing by hand, or other specialty services that need not be provided. A resident may be charged for these specialty services if he or she requests and receives them.

Interpretive Guidelines §483.10(c)(8)(ii)(I) Social Events

Facilities are required by §483.15(f) to provide an ongoing program of activities designed to meet, in accordance with the comprehensive assessment, the interests and physical, mental, and psychosocial well-being of each resident, and cannot charge residents for these services, whether they occur at the facility or off-site. Resident funds should not be charged for universal items such as bookmobile services or local newspaper subscriptions intended for use by more than one resident. However, if a resident requests and attends a social event or entertainment that is not part of the activities assessment and care plan for that resident, a facility may charge that resident's account only for actual expenses. Further, because of expenses associated with transportation, escorts, and other related costs, a resident may be charged for actual expenses for an event or entertainment he or she requests and attends that may be free to the public.

Interpretive Guidelines §483.10(c)(8)(ii)(L) Specially Prepared Foods

A resident may refuse food usually prepared and food substitutions of similar nutritive value because of personal, religious, cultural, or ethnic preference. If the resident requests and receives food that is either not commonly purchased by the facility or easily prepared, then the facility may charge the resident. For example, the facility may charge the resident's account for specially prepared food if the facility has a restricted diet policy and notified the resident on admission of the fact, in accordance with §483.10(b). The facility may not charge the resident's account for specially prepared foods that are required by the physician's order of a therapeutic diet. If a facility changes its menu so that the menu no longer reflects the food preferences of residents, see F165, F242, and F243 to determine compliance with these requirements.

(iii) Requests for items and services.

(A) The facility must not charge a resident (or his or her representative) for any item or service not requested by the resident.

(B) The facility must not require a resident (or his or her representative) to request any item or service as a condition of admission or continued stay.

(C) The facility must inform the resident (or his or her representative) requesting an item or service for which a charge will be made that there will be a charge for the item or service and what the charge will be.

Interpretive Guidelines §483.10(c)(8)(iii) Requests for Items and Services

A facility may not charge a resident or the resident's representative for items and services that are not requested by the resident or representative, whether or not the item or services are requested by a physician. The item or service ordered by the physician should fit in with the resident's care plan.

F163 Free choice in physician, treatments

§483.10(d)(1) — Choose a personal attending physician

Interpretive Guidelines §483.10(d)(1)

The right to choose a personal physician does not mean that the physician must or will serve the resident, or that a resident must designate a personal physician. If a physician of the resident's choosing fails to fulfill a given requirement, such as §483.25(l)(1), Unnecessary drugs; §483.25(l)(2), Antipsychotic drugs; or §483.40, frequency of physician visits, the facility will have the right, after informing the resident, to seek alternate physician participation to assure provision of appropriate and adequate care and treatment. A facility may not place barriers in the way of residents choosing their own physicians. For example, if a resident does not have a physician, or if the resident's physician becomes unable or unwilling to continue providing care to the resident, the facility must assist the resident in exercising his or her choice in finding another physician.

Before consulting an alternate physician, one mechanism to alleviate a possible problem could involve the facility's utilization of a peer review process for cases which cannot be satisfactorily resolved by discussion between the medical director and the attending physician. Only after a failed attempt to work with the attending physician or mediate differences in delivery of care should the facility request an alternate physician when requested to do so by the resident or when the physician will not adhere to the regulations.

If it is a condition for admission to a continuing care retirement center, the requirement for free choice is met if a resident is allowed to choose a personal physician from among those who have practice privileges at the retirement center.

A resident in a distinct part of a general acute care hospital can choose his/her own physician, unless the hospital requires that physicians with residents in the distinct part have hospital admitting privileges. If this is so, the resident can choose his/her own physician, but cannot have a physician who does not have hospital admitting privileges.

If residents appear to have problems in choosing physicians, determine how the facility makes physician services available to residents.

F164 Privacy and confidentiality in records, treatments, visits, accommodations, communications, meetings

(Rev. 5, Issued: 11-19-04, Effective: 11-19-04, Implementation: 11-19-04)

§483.10(e) Privacy and Confidentiality

The resident has the right to personal privacy and confidentiality of his or her personal and clinical records.

(1) Personal privacy includes accommodations, medical treatment, written and telephone communications, personal care, visits, and meetings of family and resident groups, but this does not require the facility to provide a private room for each resident;

(2) Except as provided in paragraph (e)(3) of this section, the resident may approve or refuse the release of personal and clinical records to any individual outside the facility;

(3) The resident's right to refuse release of personal and clinical records does not apply when—

(i) The resident is transferred to another health care institution; or

(ii) Record release is required by law.

Interpretive Guidelines §483.10(e)

"Right to privacy" means that the resident has the right to privacy with whomever the resident wishes to be private and that this privacy should include full visual, and, to the extent desired, for visits or other activities, auditory privacy. Private space may be created flexibly and need not be dedicated solely for visitation purposes.

For example, privacy for visitation or meetings might be arranged by using a dining area between meals, a vacant chapel, office, or room; or an activities area when activities are not in progress. Arrangements for private space could be accomplished through cooperation between the facility's administration and resident or family groups so that private space is provided for those requesting it without infringement on the rights of other residents.

With the exception of the explicit requirement for privacy curtains in all initially certified facilities (see §483.70(d)(1)(v)), the facility is free to innovate to provide privacy for its residents, as exemplified in the preceding paragraph. This may, but need not, be through the provision of a private room.

Facility staff must examine and treat residents in a manner that maintains the privacy of their bodies. A resident must be granted privacy when going to the bathroom and in other activities of personal hygiene. If an individual requires assistance, authorized staff should respect the individual's need for privacy. Only authorized staff directly involved in treatment should be present when treatments are given. People not involved in the care of the individual should not be present without the individual's consent while he/she is being examined or treated. Staff should pull privacy curtains, close doors, or otherwise remove residents from public view and provide clothing or draping to prevent unnecessary exposure of body parts during the provision of personal care and services.

Personal and clinical records include all types of records the facility might keep on a resident, whether they are medical, social, fund accounts, automated or other.

Additional guidelines on mail, visitation rights, and telephone communication are addressed in §483.10(i), (j), and (k). See §483.70(d)(1)(iv) for full visual privacy around beds.

Procedures §483.10(e)(1) - (3)

Document any instances where you observe a resident's privacy being violated. Completely document how the resident's privacy was violated (e.g., Resident #12 left without gown or bed covers and unattended), and where and when this occurred (e.g., 2B Corridor, 3:30 pm, February 25). If possible, identify the responsible party.

§483.75(l)(4) The facility must keep confidential all information contained in the resident's records, regardless of the form or storage method of the records, except when release is required by—

(i) Transfer to another health care institution;

(ii) Law;

(iii) Third party payment contract; or

(iv) The resident.

Interpretive Guidelines §483.75(l)(4)

"Keep confidential" is defined as safeguarding the content of information including video, audio, or other computer stored information from unauthorized disclosure without the consent of the individual and/or the individual's surrogate or representative.

If there is information considered too confidential to place in the record used by all staff, such as the family's financial assets or sensitive medical data, it may be retained in a secure place in the facility, such as a locked cabinet in the administrator's office. The record should show the location of this confidential information.

F165 Voice grievances without reprisal

A resident has the right to—

§483.10(f)(1) — Voice grievances without discrimination or reprisal. Such grievances include those with respect to treatment which has been furnished as well as that which has not been furnished; and

(SEE TAG 166 FOR GUIDANCE)

F166 Prompt facility effort to resolve grievances

A resident has the right to—

§483.10(f)(2) — Prompt efforts by the facility to resolve grievances the resident may have, including those with respect to the behavior of other residents.

Intent §483.10(f)

The intent of the regulation is to support each resident's right to voice grievances (e.g., those about treatment, care, management of funds, lost clothing, or violation of rights) and to assure that after receiving a complaint/grievance, the facility actively seeks a resolution and keeps the resident appropriately apprised of its progress toward resolution.

Interpretive Guidelines §483.10(f)

"Voice grievances" is not limited to a formal, written grievance process but may include a resident's verbalized complaint to facility staff.

"Prompt efforts . . . to resolve" include facility acknowledgement of complaint/grievances and actively working toward resolution of that complaint/grievance.

If residents' responses indicate problems in voicing grievances and getting grievances resolved, determine how the facility deals with and makes prompt efforts to resolve resident complaints and grievances.

- With permission, review resident council minutes.
- Interview staff about how grievances are handled.
- Interview staff about communication (to resident) of progress toward resolution of complaint/grievance.

If problems are identified, also investigate compliance with §483.10(b)(7)(iii).

F167 Examination of survey results by residents

§483.10(g) Examination of Survey Results

A resident has the right to—

(1) Examine the results of the most recent survey of the facility conducted by Federal or State surveyors and any plan of correction in effect with respect to the facility. The facility must make the results available for examination in a place readily accessible to residents and must post a notice of their availability; and

SEE GUIDANCE UNDER TAG 168

F168 Information reception by residents from client advocate agencies

A resident has the right to:

§483.10(g)(2) — Receive information from agencies acting as client advocates, and be afforded the opportunity to contact these agencies.

Interpretive Guidelines §483.10(g)(1)-(2)

"Results of the most recent survey" means the Statement of Deficiencies (Form CMS-2567) and the Statement of Isolated Deficiencies generated by the most recent standard survey and any subsequent extended surveys, and any deficiencies resulting from any subsequent complaint investigation(s).

"Made available for examination" means that survey results and approved plan of correction, if applicable, are available in a readable form, such as a binder, large print, or are provided with a magnifying glass; have not been altered by the facility unless authorized by the State agency; and are available to residents without having to ask a staff person.

"Place readily accessible to residents" is a place (such as a lobby or other area frequented by most residents) where individuals wishing to examine survey results do not have to ask to see them.

F169 Work

§483.10(h) Work

The resident has the right to—

(1) Refuse to perform services for the facility;

(2) Perform services for the facility, if he or she chooses, when—

(i) The facility has documented the need or desire for work in the plan of care;

(ii) The plan specifies the nature of the services performed and whether the services are voluntary or paid;

(iii) Compensation for paid services is at or above prevailing rates; and

(iv) The resident agrees to the work arrangement described in the plan of care.

Interpretive Guidelines §483.10(h)(1)-(2)

"Prevailing rate" is the wage paid to workers in the community surrounding the facility for essentially the same type, quality, and quantity of work requiring comparable skills.

All resident work, whether of a voluntary or paid nature, must be part of the plan of care. A resident's desire for work is subject to discussion of medical appropriateness. As part of the plan of care, a therapeutic work assignment must be agreed to by the resident. The resident also has the right to refuse such treatment at any time that he or she wishes. At the time of development or review of the plan, voluntary or paid work can be negotiated.

Procedures §483.10(h)(1)-(2)

Are residents engaged in what may be paid or volunteer work (e.g., doing housekeeping, doing laundry, preparing meals)? Pay special attention to the possible work activities of residents with mental retardation or mental illness. If you observe such a situation, determine if the resident is in fact performing work and, if so, is this work, whether voluntary or paid, described in the plan of care?

F170 Mail rights in sending and receiving

§483.10(i)(1) Send and promptly receive mail that is unopened; and

SEE GUIDANCE UNDER TAG 171

F171 Access to stationery, postage, writing implements

§483.10(i)(2) Have access to stationery, postage, and writing implements at the resident's own expense.

Interpretive Guidelines §483.10(i)(1)-(2)

"Promptly" means delivery of mail or other materials to the resident within 24 hours of delivery by the postal service (including a post office box) and delivery of outgoing mail to the postal service within 24 hours, except when there is no regularly scheduled postal delivery and pick-up service.

F172 Access and visitation rights

(Rev. 12, Issued: 10-14-05, Effective: 10-14-05, Implementation: 10-14-05)

§483.10(j) Access and Visitation Rights

§483.10(j)(1) The resident has the right and the facility must provide immediate access to any resident by the following:

(i) Any representative of the Secretary;

(ii) Any representative of the State;

(iii) The resident's individual physician;

(iv) The State long-term care ombudsman (established under section 307 (a)(12) of the Older Americans Act of 1965);

(v) The agency responsible for the protection and advocacy system for developmentally disabled individuals (established under part C of the Developmental Disabilities Assistance and Bill of Rights Act);

(vi) The agency responsible for the protection and advocacy system for mentally ill individuals (established under the Protection and Advocacy for Mentally Ill Individuals Act);

(vii) Subject to the resident's right to deny or withdraw consent at any time, immediate family or other relatives of the resident; and

(viii) Subject to reasonable restrictions and the resident's right to deny or withdraw consent at any time, others who are visiting with the consent of the resident.

§483.10(j)(2) The facility must provide reasonable access to any resident by any entity or individual that provides health, social, legal, or other services to the resident, subject to the resident's right to deny or withdraw consent at any time.

Interpretive Guidelines §483.10(j)(1) and (2)

The facility must provide immediate access to any representative of the Secretary of the Department of Health and Human Services, the State, the resident's individual physician, the State long-term care ombudsman, or the agencies responsible for the protection and advocacy of developmentally disabled or mentally ill individuals. The facility cannot refuse to permit residents to talk with surveyors. Representatives of the Department of Health and Human Services, the State, the State ombudsman system, and protection and advocacy agencies for mentally ill and mentally retarded individuals are not subject to visiting hour limitations.

Immediate family or other relatives are not subject to visiting hour limitations or other restrictions not imposed by the resident. However, the facility may try to change the location of visits to assist care giving or protect the privacy of other residents, if these visitation rights infringe upon the rights of other residents in the facility. For example, a resident's family visits in the late evening, which prevents the resident's roommate from sleeping.

Non-family visitors must also be granted "immediate access" to the resident. The facility may place reasonable restrictions upon the exercise of this right such as reasonable visitation hours to facilitate care giving for the resident or to protect the privacy of other residents, such as requiring that visits not take place in the resident's room if the roommate is asleep or receiving care.

An individual or representative of an agency that provides health, social, legal, or other services to the resident has the right of "reasonable access" to the resident, which means that the facility may establish guidelines regarding the timing or other circumstances of the visit, such as location. These guidelines must allow for ready access of residents to these services.

Procedures §483.10(j)(1) and (2)

If you identify problems during interviews, determine how the facility ensures access to:

- Representatives of the State;
- Representatives of the U.S. Department of Health and Human Services;
- The resident's individual physician;
- Representatives of the State long-term care ombudsman;
- Representatives of agencies responsible for protecting and advocating rights of persons with mental illness or developmental disabilities;
- Family or relatives; and
- Other visitors.

F173 State Ombudsman access to patient's clinical records

§483.10(j)(3) — The facility must allow representatives of the State Ombudsman, described in paragraph (j)(1)(iv) of this section, to examine a resident's clinical records with the permission of the resident or the resident's legal representative, and consistent with State law.

Procedures §483.10(j)(3)

Ask the ombudsman if the facility allows him/her to examine resident's clinical records with the permission of the resident, and to the extent allowed by State law.

F174 Resident access to telephone
Personal property rights (Refer to F252)

§483.10(k) Telephone

The resident has the right to have reasonable access to the use of a telephone where calls can be made without being overheard.

Interpretive Guidelines §483.10(k)

Telephones in staff offices or at nurses' stations do not meet the provisions of this requirement. Examples of facility accommodations to provide reasonable access to the use of a telephone without being overheard include providing cordless telephones or having telephone jacks in residents' rooms.

"Reasonable access" includes placing telephones at a height accessible to residents who use wheelchairs and adapting telephones for use by the residents with impaired hearing.

(Rev. 12, Issued: 10-14-05, Effective: 10-14-05, Implementation: 10-14-05)

§483.10(l) Personal Property

The resident has the right to retain and use personal possessions, including some furnishings, and appropriate clothing, as space permits, unless to do so would infringe upon the rights or health and safety of other residents.

Intent §483.10(l)

The intent of this regulation is to encourage residents to bring personal possessions into the facility, as space, safety considerations, and fire code permits.

Interpretive Guidelines §483.10(l)

All residents' possessions, regardless of their apparent value to others, must be treated with respect, for what they are and for what they may represent to the resident. The right to retain and use personal possessions assures that the residents' environment be as homelike as possible and that residents retain as much control over their lives as possible. The facility has the right to limit the residents' exercise of this right on grounds of space and health or safety.

Procedures §483.10(l)

If residents' rooms have few personal possessions, ask residents, families, and the local ombudsman if:

- Residents are encouraged to have and to use them;
- The facility informs residents not to bring in certain items and for what reason; and
- Personal property is safe in the facility.

Ask staff if the facility sets limits on the value of the property that residents may have in their possession or requires that residents put personal property in the facility's safe.

F175 Married couples sharing a room

§483.10(m) Married Couples

The resident has the right to share a room with his or her spouse when married residents live in the same facility and both spouses consent to the arrangement.

Interpretive Guidelines §483.10(m)

The right of residents who are married to each other to share a room does not give a resident the right, or the facility the responsibility, to compel another resident to relocate to accommodate a spouse. The requirement means that when a room is available for a married couple to share, the facility must permit them to share it if they choose. If a married resident's spouse is admitted to the facility later and the couple want to share a room, the facility must provide a shared room as quickly as possible. However, a couple is not able to share a room if one of the spouses has a different payment source for which the facility is not certified (if the room is in a distinct part, unless one of the spouses elects to pay for his or her care).

F176 Self-administration of drugs (requirements)

§483.10(n) Self-Administration of Drugs

An individual resident may self-administer drugs if the interdisciplinary team, as defined by §483.20(d)(2)(ii), has determined that this practice is safe.

Interpretive Guidelines §483.10(n)

If a resident requests to self-administer drugs, it is the responsibility of the interdisciplinary team to determine that it is safe for the resident to self-administer drugs before the resident may exercise that right. The interdisciplinary team must also determine who will be responsible (the resident or the nursing staff) for storage and documentation of the administration of drugs, as well as the location of the drug administration (e.g., resident's room, nurses' station, or activities room). Appropriate notation of these determinations should be placed in the resident's care plan.

The decision that a resident has the ability to self-administer medication(s) is subject to periodic re-evaluation based on change in the resident's status. The facility may require that drugs be administered by the nurse or medication aide, if allowed by State law, until the care planning team has the opportunity to obtain information necessary to make an assessment of the resident's ability to safely self-administer medications. If the resident chooses to self-administer drugs, this decision should be made at least by the time the care plan is completed within seven days after completion of the comprehensive assessment.

Medication errors occurring with residents who self-administer drugs should not be counted in the facility's medication error rate (see Guidelines for §483.25(m)), but should call into question the judgment made by the facility in allowing self-administration for those residents.

Probes §483.10(n)

For residents selected for a comprehensive review or a focused review, as appropriate:

- Does resident self-administer drugs? Which ones? How much? How often?
- Does the care plan reflect self-administration?

F177 Refusal of certain transfers. Admission, transfer, and discharge rights

§483.10(o) Refusal of Certain Transfers

(1) An individual has the right to refuse a transfer to another room within the institution, if the purpose of the transfer is to relocate—

(i) A resident of a SNF, from the distinct part of the institution that is a SNF to a part of the institution that is not a SNF, or

(ii) A resident of a NF, from the distinct part of the institution that is a NF to a distinct part of the institution that is a SNF.

(2) A resident's exercise of the right to refuse transfer under paragraph (o)(1) of this section does not affect the individual's eligibility or entitlement to Medicare or Medicaid benefits.

Interpretive Guidelines §483.10(o)

This requirement applies to transfer within a physical plant.

These provisions allow a resident to refuse transfer from a room in one distinct part of an institution to a room in another distinct part of the institution for purposes of obtaining Medicare or Medicaid eligibility. If a resident refuses to transfer from a portion of the institution that is not Medicare certified, the resident forgoes the possibility of Medicare coverage for the care received there. If that portion of the institution is Medicaid certified and the resident is Medicaid-eligible, then Medicaid covered services would be paid by Medicaid. If the resident is Medicaid-eligible, but that portion of the institution is not Medicaid certified, then the resident would assume responsibility for payment for the services. If the resident is unable to pay for those services, then the facility may, after giving the resident a 30-day notice, transfer the resident under the provisions of §483.12(a).

When a resident occupies a bed in a distinct part of a NF that participates in Medicaid and not in Medicare, he or she may not be moved involuntarily to another part of the institution by the facility (or required to be moved by the State) solely for the purpose of assuring Medicare eligibility for payment. Such moves are only appropriate when they occur at the request of a resident (for example, when a privately paying Medicare beneficiary believes that admission to a bed in a Medicare-participating distinct part of the institution may result in Medicare payment).

See Interpretive Guidelines, §483.12 for further discussion regarding transfers.

For transfers of residents between Medicare or Medicaid approved distinct parts:

- Is there a documented medical reason for the transfer?
- Was the resident transferred because of a change in payment source?
- If a Medicare or Medicaid resident is notified that he/she is no longer eligible, does the facility transfer the resident? Did the facility give the resident the opportunity to refuse the transfer? How? What happened?
- Ask the local ombudsman about facility compliance with transfer requirements. See also §483.12, Criteria for Transfer.

§483.12 Admission, Transfer, and Discharge Rights

§483.12(a) Transfer and Discharge

(1) Definition

Transfer and discharge includes movement of a resident to a bed outside of the certified facility whether that bed is in the same physical plant or not. Transfer and discharge does not refer to movement of a resident to a bed within the same certified facility.

Interpretive Guidelines §483.12

This requirement applies to transfers or discharges that are initiated by the facility, not by the resident. Whether or not a resident agrees to the facility's decision, these requirements apply whenever a facility initiates the transfer or discharge. "Transfer" is moving the resident from the facility to another legally responsible institutional setting, while "discharge" is moving the resident to a non-institutional setting when the releasing facility ceases to be responsible for the resident's care.

If a resident is living in an institution participating in both Medicare and Medicaid (SNF/NF) under separate provider agreements, a move from either the SNF or NF would constitute a transfer.

Transfer and discharge provisions significantly restrict a facility's ability to transfer or discharge a resident once that resident has been admitted to the facility. The facility may not transfer or discharge the resident unless:

1. The transfer or discharge is necessary to meet the resident's welfare and the resident's welfare cannot be met in the facility;

2. The transfer or discharge is appropriate because the resident's health has improved sufficiently so the resident no longer needs the services provided by the facility;

3. The safety of individuals in the facility is endangered;

4. The health of individuals in the facility would otherwise be endangered;

5. The resident has failed, after reasonable and appropriate notice, to pay for a stay at the facility; or

6. The facility ceases to operate.

To demonstrate that any of the events specified in 1–5 have occurred, the law requires documentation in the resident's clinical record. To demonstrate situations 1 and 2, the resident's physician must provide the documentation. In situation 4, the documentation must be provided by any physician. (See §483.12(a)(2).)

Moreover, before the transfer or discharge occurs, the law requires that the facility notify the resident and, if known, the family member, surrogate, or representative of the transfer and the reasons for the transfer, and record the reasons in the clinical record. The facility's notice must include an explanation of the right to appeal the transfer to the State as well as the name, address, and phone number of the State long-term care ombudsman. In the case of a developmentally disabled individual, the notice must include the name, address, and phone number of the agency responsible for advocating for the developmentally disabled, and in the case of a mentally ill individual, the name, address, and phone number of the agency responsible for advocating for mentally ill individuals. (See §483.12(a)(3) and (5).)

Generally, this notice must be provided at least 30 days prior to the transfer. Exceptions to the 30-day requirement apply when the transfer is effected because of:

• Endangerment to the health or safety of others in the facility;
• When a resident's health has improved to allow a more immediate transfer or discharge;

- When a resident's urgent medical needs require more immediate transfer; and
- When a resident has not resided in the facility for 30 days.

In these cases, the notice must be provided as soon as practicable before the discharge. (See §483.12(a)(4).)

Finally, the facility is required to provide sufficient preparation and orientation to residents to ensure safe and orderly discharge from the facility. (See §483.12(a)(6).)

Under Medicaid, a participating facility is also required to provide notice to its residents of the facility's bed-hold policies and readmission policies prior to transfer of a resident for hospitalization or therapeutic leave. Upon such transfer, the facility must provide written notice to the resident and an immediate family member, surrogate, or representative of the duration of any bed-hold. With respect to readmission in a Medicaid participating facility, the facility must develop policies that permit residents eligible for Medicaid, who were transferred for hospitalization or therapeutic leave, and whose absence exceeds the bed-hold period as defined by the State plan, to return to the facility in the first available bed. (See §483.12(b).)

A resident cannot be transferred for non-payment if he or she has submitted to a third party payor all the paperwork necessary for the bill to be paid. Non-payment would occur if a third party payor, including Medicare or Medicaid, denies the claim and the resident refused to pay for his or her stay.

§483.10(o), Tag F177, addresses the right of residents to refuse certain transfers within an institution on the basis of payment status.

§483.12 Admission, Transfer, and Discharge Rights   Tags 201 – 208

§483.12(a) Transfer and Discharge
§483.12(b) Notice of Bed-Hold Policy and Readmission
§483.12(c) Equal Access to Quality Care
§483.12(d) Admissions Policy

F201 Transfer and discharge requirements

§483.12(a)(2) Transfer and Discharge Requirements

The facility must permit each resident to remain in the facility, and not transfer or discharge the resident from the facility unless—

(i) The transfer or discharge is necessary for the resident's welfare and the resident's needs cannot be met in the facility;

(ii) The transfer or discharge is appropriate because the resident's health has improved sufficiently so the resident no longer needs the services provided by the facility;

(iii) The safety of individuals in the facility is endangered;

(iv) The health of individuals in the facility would otherwise be endangered;

(v) The resident has failed, after reasonable and appropriate notice, to pay for (or to have paid under Medicare or Medicaid) a stay at the facility. For a resident who becomes eligible for Medicaid after admission to a nursing facility, the nursing facility may charge a resident only allowable charges under Medicaid; or

(vi) The facility ceases to operate.

SEE GUIDANCE UNDER TAG 202

F202 Documentation of transfer by specified physician

§483.12(a)(3) Documentation

When the facility transfers or discharges a resident under any of the circumstances specified in paragraphs (a)(2)(i) through (v) of this section, the resident's clinical record must be documented. The documentation must be made by—

(i) The resident's physician when transfer or discharge is necessary under paragraph (a)(2)(i) or paragraph (a)(2)(ii) of this section; and

(ii) A physician when transfer or discharge is necessary under paragraph (a)(2)(iv) of this section.

Interpretive Guidelines §483.12(a)(2) and (3)

If transfer is due to a significant change in the resident's condition, but not an emergency requiring an immediate transfer, then prior to any action, the facility must conduct the appropriate assessment to determine if a new care plan would allow the facility to meet the resident's needs. (See §483.20(b)(4)(iv), F274, for information concerning assessment upon significant change.)

Conversion from a private pay rate to payment at the Medicaid rate does not constitute non-payment.

Refusal of treatment would not constitute grounds for transfer, unless the facility is unable to meet the needs of the resident or protect the health and safety of others.

Documentation of the transfer/discharge may be completed by a physician extender unless prohibited by State law or facility policy.

Procedures §483.12(a)(2) and (3)

During closed record review, determine the reasons for transfer/discharge.

- Do records document accurate assessments and attempts through care planning to address resident's needs through multi-disciplinary interventions, accommodation of individual needs, and attention to the resident's customary routines?
- Did the resident's physician document the record if:

    ✧ The resident was transferred/discharged for the sake of the resident's welfare and the resident's needs could not be met in the facility (e.g., a resident develops an acute condition requiring hospitalization)? or
    ✧ The resident's health improved to the extent that the transferred/discharged resident no longer needed the services of the facility?

- Did a physician document the record if residents were transferred because the health of individuals in the facility are endangered?
- Do the records of residents transferred/discharged due to safety reasons reflect the process by which the facility concluded that in each instance transfer or discharge was necessary? Did the survey team observe residents with similar safety concerns in the facility? If so, determine differences between these residents and those who were transferred or discharged.

- Look for changes in source of payment coinciding with transfer. If you find such transfer, determine if the transfers were triggered by one of the criteria specified in §483.12(a)(2).
- Ask the ombudsman if there were any complaints regarding transfer and/or discharge. If there were, what was the result of the ombudsman's investigation?
- If the entity to which the resident was discharged is another long-term care facility, evaluate the extent to which the discharge summary and the resident's physician justify why the facility could not meet the needs of this resident.

F203 Notice to resident before transfer

§483.12(a)(4) Notice Before Transfer

Before a facility transfers or discharges a resident, the facility must—

(i) Notify the resident and, if known, a family member or legal representative of the resident of the transfer or discharge and the reasons for the move in writing and in a language and manner they understand.

(ii) Record the reasons in the resident's clinical record; and

(iii) Include in the notice the items described in paragraph (a)(6) of this section.

§483.12(a)(5) Timing of the Notice

(i) Except when specified in paragraph (a)(5)(ii) of this section, the notice of transfer or discharge required under paragraph (a)(4) of this section must be made by the facility at least 30 days before the resident is transferred or discharged.

(ii) Notice may be made as soon as practicable before transfer or discharge when—

(A) The safety of the individuals in the facility would be endangered under paragraph (a)(2)(iii) of this section;

(B) The health of individuals in the facility would be endangered, under (a)(2)(iv) of this section;

(C) The resident's health improves sufficiently to allow a more immediate transfer or discharge, under paragraph (a)(2)(ii) of this section;

(D) An immediate transfer or discharge is required by the resident's urgent medical needs, under paragraph (a)(2)(i) of this section; or

(E) A resident has not resided in the facility for 30 days.

§483.12(a)(6) Contents of the Notice

The written notice specified in paragraph (a)(4) of this section must include the following:

(i) The reason for transfer or discharge;

(ii) The effective date of transfer or discharge;

(iii) The location to which the resident is transferred or discharged;

(iv) A statement that the resident has the right to appeal the action to the State;

(v) The name, address, and telephone number of the State long-term care ombudsman;

(vi) For nursing facility residents with developmental disabilities, the mailing address and telephone number of the agency responsible for the protection and advocacy of developmentally disabled individuals established under Part C of the Developmental Disabilities Assistance and Bill of Rights Act; and

(vii) For nursing facility residents who are mentally ill, the mailing address and telephone number of the agency responsible for the protection and advocacy of mentally ill individuals established under the Protection and Advocacy for Mentally Ill Individuals Act.

Procedures §483.12(a)(4)-(6)

If the team determines that there are concerns about the facility's transfer and discharge actions, during closed record review, look at notices to determine if the notice requirements are met, including:

- Advance notice (either 30 days or, as soon as practicable, depending on the reason for transfer/discharge);
- Reason for transfer/discharge;
- The effective date of the transfer or discharge;
- The location to which the resident was transferred or discharged;
- Right of appeal;
- How to notify the ombudsman (name, address, and telephone number); and
- How to notify the appropriate protection and advocacy agency for residents with mental illness or mental retardation (mailing address and telephone numbers).
- Determine whether the facility notified a family member or legal representative of the proposed transfer or discharge.

F204 Resident orientation for transfer or discharge

§483.12(a)(7) Orientation for Transfer or Discharge

A facility must provide sufficient preparation and orientation to residents to ensure safe and orderly transfer or discharge from the facility.

Interpretive Guidelines §483.12(a)(7)

"Sufficient preparation" means the facility informs the resident where he or she is going and takes steps under its control to assure safe transportation. The facility should actively involve, to the extent possible, the resident and the resident's family in selecting the new residence. Some examples of orientation may include trial visits, if possible, by the resident to a new location; working with family to ask their assistance in assuring the resident that valued possessions are not left behind or lost; orienting staff in the receiving facility to resident's daily patterns; and reviewing with staff routines for handling transfers and discharges in a manner that minimizes unnecessary and avoidable anxiety or depression and recognizes characteristic resident reactions identified by the resident assessment and care plan.

Procedures §483.12(a)(7)

During Resident Review, check social service notes to see if appropriate referrals have been made and, if necessary, if resident counseling has occurred.

F205 Two notices of bed-hold policy and readmission

§483.12(b) Notice of Bed-Hold Policy and Readmission

§483.12(b)(1) Notice before transfer. Before a nursing facility transfers a resident to a hospital or allows a resident to go on therapeutic leave, the nursing facility must provide written information to the resident and a family member or legal representative that specifies—

(i) The duration of the bed-hold policy under the State plan, if any, during which the resident is permitted to return and resume residence in the nursing facility; and

(ii) The nursing facility's policies regarding bed-hold periods, which must be consistent with paragraph (b)(3) of this section, permitting a resident to return.

§483.12(b)(2) Bed-hold notice upon transfer. At the time of transfer of a resident for hospitalization or therapeutic leave, a nursing facility must provide to the resident and a family member or legal representative written notice which specifies the duration of the bed-hold policy described in paragraph (b)(1) of this section.

Interpretive Guidelines §483.12(b)(1) and (2)

The nursing facility's bed-hold policies apply to all residents.

These sections require two notices related to the facility's bed-hold policies to be issued. The first notice of bed-hold policies could be given well in advance of any transfer. However, reissuance of the first notice would be required if the bed-hold policy under the State plan or the facility's policy were to change. The second notice, which specifies the duration of the bed-hold policy, must be issued at the time of transfer.

In cases of emergency transfer, notice "at the time of transfer" means that the family, surrogate, or representative are provided with written notification within 24 hours of the transfer. The requirement is met if the resident's copy of the notice is sent with other papers accompanying the resident to the hospital.

Bed-hold for days of absence in excess of the State's bed-hold limit are considered non-covered services which means that the resident could use his/her own income to pay for the bed-hold. However, if such a resident does not elect to pay to hold the bed, readmission rights to the next available bed are specified at §483.12(b)(3). Non-Medicaid residents may be requested to pay for all days of bed-hold.

If residents (or their representatives in the case of residents who are unable to understand their rights) are unsure or unclear about their bed-hold rights, review facility bed-hold policies.

- Do policies specify the duration of the bed-hold?
- Is this time period consistent with that specified in the State plan?
- During closed record review, look at records of residents transferred to a hospital or on therapeutic leave to determine if bed-hold requirements were followed. Was notice given before and at the time of transfer?
- During closed record review, look at records of residents transferred to a hospital or on therapeutic leave to determine if bed-hold requirements were followed. Was notice given before and at the time of transfer?

F206 Policy permitting resident to return to facility

§483.12(b)(3) Permitting Resident to Return to Facility

A nursing facility must establish and follow a written policy under which a resident whose hospitalization or therapeutic leave exceeds the bed-hold period under the State plan, is readmitted to the facility immediately upon the first availability of a bed in a semi-private room if the resident—

(i) Requires the services provided by the facility; and

(ii) Is eligible for Medicaid nursing facility services.

Interpretive Guidelines §483.12(b)(3)

"First available bed in a semi-private room" means a bed in a room shared with another resident of the same sex. (See §483.10(m) for the right of spouses to share a room.)

Medicaid-eligible residents who are on therapeutic leave or are hospitalized beyond the State's bed-hold policy must be readmitted to the first available bed even if the residents have outstanding Medicaid balances. Once readmitted, however, these residents may be transferred if the facility can demonstrate that non-payment of charges exists and documentation and notice requirements are followed. The right to readmission is applicable to individuals seeking to return from a transfer or discharge as long as all of the specific qualifications set out in §483.12(b)(3) are met.

Procedures §483.12(b)(3)

For Medicaid recipients whose hospitalization or therapeutic leave exceeds the bed-hold period, do facility policies specify readmission rights?

Refer to the Minimum Data Set (MDS), section A.10, Discharge Planned; MDS 2.0, section Q, Discharge Potential and Overall Status.

Review the facility's written bed-hold policy to determine if it specifies legal readmission rights. Ask the local ombudsman if there are any problems with residents being readmitted to the facility following hospitalization. In closed record review, determine why the resident did not return to the facility.

Ask the social worker or other appropriate staff what he/she tells Medicaid-eligible residents about the facility's bed-hold policies and the right to return and how Medicaid-eligible residents are assisted in returning to the facility.

If potential problems are identified, talk to discharge planners at the hospital to which residents are transferred to determine their experience with residents returning to the facility.

F207 Equal access to quality care

§483.12(c) Equal Access to Quality Care

§483.12(c)(1) A facility must establish and maintain identical policies and practices regarding transfer, discharge, and the provision of services under the State plan for all individuals regardless of source of payment;

§483.12(c)(2) The facility may charge any amount for services furnished to non-Medicaid residents consistent with the notice requirement in §483.10(b)(5)(i) and (b)(6) describing the charges; and

§483.12(c)(3) The State is not required to offer additional services on behalf of a resident other than services provided in the State plan.

Interpretive Guidelines §483.12(c)

Facilities must treat all residents alike when making transfer and discharge decisions. "Identical policies and practices" concerning services means that facilities must not distinguish between residents based on their source of payment when providing services that are required to be provided under the law. All nursing services, specialized rehabilitative services, social services, dietary services, pharmaceutical services, or activities that are mandated by the law must be provided to residents according to residents' individual needs, as determined by assessments and care plans.

Procedures §483.12(c)

Determine if residents are grouped in separate wings or floors for reasons other than care needs.

F208 Admission and placement policies; permissible charges

§483.12(d) Admissions Policy

(1) The facility must—

(i) Not require residents or potential residents to waive their rights to Medicare or Medicaid; and

(ii) Not require oral or written assurance that residents or potential residents are not eligible for, or will not apply for, Medicare or Medicaid benefits.

Interpretive Guidelines §483.12(d)(1)

This provision prohibits both direct and indirect request for waiver of rights to Medicare or Medicaid. A direct request for waiver, for example, requires residents to sign admissions documents explicitly promising or agreeing not to apply for Medicare or Medicaid. An indirect request for waiver includes requiring the resident to pay private rates for a specified period of time, such as two years ("private pay duration of stay contract") before Medicaid will be accepted as a payment source for the resident. Facilities must not seek or receive any kind of assurances that residents are not eligible for, or will not apply for, Medicare or Medicaid benefits.

Procedures §483.12(d)(1)

If concerns regarding admissions procedures arise during interviews, review admissions packages and contracts to determine if they contain prohibited requirements (e.g., "side agreements" for the resident to be private pay or to supplement the Medicaid rate).

Ask staff what factors lead to decisions to place residents in different wings or floors. Note if factors other than medical and nursing needs affect these decisions. Do staff know the source of payment for the residents they take care of?

Ask the ombudsman if the facility treats residents differently in transfer, discharge, and covered services based on source of payment.

With respect to transfer and discharge, if the facility appears to be sending residents to hospitals at the time (or shortly before) their payment source changes from private-pay or Medicare to Medicaid, call the hospitals and ask their discharge planners if they have detected any pattern of dumping. Also, ask discharge planners if the facility readmits Medicaid recipients who are ready to return to the facility. During the tour, observe possible differences in services.

- Observe if there are separate dining rooms. If so, are different foods served in these dining rooms? For what reasons? Are residents excluded from some dining rooms because of source of payment?
- Observe the placement of residents in rooms in the facility. If residents are segregated on floors or wings by source of payment, determine if the facility is providing different services based on source of payment. Be particularly alert to differences in treatment and services. For example, determine whether less experienced aides and nursing staff are assigned to Medicaid portions of the facility. Notice the condition of the rooms (e.g., carpeted in private-pay wings, tile in Medicaid wings, proximity to the nurses' station, quality of food served as evening snacks).

As part of closed record review, determine if residents have been treated differently in transfers or discharges because of payment status. For example, determine if the facility is sending residents to acute care hospitals shortly before they become eligible for Medicaid as a way of getting rid of Medicaid recipients.

Ask social services staff to describe the facility's policy and practice on providing services, such as rehabilitative services. Determine if services are provided based on source of payment, rather than on need for services to attain or maintain functioning.

§483.12(d)(2) The facility must not require a third party guarantee of payment to the facility as a condition of admission or expedited admission, or continued stay in the facility. However, the facility may require an individual who has legal access to a resident's income or resources available to pay for facility care to sign a contract, without incurring personal financial liability, to provide facility payment from the resident's income or resources.

Interpretive Guidelines §483.12(d)(2)

The facility may not require a third person to accept personal responsibility for paying the facility bill out of his or her own funds. However, he or she may use the resident's money to pay for care. A third party guarantee is not the same as a third party payor, e.g., an insurance company; and this provision does not preclude the facility from obtaining information about Medicare or Medicaid eligibility or the availability of private insurance. The prohibition against third-party guarantees applies to all residents and prospective residents in all certified long-term care facilities, regardless of payment source.

§483.12(d)(3) In the case of a person eligible for Medicaid, a nursing facility must not charge, solicit, accept, or receive, in addition to any amount otherwise required to be paid under the State plan, any gift, money, donation, or other consideration as a precondition of admission, expedited admission, or continued stay in the facility. However,—

(i) A nursing facility may charge a resident who is eligible for Medicaid for items and services the resident has requested and received, and that are not specified in the State plan as included in the term "nursing facility services" so long as the facility gives proper notice of the availability and cost of these services to residents and does not condition the resident's admission or continued stay on the request for and receipt of such additional services; and

(ii) A nursing facility may solicit, accept, or receive a charitable, religious, or philanthropic contribution from an organization or from a person unrelated to a Medicaid-eligible resident or potential resident, but only to the extent that the contribution is not a condition of admission, expedited admission, or continued stay in the facility for a Medicaid-eligible resident.

Interpretive Guidelines §483.12(d)(3)

This requirement applies only to Medicaid-certified nursing facilities.

Facilities may not charge for any service that is included in the definition of "nursing facility services" and, therefore, required to be provided as part of the daily rate. Facilities may not accept additional payment from residents or their families as a prerequisite to admission or to continued stay in the facility. Additional payment includes deposits from Medicaid-eligible residents or their families, or any promise to pay private rates for a specified period of time.

A nursing facility may charge a Medicaid beneficiary for a service the beneficiary has requested and received, only if:

- That service is not defined in the State plan as a "nursing facility" service;
- The facility informs the resident and the resident's representative in advance that this is not a covered service to allow them to make an informed choice regarding the fee; and
- The resident's admission or continued stay is not conditioned on the resident's requesting and receiving that service.

Procedures §483.12(d)(3)

Review State covered services. Compare with the list of items for which the facility charges to determine if the facility is charging for covered services.

Determine if the facility requires deposits from residents. If you identify potential problems with discrimination, review the files of one or more residents selected for a focused or comprehensive review to determine if the facility requires residents to submit deposits as a precondition of admission besides what may be paid under the State plan.

If interviews with residents suggest that the facility may have required deposits from Medicaid recipients at admission, except those admitted when Medicaid eligibility is pending, corroborate by, for example, reviewing the facility's admissions documents or interviewing family members.

§483.12(d)(4) States or political subdivisions may apply stricter admissions standards under State or local laws than are specified in this section, to prohibit discrimination against individuals entitled to Medicaid.

§483.13 Resident Behavior and Facility Practices   Tags 221 – 226

§483.13(a) Restraints

§483.13(b) Abuse

§483.13(c) Staff Treatment of Residents (F224 and F226)

F221 Deficiencies concerning physical restraints

Use Tag F221 for deficiencies concerning physical restraints.

USE GUIDANCE UNDER TAG F222

F222 Deficiencies concerning chemical restraints

Use Tag F222 for deficiencies concerning chemical restraints.

§483.13(a) Restraints

The resident has the right to be free from any physical or chemical restraints imposed for purposes of discipline or convenience, and not required to treat the resident's medical symptoms.

Intent §483.13(a)

The intent of this requirement is for each person to attain and maintain his/her highest practicable well-being in an environment that prohibits the use of restraints for discipline or convenience and limits restraint use to circumstances in which the resident has medical symptoms that warrant the use of restraints.

Interpretive Guidelines §483.13(a)

Definitions of Terms

"Physical Restraints" are defined as any manual method or physical or mechanical device, material, or equipment attached or adjacent to the resident's body that the individual cannot remove easily which restricts freedom of movement or normal access to one's body.

"Chemical Restraints" is defined as any drug that is used for discipline or convenience and not required to treat medical symptoms.

"Discipline" is defined as any action taken by the facility for the purpose of punishing or penalizing residents.

"Convenience" is defined as any action taken by the facility to control a resident's behavior or manage a resident's behavior with a lesser amount of effort by the facility and not in the resident's best interest.

"Medical Symptom" is defined as an indication or characteristic of a physical or psychological condition.

"Convenience" is defined as any action taken by the facility to control a resident's behavior or manage a resident's behavior with a lesser amount of effort by the facility and not in the resident's best interest.

Restraints may not be used for staff convenience. However, if the resident needs emergency care, restraints may be used for brief periods to permit medical treatment to proceed unless the facility has a notice indicating that the resident has previously made a valid refusal of the treatment in question. If a resident's unanticipated violent or aggressive behavior places him/her or others in imminent danger, the resident does not have the right to refuse the use of restraints. In this situation, the use of restraints is a measure of last resort to protect the safety of the resident or others and must not extend beyond the immediate episode. The resident's right to participate in care planning and the right to refuse treatment are addressed at §§483.20(k)(2)(ii) and 483.10(b)(4), respectively, and include the right to accept or refuse restraints.

Physical Restraints are defined as any manual method or physical or mechanical device, material, or equipment attached or adjacent to the resident's body that the individual cannot remove easily which restricts freedom of movement or normal access to one's body.

"Physical restraints" include, but are not limited to, leg restraints, arm restraints, hand mitts, soft ties or vests, lap cushions, and lap trays the resident cannot remove easily. Also included as restraints are facility practices that meet the definition of a restraint, such as:

- Using side rails that keep a resident from voluntarily getting out of bed;
- Tucking in or using velcro to hold a sheet, fabric, or clothing tightly so that a resident's movement is restricted;
- Using devices in conjunction with a chair, such as trays, tables, bars, or belts, that the resident cannot remove easily, that prevent the resident from rising;
- Placing a resident in a chair that prevents a resident from rising; and
- Placing a chair or bed so close to a wall that the wall prevents the resident from rising out of the chair or voluntarily getting out of bed.

Side rails sometimes restrain residents. The use of side rails as restraints is prohibited unless they are necessary to treat a resident's medical symptoms. Residents who attempt to exit a bed through, between, over, or around side rails are at risk of injury or death.

The potential for serious injury is more likely from a fall from a bed with raised side rails than from a fall from a bed where side rails are not used. They also potentially increase the likelihood that the resident will spend more time in bed and fall when attempting to transfer from the bed.

As with other restraints, for residents who are restrained by side rails, it is expected that the process facilities employ to reduce the use of side rails as restraints is systematic and gradual to ensure the resident's safety while treating the resident's medical symptom.

The same device may have the effect of restraining one individual but not another, depending on the individual resident's condition and circumstances. For example, partial rails may assist one resident to enter and exit the bed independently while acting as a restraint for another.

Orthotic body devices may be used solely for therapeutic purposes to improve the overall functional capacity of the resident.

An enclosed framed wheeled walker, with or without a posterior seat, would not meet the definition of a restraint if the resident could easily open the front gate and exit the device. If the resident cannot open the front gate (due to cognitive or physical limitations that prevent him or her from exiting the device or because the device has been altered to prevent the resident from exiting the device), the enclosed framed wheeled walker would meet the definition of a restraint since the device would restrict the resident's freedom of movement (e.g. transferring to another chair, to the commode, or into the bed). The decision on whether framed wheeled walkers are a restraint must be made on an individual basis.

"Medical Symptom" is defined as an indication or characteristic of a physical or psychological condition.

The resident's medical symptoms should not be viewed in isolation, rather the symptoms should be viewed in the context of the resident's condition, circumstances, and environment. Objective findings derived from clinical evaluation and the resident's subjective symptoms should be considered to determine the presence of the medical symptom. The resident's subjective symptoms may not be used as the sole basis for using a restraint. Before a resident is restrained, the facility must determine the presence of a specific medical symptom that would require the use of restraints, and how the use of restraints would treat the medical symptom, protect the resident's safety, and assist the resident in attaining or maintaining his or her highest practicable level of physical and psychosocial well-being.

Medical symptoms that warrant the use of restraints must be documented in the resident's medical record, ongoing assessments, and care plans. While there must be a physician's order reflecting the presence of a medical symptom, CMS will hold the facility ultimately accountable for the appropriateness of that determination. The physician's order alone is not sufficient to warrant the use of the restraint. It is further expected, for those residents whose care plans indicate the need for restraints, that the facility engage in a systematic and gradual process toward reducing restraints (e.g., gradually increasing the time for ambulation and muscle-strengthening activities). This systematic process would also apply to recently admitted residents for whom restraints were used in the previous setting.

Consideration of Treatment Plan

In order for the resident to be fully informed, the facility must explain, in the context of the individual resident's condition and circumstances, the potential risks and benefits of all options under consideration including using a restraint, not using a restraint, and alternatives to restraint use. Whenever restraint use is considered, the facility must explain to the resident how the use of restraints would treat the resident's medical symptoms and assist the resident in attaining or maintaining his/her highest practicable level of physical or psychological well-being. In addition, the facility must also explain the potential negative outcomes of restraint use which include, but are not limited to, declines in the resident's physical functioning (e.g., ability to ambulate) and muscle condition, contractures, increased incidence of infections and development of pressure sores/ulcers, delirium, agitation, and incontinence. Moreover, restraint use may constitute an accident hazard. Restraints have been found in some cases to increase the incidence of falls or head trauma due to falls and other accidents (e.g., strangulation, entrapment). Finally, residents who are restrained may face a loss of autonomy, dignity, and self respect, and may show symptoms of withdrawal, depression, or reduced social contact. In effect, restraint use can reduce independence, functional capacity, and quality of life. Alternatives to restraint use should be considered and discussed with the resident. Alternatives to restraint use might include modifying the resident's environment and/or routine.

In the case of a resident who is incapable of making a decision, the legal surrogate or representative may exercise this right based on the same information that would have been provided to the resident. (See §483.10(a)(3) and (4).) However, the legal surrogate or representative cannot give permission to use restraints for the sake of discipline or staff convenience or when the restraint is not necessary to treat the resident's medical symptoms. That is, the facility may not use restraints in violation of the regulation solely based on a legal surrogate or representative's request or approval.

Assessment and Care Planning for Restraint Use

There are instances where, after assessment and care planning, a least restrictive restraint may be deemed appropriate for an individual resident to attain or maintain his or her highest practicable physical and psychosocial well-being. This does not alter the facility's responsibility to assess and care plan restraint use on an ongoing basis.

Before using a device for mobility or transfer, assessment should include a review of the resident's:

- Bed mobility (e.g., would the use of a device assist the resident to turn from side to side? Is the resident totally immobile and unable to change position without assistance?); and
- Ability to transfer between positions, to and from bed or chair, to stand and toilet (e.g., does the raised side rail add risk to the resident's ability to transfer?).

The facility must design its interventions not only to minimize or eliminate the medical symptom, but also to identify and address any underlying problems causing the medical symptom.

- Interventions that the facility might incorporate in care planning include:

    ✧ Providing restorative care to enhance abilities to stand, transfer, and walk safely;
    ✧ Providing a device such as a trapeze to increase a resident's mobility in bed; moving the bed lower to the floor and surrounding the bed with a soft mat;

✧ Equipping the resident with a device that monitors his/her attempts to arise;

✧ Providing frequent monitoring by staff with periodic assisted toileting for residents who attempt to arise to use the bathroom;

✧ Furnishing visual and verbal reminders to use the call bell for residents who are able to comprehend this information and are able to use the call bell device; and/or

✧ Providing exercise and therapeutic interventions, based on individual assessment and care planning, that may assist the resident in achieving proper body position, balance, and alignment, without the potential negative effects associated with restraint use.

Procedures §483.13(a)

Determine if the facility follows a systematic process of evaluation and care planning prior to using restraints. Since continued restraint use is associated with a potential for a decline in functioning if the risk is not addressed, determine if the interdisciplinary team addressed the risk of decline at the time restraint use was initiated and that the care plan reflected measures to minimize a decline. Also determine if the plan of care was consistently implemented. Determine whether the decline can be attributed to a disease progression or inappropriate use of restraints.

For sampled residents observed as physically restrained during the survey or whose clinical records show the use of physical restraints within 30 days of the survey, determine whether the facility used the restraint for convenience or discipline, or a therapeutic intervention for specific periods to attain and maintain the resident's highest practicable physical, mental, or psychosocial well-being.

Probes §483.13(a)

This systematic approach should answer these questions:

1. What are the medical symptoms that led to the consideration of the use of restraints?

2. Are these symptoms caused by failure to:

   a. Meet individual needs in accordance with the resident assessments including, but not limited to, section III of the MDS, Customary Daily Routines (MDS Version 2.0, section AC), in the context of relevant information in sections I and II of the MDS (MDS Version 2.0, sections AA and AB)?

   b. Use rehabilitative/restorative care?

   c. Provide meaningful activities?

   d. Manipulate the resident's environment, including seating?

3. Can the cause(s) of the medical symptoms be eliminated or reduced?

4. If the cause(s) cannot be eliminated or reduced, then has the facility attempted to use alternatives in order to avoid a decline in physical functioning associated with restraint use? (See Physical Restraints Resident Assessment Protocol (RAP), paragraph I.)

5. If alternatives have been tried and deemed unsuccessful, does the facility use the least restrictive restraint for the least amount of time? Does the facility monitor and adjust care to reduce the potential for negative outcomes while continually trying to find and use less restrictive alternatives?

6. Did the resident or legal surrogate make an informed choice about the use of restraints? Were risks, benefits, and alternatives explained?

7. Does the facility use the Physical Restraints RAP to evaluate the appropriateness of restraint use?

8. Has the facility re-evaluated the need for the restraint, made efforts to eliminate its use, and maintained resident's strength and mobility?

F223 Abuse

(Rev. 12, Issued: 10-14-05, Effective: 10-14-05, Implementation: 10-14-05)

§483.13(b) Abuse

The resident has the right to be free from verbal, sexual, physical, and mental abuse; corporal punishment; and involuntary seclusion.

Intent §483.13(b)

Each resident has the right to be free from abuse, corporal punishment, and involuntary seclusion. Residents must not be subjected to abuse by anyone, including, but not limited to, facility staff, other residents, consultants or volunteers, staff of other agencies serving the resident, family members or legal guardians, friends, or other individuals.

Interpretive Guidelines §483.13(b) and (c)

"Abuse" means the willful infliction of injury, unreasonable confinement, intimidation, or punishment with resulting physical harm, pain, or mental anguish." (42 CFR §488.301)

This also includes the deprivation by an individual, including a caretaker, of goods or services that are necessary to attain or maintain physical, mental, and psychosocial well-being. This presumes that instances of abuse of all residents, even those in a coma, cause physical harm, pain, or mental anguish.

"Verbal abuse" is defined as the use of oral, written, or gestured language that willfully includes disparaging and derogatory terms to residents or their families, or within their hearing distance, regardless of their age, ability to comprehend, or disability. Examples of verbal abuse include, but are not limited to: threats of harm; saying things to frighten a resident, such as telling a resident that he/she will never be able to see his/her family again.

"Sexual abuse" includes, but is not limited to, sexual harassment, sexual coercion, or sexual assault.

"Physical abuse" includes hitting, slapping, pinching, and kicking. It also includes controlling behavior through corporal punishment.

"Mental abuse" includes, but is not limited to, humiliation, harassment, threats of punishment or deprivation.

"Involuntary seclusion" is defined as separation of a resident from other residents or from her/his room or confinement to her/his room (with or without roommates) against the resident's will, or the will of the resident's legal representative. Emergency or short-term monitored separation from other residents will not be considered involuntary seclusion and may be permitted if used for a limited period of time as a therapeutic intervention to reduce agitation until professional staff can develop a plan of care to meet the resident's needs.

Investigation of possible involuntary seclusion, may involve one of two types of situations: that in which residents are living in an area of the facility that restricts their freedom of movement throughout the facility, or that in which a resident is temporarily separated from other residents.

- If the stated purpose of a unit which prevents residents from free movement throughout the facility is to provide specialized care for residents who are cognitively impaired, then placement in the unit is not considered involuntary seclusion, as long as care and services are provided in accordance with each resident's individual needs and preferences rather than for staff convenience, and as long as the resident, surrogate, or representative (if any) participates in the placement decision, and is involved in continuing care planning to assure placement continues to meet resident needs and preferences.
- If a resident is receiving emergency short-term monitored separation due to temporary behavioral symptoms (such as brief catastrophic reactions or combative or aggressive behaviors which pose a threat to the resident, other residents, staff, or others in the facility), this is not considered involuntary seclusion as long as this is the least restrictive approach for the minimum amount of time, and is being done according to resident needs and not for staff convenience.

If a resident is being temporarily separated from other residents, i.e., for less than 24 hours, as an emergency short-term intervention, answer these questions:

1. What are the symptoms that led to the consideration of the separation?

2. Are these symptoms caused by failure to:

   a. Meet individual needs?

   b. Provide meaningful activities?

   c. Manipulate the resident's environment?

3. Can the cause(s) be removed?

4. If the cause(s) cannot be removed, has the facility attempted to use alternatives short of separation?

5. If these alternatives have been tried and found ineffective, does the facility use separation for the least amount of time?

6. To what extent has the resident, surrogate, or representative (if any) participated in care planning and made an informed choice about separation?

7. Does the facility monitor and adjust care to reduce negative outcomes, while continually trying to find and use less restrictive alternatives?

If, during the course of the survey, you identify the possibility of abuse according to the definitions above, investigate through interviews, observations, and record review. (For investigative options, refer to the Guidelines for Complaint Investigation which outlines the steps of investigations for various types of suspected abuse and misappropriation of property.)

Report and record any instances where the survey team observes an abusive incident. Completely document who committed the abusive act, the nature of the abuse, and where and when it occurred. Ensure that the facility addresses the incident immediately.

Properly trained staff should be able to respond appropriately to resident behavior. The CMS does not consider striking a combative resident an appropriate response in any situation. Retaliation by staff is abuse and should be cited as such.

---

§483.13(c) Staff Treatment of Residents

F224* and F226**

The facility must develop and implement written policies and procedures that prohibit mistreatment, neglect, and abuse of residents and misappropriation of resident property.

§483.13(c)(1)(i) Staff Treatment of Residents

(1) The facility must—

(i) Not use verbal, mental, sexual, or physical abuse; corporal punishment; or involuntary seclusion;

F224 Staff treatment of residents

* Intent §483.13(c) (F224)

Each resident has the right to be free from mistreatment, neglect, and misappropriation of property. This includes the facility's identification of residents whose personal histories render them at risk for abusing other residents, and development of intervention strategies to prevent occurrences, monitoring for changes that would trigger abusive behavior, and reassessment of the interventions on a regular basis.

* Use tag F224 for deficiencies concerning mistreatment, neglect, or misappropriation of resident property.

* Guidelines §483.13(c) (F224)

"Neglect" means failure to provide goods and services necessary to avoid physical harm, mental anguish, or mental illness. (42 CFR 488.301)

"Misappropriation of resident property" means the deliberate misplacement; exploitation; or wrongful, temporary or permanent use of a resident's belongings or money without the resident's consent. (42 CFR 488.301)

F226 Employee screening and training policies

(Rev. 12, Issued: 10-14-05, Effective: 10-14-05, Implementation: 10-14-05)

** Intent §483.13(c), F226

The facility must develop and operationalize policies and procedures for screening and training employees; protection of residents; and for the prevention, identification, investigation, and reporting of abuse, neglect, mistreatment, and misappropriation of property. The purpose is to assure that the facility is doing all that is within its control to prevent occurrences.

** Use tag F226 for deficiencies concerning the facility's development and implementation of policies and procedures.

** Guidelines §483.13(c), F226

The facility must develop and implement policies and procedures that include the seven components: screening, training, prevention, identification, investigation, protection, and reporting/ response. The items under each component listed below are examples of ways in which the facility could operationalize each component.

I. Screening (483.13(c)(1)(ii)(A)&(B)): Have procedures to:

- Screen potential employees for a history of abuse, neglect, or mistreating residents as defined by the applicable requirements at 483.13(c)(1)(ii)(A) and (B). This includes attempting to obtain information from previous employers and/or current employers, and checking with the appropriate licensing boards and registries.

II. Training (42 CFR 483.74(e)): Have procedures to:

- Train employees, through orientation and on-going sessions on issues related to abuse prohibition practices such as:

  ✧ Appropriate interventions to deal with aggressive and/or catastrophic reactions of residents;
  ✧ How staff should report their knowledge related to allegations without fear of reprisal;
  ✧ How to recognize signs of burnout, frustration, and stress that may lead to abuse; and
  ✧ What constitutes abuse, neglect, and misappropriation of resident property.

III. Prevention (483.13(b) and 483.13(c)): Have procedures to:

- Provide residents, families, and staff information on how and to whom they may report concerns, incidents, and grievances without the fear of retribution; and provide feedback regarding the concerns that have been expressed. (See 483.10(f) for further information regarding grievances.)
- Identify, correct, and intervene in situations in which abuse, neglect, and/or misappropriation of resident property is more likely to occur.
- This includes an analysis of:

  ✧ Features of the physical environment that may make abuse and/or neglect more likely to occur, such as secluded areas of the facility;
  ✧ The deployment of staff on each shift in sufficient numbers to meet the needs of the residents, and assure that the staff assigned have knowledge of the individual resident's care needs;
  ✧ The supervision of staff to identify inappropriate behaviors, such as using derogatory language, rough handling, ignoring residents while giving care, directing residents who need toileting assistance to urinate or defecate in their beds; and
  ✧ The assessment, care planning, and monitoring of residents with needs and behaviors which might lead to conflict or neglect, such as residents with a history of aggressive behaviors, residents who have behaviors such as entering other residents' rooms, residents with self-injurious behaviors, residents with communication disorders, those that require heavy nursing care and/or are totally dependent on staff.

IV. Identification (483.13(c)(2)): Have procedures to:

- Identify events, such as suspicious bruising of residents, occurrences, patterns, and trends that may constitute abuse; and to determine the direction of the investigation.

V. Investigation (483.13(c)(3)): Have procedures to:

- Investigate different types of incidents; and
- Identify the staff member responsible for the initial reporting, investigation of alleged violations and reporting of results to the proper authorities. (See §483.13 (c)(2), (3), and (4).)

VI. Protection (483.13(c)(3): Have procedures to:

- Protect residents from harm during an investigation.

VII. Reporting/Response (483.13(c)(1)(iii), 483.13(c)(2), and 483.13(c)(4)): Have procedures to:

- Report all alleged violations and all substantiated incidents to the state agency and to all other agencies as required, and take all necessary corrective actions depending on the results of the investigation;
- Report to the State nurse aide registry or licensing authorities any knowledge it has of any actions by a court of law which would indicate an employee is unfit for service; and
- Analyze the occurrences to determine what changes are needed, if any, to policies and procedures to prevent further occurrences.

F225 Not employ certain individuals

(Rev. 12, Issued: 10-14-05, Effective: 10-14-05, Implementation: 10-14-05)

The facility must—

§483.13(c)(1)(ii) Not employ individuals who have been—

(A) Found guilty of abusing, neglecting, or mistreating residents by a court of law; or

(B) Have had a finding entered into the State nurse aide registry concerning abuse, neglect, mistreatment of residents or misappropriation of their property; and

(iii) Report any knowledge it has of actions by a court of law against an employee, which would indicate unfitness for service as a nurse aide or other facility staff to the State nurse aide registry or licensing authorities.

§483.13(c)(2) The facility must ensure that all alleged violations involving mistreatment, neglect, or abuse, including injuries of unknown source and misappropriation of resident property are reported immediately to the administrator of the facility and to other officials in accordance with State law through established procedures (including to the State survey and certification agency).

§483.13(c)(3) The facility must have evidence that all alleged violations are thoroughly investigated, and must prevent further potential abuse while the investigation is in progress.

§483.13(c)(4) The results of all investigations must be reported to the administrator or his designated representative and to other officials in accordance with State law (including to the

State survey and certification agency) within 5 working days of the incident, and if the alleged violation is verified, appropriate corrective action must be taken.

Intent §483.13(c)(1)(ii) and (iii)

The facility must not hire a potential employee with a history of abuse, if that information is known to the facility. The facility must report knowledge of actions by a court of law against an employee that indicates the employee is unfit for duty. The facility must report alleged violations, conduct an investigation of all alleged violations, report the results to proper authorities, and take necessary corrective actions.

Interpretive Guidelines §483.13(c)(1)(ii) and (iii)

Facilities must be thorough in their investigations of the past histories of individuals they are considering hiring. In addition to inquiry of the State nurse aide registry or licensing authorities, the facility should check information from previous and/or current employers and make reasonable efforts to uncover information about any past criminal prosecutions.

"Found guilty . . . by a court of law" applies to situations where the defendant pleads guilty, is found guilty, or pleads nolo contendere.

"Finding" is defined as a determination made by the State that validates allegations of abuse, neglect, mistreatment of residents, or misappropriation of their property.

A certified nurse aide found guilty of neglect, abuse, or mistreating residents or misappropriation of property by a court of law, must have her/his name entered into the nurse aide registry. A licensed staff member found guilty of the above must be reported to their licensing board. Further, if a facility determines that actions by a court of law against an employee are such that they indicate that the individual is unsuited to work in a nursing home (e.g., felony conviction of child abuse, sexual assault, or assault with a deadly weapon), then the facility must report that individual to the nurse aide registry (if a nurse aide) or to the State licensing authorities (if a licensed staff member). Such a determination by the facility is not limited to mistreatment, neglect, and abuse of residents and misappropriation of their property, but to any treatment of residents or others inside or outside the facility which the facility determines to be such that the individual should not work in a nursing home environment.

A State must not make a finding that an individual has neglected a resident if the individual demonstrates that such neglect was caused by factors beyond the control of the individual.

Interpretive Guidelines §483.13(c)(2) and (4)

The facility's reporting requirements under 483.13(c)(2) and (4) include reporting both alleged violations and the results of investigations to the State survey agency.

"Injuries of unknown source" — An injury should be classified as an "injury of unknown source" when both of the following conditions are met:

- The source of the injury was not observed by any person or the source of the injury could not be explained by the resident; and
- The injury is suspicious because of the extent of the injury or the location of the injury (e.g., the injury is located in an area not generally vulnerable to trauma) or the number of injuries observed at one particular point in time or the incidence of injuries over time.

"Immediately" means as soon as possible, but ought not exceed 24 hours after discovery of the incident, in the absence of a shorter State time frame requirement. Conformance with this definition requires that each State has a means to collect reports, even on off-duty hours (e.g., answering machine, voice mail, fax).

The phrase "in accordance with State law" modifies the word "officials" only. As such, State law may stipulate that alleged violations and the results of the investigations be reported to additional State officials beyond those specified in Federal regulations. This phrase does not modify what types of alleged violations must be reported or the time frames in which the reports are to be made. As such, States may not eliminate the obligation for any of the alleged violations (i.e., mistreatment, neglect, abuse, injuries of unknown source, and misappropriation of resident property) to be reported, nor can the State establish longer time frames for reporting than mandated in the regulations at §§483.13(c)(2) and (4). No State can override the obligation of the nursing home to fulfill the requirements under §483.13(c), so long as the Medicare/ Medicaid certification is in place.

§483.15 Quality of Life   Tags 240 – 258

§483.15(a) Dignity
§483.15(b) Self-Determination and Participation
§483.15(c) Participation in Resident and Family Groups
§483.15(d) Participation in Other Activities
§483.15(e) Accommodation of Needs
§483.15(f) Activities
§483.15(g) Social Services
§483.15(h) Environment

F240 Quality of life

§483.15 Quality of Life

A facility must care for its residents in a manner and in an environment that promotes maintenance or enhancement of each resident's quality of life.

Interpretive Guidelines §483.15

The intention of the quality of life requirements is to specify the facility's responsibilities toward creating and sustaining an environment that humanizes and individualizes each resident. Compliance decisions here are driven by the quality of life each resident experiences.

F241 Quality of life: dignity

§483.15(a) Dignity

The facility must promote care for residents in a manner and in an environment that maintains or enhances each resident's dignity and respect in full recognition of his or her individuality.

Interpretive Guidelines §483.15(a)

"Dignity" means that in their interactions with residents, staff carries out activities that assist the resident to maintain and enhance his/her self-esteem and self-worth. For example:

- Grooming residents as they wish to be groomed (e.g., hair combed and styled, beards shaved/trimmed, nails clean and clipped);
- Assisting residents to dress in their own clothes appropriate to the time of day and individual preferences;

- Assisting residents to attend activities of their own choosing;
- Labeling each resident's clothing in a way that respects his or her dignity;
- Promoting resident independence and dignity in dining (such as avoidance of day-to-day use of plastic cutlery and paper/plastic dishware, bibs instead of napkins, dining room conducive to pleasant dining, aides not yelling);
- Respecting resident's private space and property (e.g., not changing radio or television station without resident's permission, knocking on doors and requesting permission to enter, closing doors as requested by the resident, not moving or inspecting resident's personal possessions without permission);
- Respecting resident's social status, speaking respectfully, listening carefully, treating residents with respect (e.g., addressing the resident with a name of the resident's choice, not excluding residents from conversations or discussing residents in community setting); and
- Focusing on residents as individuals when they talk to them and addressing residents as individuals when providing care and services.

Procedures §483.15(a)

For sampled residents, use the Resident Assessment Instrument (RAI) and comprehensive care plan to consider the resident's former lifestyle and personal choices made while in the facility to obtain a picture of characteristic resident behaviors. As part of the team's information gathering and decision-making, look at the actions and omissions of staff and the uniqueness of the individual sampled resident and on the needs and preferences of the resident, not on the actions and omissions themselves.

Throughout the survey, observe: Do staff show respect for residents? When staff interact with a resident, do staff pay attention to the resident as an individual? Do staff respond in a timely manner to the resident's requests for assistance? In group activities, do staff focus attention on the group of residents? Or, do staff appear distracted when they interact with residents? For example, do staff continue to talk with each other while doing a "task" for a resident(s) as if she/he were not present?

If the survey team identifies potential compliance issues regarding the privacy of residents during treatment, refer to §483.10(e), F164.

F242 Quality of life: self-determination and participation

§483.15(b) Self-Determination and Participation

The resident has the right to—

(1) Choose activities, schedules, and health care consistent with his or her interests, assessments, and plans of care;

(2) Interact with members of the community both inside and outside the facility; and

(3) Make choices about aspects of his or her life in the facility that are significant to the resident.

Procedures §483.15(b)

Observe how well staff knows each resident and what aspects of life are important to him/her. Determine if staff makes adjustments to allow residents to exercise choice and self-determination.

Review MDS Background Information III (MDS version 2.0 section AC) for customary routines. For sampled residents, review MDS to determine level of participation in assessment and care planning by resident and family members. Review MDS, section G (MDS version 2.0 section F) for Psychosocial Well-Being and Care Planning.

If the facility has failed to reasonably accommodate the preferences of the resident consistent with interests, assessments, and plan of care, see §483.15(e), F246.

Interpretive Guidelines §483.15(b)(3)

The intent of this requirement is to specify that the facility must create an environment that is respectful of the right of each resident to exercise his or her autonomy regarding what the resident considers to be important facets of his or her life. For example, if a facility changes its policy and prohibits smoking, it must allow current residents who smoke to continue smoking in an area that maintains the quality of life for these residents. Weather permitting, this may be an outside area. Residents admitted after the facility changes its policy must be informed of this policy at admission. (See §483.10(b)(1).) Or, if a resident mentions that her therapy is scheduled at the time of her favorite television program, the facility should accommodate the resident to the extent that it can.

F243 Quality of life: participation in resident and family groups

§483.15(c) Participation in Resident and Family Groups

(1) A resident has the right to organize and participate in resident groups in the facility;

(2) A resident's family has the right to meet in the facility with the families of other residents in the facility;

(3) The facility must provide a resident or family group, if one exists, with private space;

(4) Staff or visitors may attend meetings at the group's invitation;

(5) The facility must provide a designated staff person responsible for providing assistance and responding to written requests that result form group meetings;

SEE INTERPRETIVE GUIDANCE FOR §483.15(c) AT TAG F244

F244 Quality of life: required facility responses to resident or family groups

§483.15(c)(6) When a resident or family group exists, the facility must listen to the views and act upon the grievances and recommendations of residents and families concerning proposed policy and operational decisions affecting resident care and life in the facility.

Interpretive Guidelines §483.15(c)

This requirement does not require that residents' organize a residents or family group. However, whenever residents or their families wish to organize, facilities must allow them to do so without interference. The facility must provide the group with space, privacy for meetings, and staff support. Normally, the designated staff person responsible for assistance and liaison between the group and the facility's administration and any other staff members attend the meeting only if requested.

- "A resident's or family group" is defined as a group that meets regularly to:

    ◇ Discuss and offer suggestions about facility policies and procedures affecting residents' care, treatment, and quality of life;
    ◇ Support each other;
    ◇ Plan resident and family activities;
    ◇ Participate in educational activities; or
    ◇ For any other purpose.

The facility is required to listen to resident and family group recommendations and grievances. Acting upon these issues does not mean that the facility must accede to all group recommendations, but the facility must seriously consider the group's recommendations and must attempt to accommodate those recommendations, to the extent practicable, in developing and changing facility policies affecting resident care and life in the facility. The facility should communicate its decisions to the resident and/or family group.

Procedures §483.15(c)

If no organized group exists, determine if residents have attempted to form one and have been unsuccessful, and, if so, why.

F245 Quality of life: resident participation in outside community

§483.15(d) Participation in Other Activities

A resident has the right to participate in social, religious, and community activities that do not interfere with the rights of other residents in the facility.

Interpretive Guidelines §483.15(d)

The facility, to the extent possible, should accommodate an individual's needs and choices for how he/she spends time, both inside and outside the facility.

Ask the social worker or other appropriate staff how they help residents pursue activities outside the facility.

F246 Quality of life: accommodations of individual needs and preferences

(Rev. 5, Issued: 11-19-04, Effective: 11-19-04, Implementation: 11-19-04)

§483.15(e) Accommodation of Needs

A resident has a right to—

§483.15(e)(1) Reside and receive services in the facility with reasonable accommodations of individual needs and preferences, except when the health or safety of the individual or other residents would be endangered; and

ALSO SEE INTERPRETIVE GUIDANCE AT TAG F247

F247 Quality of life: receive notice before resident's room or roommate is changed

A resident has a right to—

§483.15(e)(2) Receive notice before the resident's room or roommate in the facility is changed.

Interpretive Guidelines §483.15(e)

"Reasonable accommodations of individual needs and preferences," is defined as the facility's efforts to individualize the resident's environment. The facility's physical environment and staff behaviors should be directed toward assisting the resident in maintaining and/or achieving independent functioning, dignity, and well-being to the extent possible in accordance with the resident's own preferences, assessment, and care plans. The facility should attempt to adapt such things as schedules, call systems, and room arrangements to accommodate resident's preferences, desires, and unique needs.

This requirement applies to areas and environment in accordance with needs and preferences NOT addresses at: §§483.10(k), Telephone; 483.10(1), Personal Property; 483.10(m), Married Couples; 483.15(b), Self-Determination and Participation; 483.15(f)(1), Activities; 483.15(g)(1), Social Services; 483.15(h)(1), Homelike Environment; 483.25(a)(2) and (3), Activities of Daily Living; 483.25(f)(1), Psychosocial functioning; 483.25(h)(2), Accidents, Prevention-Assistive devices; 483.35(d)(3), Food prepared in a form designed to meet individual needs.

The facility must demonstrate that it accommodates resident's needs. For example, if the resident refuses a bath because he or she prefers a shower, prefers it at a different time of day or on a different day, does not feel well that day, is uneasy about the aide assigned to help or is worried about falling, the staff should make the necessary adjustments realizing the resident is not refusing to be clean but refusing the bath under the circumstance provided. The facility staff should meet with the resident to make adjustments in the care plan to accommodate his or her needs.

This includes learning the residents' preferences and taking them into account when discussing changes of rooms or roommates and the timing of such changes. In addition, this also includes making necessary adjustments to ensure that residents are able to reach call cords, buttons, or other communication mechanisms, as well as accommodating food activities or room choices.

Procedures §483.15(e)

Observe resident-staff interaction and determine to what extent staff attempt to accommodate resident's preferences. For those areas not addressed in other regulations, determine what happens when a resident states a preference in the form of a refusal. How does the staff attempt to learn what the resident is refusing, and why, and make adjustments to an extent practicable to meet the resident's needs?

Probes §483.15(e)

- Are rooms arranged such that residents in wheel chairs can easily access personal items and transfer in and out of bed?
- Does the facility respond to resident's stated needs and preferences?
- If the resident is unable to express needs and preferences that would individualize care, has the family expressed the resident's routine and has the facility responded?

Interpretive Guidelines §483.15(e)(1)

Review the extent to which the facility adapts the physical environment to enable residents to maintain unassisted functioning. These adaptations include, but are not limited to:

1. Furniture and adaptive equipment that enable residents to:

   a. Stand independently;

   b. Transfer without assistance (e.g., arm supports, correct chair height, firm support);

   c. Maintain body symmetry; and

   d. Participate in resident-preferred activities.

2. Measures that:

   a. Enable residents with dementia to walk freely;

   b. Reorient and remotivate residents with restorative potential (e.g., displaying easily readable calendars and clocks, wall hangings evocative of the lives of residents);

   c. Promote conversation and socialization (pictures and decorations that speak to the resident's age cohort); and

   d. Promote mobility and independence for disabled residents in going to the bathroom (e.g., grab bars, elevated toilet seats).

Determine if staff use appropriate measures to facilitate communication with residents who have difficulty communicating. For example, if necessary, does staff get at eye level, allow them to remove a resident from noisy surroundings?

Determine if staff communicate effectively with residents with cognitive impairments, such as referring in a non-contradictory way to what residents are saying, and addressing what residents are trying to express to the agenda behind their behavior.

Probes §483.15(e)(1)(2)

How have residents' needs been accommodated? Do environmental adaptations enhance residents' independence, self-control, and highest practicable well-being? Is the fit between residents' needs and environment positive?

F248 Activities

(Rev. 19, Issued: 06-01-06, Effective/Implementation: 06-01-06)

§483.15(f) Activities

§483.15(f)(1) The facility must provide for an ongoing program of activities designed to meet, in accordance with the comprehensive assessment, the interests and the physical, mental, and psychosocial well-being of each resident.

§483.15(f)(1) Intent:

Activities

The intent of this requirement is that:

- The facility identifies each resident's interests and needs; and
- The facility involves the resident in an ongoing program of activities that is designed to appeal to his or her interests and to enhance the resident's highest practicable level of physical, mental, and psychosocial well-being.

Definitions

Definitions are provided to clarify key terms used in this guidance.

- "Activities" refer to any endeavor, other than routine ADLs, in which a resident participates that is intended to enhance her/his sense of well-being and to promote or enhance physical, cognitive, and emotional health. These include, but are not limited to, activities that promote self-esteem, pleasure, comfort, education, creativity, success, and independence.

  NOTE: ADL-related activities, such as manicures/pedicures, hair styling, and makeovers, may be considered part of the activities program.

- "One-to-One Programming" refers to programming provided to residents who will not, or cannot, effectively plan their own activity pursuits, or residents needing specialized or extended programs to enhance their overall daily routine and activity pursuit needs.
- "Person Appropriate" refers to the idea that each resident has a personal identity and history that involves more than just their medical illnesses or functional impairments. Activities should be relevant to the specific needs, interests, culture, background, etc. of the individual for whom they are developed.
- "Program of Activities" includes a combination of large and small group, one-to-one, and self-directed activities; and a system that supports the development, implementation, and evaluation of the activities provided to the residents in the facility.[1]

Overview

In long term care, an ongoing program of activities refers to the provision of activities in accordance with and based upon an individual resident's comprehensive assessment. The Institute of Medicine (IOM)'s 1986 report, "Improving the Quality of Care in Nursing Homes," became the basis for the "Nursing Home Reform" part of OBRA '87 and the current OBRA long term care regulations. The IOM Report identified the need for residents in nursing homes to receive care and/or services to maximize their highest practicable quality of life. However, defining "quality of life" has been difficult, as it is subjective for each person. Thus, it is important for the facility to conduct an individualized assessment of each resident to provide additional opportunities to help enhance a resident's self-esteem and dignity.

Research findings and the observations of positive resident outcomes confirm that activities are an integral component of residents' lives. Residents have indicated that daily life and involvement should be meaningful. Activities are meaningful when they reflect a person's interests and lifestyle, are enjoyable to the person, help the person to feel useful, and provide a sense of belonging.[2]

Residents' Views on Activities

Activities are relevant and valuable to residents' quality of life. In a large-scale study commissioned by CMS, 160 residents in 40 nursing homes were interviewed about what quality of life meant to them. The study found that residents "overwhelmingly assigned priority to dignity, although they labeled this concern in many ways." The researchers determined that the two main components of dignity, in the words of these residents, were "independence" and "positive self-image." Residents listed, under the categories of independence and positive self-image, the elements of "choice of activities" and "activities that amount to something," such as those that produce or teach something; activities using skills from residents' former work; religious activities; and activities that contribute to the nursing home.

The report stated that, "Residents not only discussed particular activities that gave them a sense of purpose but also indicated that a lack of appropriate activities contributes to having no sense of purpose." "Residents rarely mentioned participating in activities as a way to just 'keep busy' or just to socialize. The relevance of the activities to the residents' lives must be considered."

According to the study, residents wanted a variety of activities, including those that are not childish, require thinking (such as word games), are gender-specific, produce something useful, relate to previous work of residents, allow for socializing with visitors and participating in community events, and are physically active. The study found that the above concepts were relevant to both interviewable and non-interviewable residents. Researchers observed that non-interviewable residents appeared "happier" and "less agitated" in homes with many planned activities for them.

Non-traditional Approaches to Activities

Surveyors need to be aware that some facilities may take a non-traditional approach to activities. In neighborhoods/households, all staff may be trained as nurse aides and are responsible to provide activities, and activities may resemble those of a private home.[3] Residents, staff, and families may interact in ways that reflect daily life, instead of in formal activities programs. Residents may be more involved in the ongoing activities in their living area, such as care-planned approaches including chores, preparing foods, meeting with other residents to choose spontaneous activities, and leading an activity. It has been reported that, "some culture changed homes might not have a traditional activities calendar, and instead focus on community life to include activities. Instead of an "activities director," some homes have a Community Life Coordinator, a Community Developer, or other title for the individual directing the activities program.[4]

For more information on activities in homes changing to a resident-directed culture, the following websites are available as resources: www.pioneernetwork.net; www.culturechangenow.com; www.qualitypartnersri.org (click on nursing homes); and www.edenalt.com.

Assessment

The information gathered through the assessment process should be used to develop the activities component of the comprehensive care plan. The ongoing program of activities should match the skills, abilities, needs, and preferences of each resident with the demands of the activity and the characteristics of the physical, social and cultural environments.[5]

In order to develop individualized care planning goals and approaches, the facility should obtain sufficient, detailed information (even if the Activities RAP is not triggered) to determine what activities the resident prefers and what adaptations, if any, are needed.[6] The facility may use, but need not duplicate, information from other sources, such as the RAI, including the RAPs, assessments by other disciplines, observation, and resident and family interviews. Other sources of relevant information include the resident's lifelong interests, spirituality, life roles, goals, strengths, needs and activity pursuit patterns and preferences.[7] This assessment should be completed by or under the supervision of a qualified professional (see F249 for definition of qualified professional).

NOTE: Some residents may be independently capable of pursuing their own activities without intervention from the facility. This information should be noted in the assessment and identified in the plan of care.

Care Planning

Care planning involves identification of the resident's interests, preferences, and abilities; and any issues, concerns, problems, or needs affecting the resident's involvement/engagement in activities.[8] In addition to the activities component of the comprehensive care plan, information may also be found in a separate activity plan, on a CNA flow sheet, in a progress note, etc. Activity goals related to the comprehensive care plan should be based on measurable objectives and focused on desired outcomes (e.g., engagement in an activity that matches the resident's ability, maintaining attention to the activity for a specified period of time, expressing satisfaction with the activity verbally or non-verbally), not merely on attendance at a certain number of activities per week.

Note: For residents with no discernable response, service provision is still expected and may include one-to-one activities such as talking to the resident, reading to the resident about prior interests, or applying lotion while stroking the resident's hands or feet.

Activities can occur at any time, are not limited to formal activities being provided only by activities staff, and can include activities provided by other facility staff, volunteers, visitors, residents, and family members. All relevant departments should collaborate to develop and implement an individualized activities program for each resident. Some medications, such as diuretics, or conditions such as pain, incontinence, etc. may affect the resident's participation in activities. Therefore, additional steps may be needed to facilitate the resident's participation in activities, such as:

- If not contraindicated, timing the administration of medications, to the extent possible, to avoid interfering with the resident's ability to participate or to remain at a scheduled activity; or
- If not contraindicated, modifying the administration time of pain medication to allow the medication to take effect prior to an activity the resident enjoys.

The care plan should also identify the discipline(s) that will carry out the approaches. For example:

- Notifying residents of preferred activities;
- Transporting residents who need assistance to and from activities (including indoor, outdoor, and outings);
- Providing needed functional assistance (such as toileting and eating assistance); and
- Providing needed supplies or adaptations, such as obtaining and returning audio books, setting up adaptive equipment, etc.

Concepts the facility should have considered in the development of the activities component of the resident's comprehensive care plan include the following, as applicable to the resident:

- A continuation of life roles, consistent with resident preferences and functional capacity (e.g., to continue work or hobbies such as cooking, table setting, repairing small appliances);[9]
- Encouraging and supporting the development of new interests, hobbies, and skills (e.g., training on using the Internet); and
- Connecting with the community, such as places of worship, veterans' groups, volunteer groups, support groups, wellness groups, athletic or educational connections (via outings or invitations to outside groups to visit the facility).

The facility may need to consider accommodations in schedules, supplies and timing in order to optimize a resident's ability to participate in an activity of choice. Examples of accommodations may include, but are not limited to:

- Altering a therapy or a bath/shower schedule to make it possible for a resident to attend a desired activity that occurs at the same time as the therapy session or bath;
- Assisting residents, as needed, to get to and participate in desired activities (e.g., dressing, toileting, transportation);
- Providing supplies (e.g., books/magazines, music, craft projects, cards, sorting materials) for activities, and assistance when needed, for residents' use (e.g., during weekends, nights, holidays, evenings, or when the activities staff are unavailable); and

- Providing a late breakfast to allow a resident to continue a lifelong pattern of attending religious services before eating.

Interventions

The concept of individualized intervention has evolved over the years. Many activity professionals have abandoned generic interventions such as "reality orientation" and large-group activities that include residents with different levels of strengths and needs. In their place, individualized interventions have been developed based upon the assessment of the resident's history, preferences, strengths, and needs. These interventions have changed from the idea of "age-appropriate" activities to promoting "person-appropriate" activities. For example, one person may care for a doll or stroke a stuffed animal, another person may be inclined to reminisce about dolls or stuffed animals they once had, while someone else may enjoy petting a dog but will not be interested in inanimate objects. The surveyor observing these interventions should determine if the facility selected them in response to the resident's history and preferences. Many activities can be adapted in various ways to accommodate the resident's change in functioning due to physical or cognitive limitations.

Some Possible Adaptations that May be Made by the Facility [10, 11]

When evaluating the provision of activities, it is important for the surveyor to identify whether the resident has conditions and/or issues for which staff should have provided adaptations. Examples of adaptations for specific conditions include, but are not limited to the following:

- For the resident with visual impairments: higher levels of lighting without glare; magnifying glasses, light-filtering lenses, telescopic glasses; use of "clock method" to describe where items are located; description of sizes, shapes, colors; large print items including playing cards, newsprint, books; audio books;
- For the resident with hearing impairments: small group activities; placement of resident near speaker/activity leader; use of amplifiers or headphones; decreased background noise; written instructions; use of gestures or sign language to enhance verbal communication; adapted TV (closed captioning, magnified screen, earphones);
- For the resident who has physical limitations, the use of adaptive equipment, proper seating and positioning, placement of supplies and materials[12] (based on clinical assessment and referral as appropriate) to enhance:

  - ✧ Visual interaction and to compensate for loss of visual field (hemianopsia);
  - ✧ Upper extremity function and range of motion (reach);
  - ✧ Hand dexterity (e.g., adapted size of items such as larger handles for cooking and woodworking equipment, built-up paintbrush handles, large needles for crocheting);
  - ✧ The ability to manipulate an item based upon the item's weight, such as lighter weight for residents with muscle weakness;[13]

- For the resident who has the use of only one hand: holders for kitchen items, magazines/books, playing cards; items (e.g., art work, bingo card, nail file) taped to the table; c-clamp or suction vise to hold wood for sanding;

- For the resident with cognitive impairment: task segmentation and simplification; programs using retained long-term memory, rather than short-term memory; length of activities based on attention span; settings that recreate past experiences or increase/decrease stimulation; smaller groups without interruption; one-to-one activities;

Note: The length, duration, and content of specific one-to-one activities are determined by the specific needs of the individual resident, such as several short interventions (rather than a few longer activities) if someone has extremely low tolerance, or if there are behavioral issues.

Examples of one-to-one activities may include any of the following:

- ◈ Sensory stimulation or cognitive therapy (e.g., touch/visual/auditory stimulation, reminiscence, or validation therapy) such as special stimulus rooms or equipment; alerting/upbeat music and using alerting aromas or providing fabrics or other materials of varying textures;
- ◈ Social engagement (e.g., directed conversation, initiating a resident to resident conversation, pleasure walk or coffee visit);
- ◈ Spiritual support, nurturing (e.g., daily devotion, Bible reading, or prayer with or for resident per religious requests/desires);
- ◈ Creative, task-oriented activities (e.g., music or pet activities/therapy, letter writing, word puzzles); or
- ◈ Support of self-directed activity (e.g., delivering of library books, craft material to rooms, setting up talking book service).

- For the resident with a language barrier: translation tools; translators; or publications and/or audio/video materials in the resident's language;
- For residents who are terminally ill: life review; quality time with chosen relatives, friends, staff, and/or other residents; spiritual support; touch; massage; music; and/or reading to the resident;[8]

Note: Some residents may prefer to spend their time alone and introspectively. Their refusal of activities does not necessarily constitute noncompliance.

- For the resident with pain: spiritual support, relaxation programs, music, massage, aromatherapy, pet therapy/pet visits, and/or touch;
- For the resident who prefers to stay in her/his own room or is unable to leave her/his room: in-room visits by staff/other residents/volunteers with similar interests/hobbies; touch and sensory activities such as massage or aromatherapy; access to art/craft materials, cards, games, reading materials; access to technology of interest (computer, DVD, hand held video games, preferred radio programs/stations, audio books); and/or visits from spiritual counselors;[14]
- For the resident with varying sleep patterns, activities are available during awake time. Some facilities use a variety of options when activities staff are not available for a particular resident: nursing staff reads a newspaper with resident; dietary staff makes finger

foods available; CNA works puzzle with the resident; maintenance staff take the resident on night rounds; and/or early morning delivery of coffee/juice to residents;

- For the resident who has recently moved-in: welcoming activities and/or orientation activities;
- For the short-stay resident: "a la carte activities" are available, such as books, magazines, cards, word puzzles, newspapers, CDs, movies, and handheld games; interesting/contemporary group activities are offered, such as dominoes, bridge, Pinochle, poker, video games, movies, and travelogues; and/or individual activities designed to match the goals of therapy, such as jigsaw puzzles to enhance fine motor skills;
- For the younger resident: individual and group music offerings that fit the resident's taste and era;
- magazines, books and movies that fit the resident's taste
- and era; computer and Internet access; and/or contemporary group activities, such as video games, and the opportunity to play musical instruments, card and board games, and sports; and
- For residents from diverse ethnic or cultural backgrounds: special events that include meals, decorations, celebrations, or music; visits from spiritual leaders and other individuals of the same ethnic background; printed materials (newspapers, magazines) about the resident's culture; and/or opportunities for the resident and family to share information about their culture with other residents, families, and staff.

Activity Approaches for Residents with Behavioral Symptoms[15, 7]

When the surveyor is evaluating the activities provided to a resident who has behavioral symptoms, they may observe that many behaviors take place at about the same time every day (e.g., before lunch or mid-afternoon). The facility may have identified a resident's pattern of behavior symptoms and may offer activity interventions, whenever possible, prior to the behavior occurring. Once a behavior escalates, activities may be less effective or may even cause further stress to the resident (some behaviors may be appropriate reactions to feelings of discomfort, pain, or embarrassment, such as aggressive behaviors exhibited by some residents with dementia during bathing).[16] Examples of activities-related interventions that a facility may provide to try to minimize distressed behavior may include, but are not limited to the following:

For the resident who is constantly walking:

- Providing a space and environmental cues that encourages physical exercise, decreases exit behavior and reduces extraneous stimulation (such as seating areas spaced along a walking path or garden; a setting in which the resident may manipulate objects; or a room with a calming atmosphere, for example, using music, light, and rocking chairs);
- Providing aroma(s)/aromatherapy that is/are pleasing and calming to the resident; and
- Validating the resident's feelings and words; engaging the resident in conversation about who or what they are seeking; and using one-to-one activities, such as reading to the resident or looking at familiar pictures and photo albums.

For the resident who engages in name-calling, hitting, kicking, yelling, biting, sexual behavior, or compulsive behavior:

- Providing a calm, non-rushed environment, with structured, familiar activities such as folding, sorting, and matching; using one-to-one activities or small group activities that comfort the resident, such as their preferred music, walking quietly with the staff, a family member, or a friend; eating a favorite snack; looking at familiar pictures;
- Engaging in exercise and movement activities; and
- Exchanging self-stimulatory activity for a more socially-appropriate activity that uses the hands, if in a public space.

For the resident who disrupts group activities with behaviors such as talking loudly and being demanding, or the resident who has catastrophic reactions such as uncontrolled crying or anger, or the resident who is sensitive to too much stimulation:

- Offering activities in which the resident can succeed, that are broken into simple steps, that involve small groups or are one-to-one activities such as using the computer, that are short and repetitive, and that are stopped if the resident becomes overwhelmed (reducing excessive noise such as from the television);
- Involving in familiar occupation-related activities. (A resident, if they desire, can do paid or volunteer work and the type of work would be included in the resident's plan of care, such as working outside the facility, sorting supplies, delivering resident mail, passing juice and snacks, refer to F169, Work);
- Involving in physical activities such as walking, exercise or dancing, games or projects requiring strategy, planning, and concentration, such as model building, and creative programs such as music, art, dance or physically resistive activities, such as kneading clay, hammering, scrubbing, sanding, using a punching bag, using stretch bands, or lifting weights; and
- Slow exercises (e.g., slow tapping, clapping or drumming); rocking or swinging motions (including a rocking chair).

For the resident who goes through others' belongings:

- Using normalizing activities such as stacking canned food onto shelves, folding laundry; offering sorting activities (e.g., sorting socks, ties or buttons); involving in organizing tasks (e.g., putting activity supplies away); providing rummage areas in plain sight, such as a dresser; and
- Using non-entry cues, such as "Do not disturb" signs or removable sashes, at the doors of other residents' rooms; providing locks to secure other resident's belongings (if requested).

For the resident who has withdrawn from previous activity interests/customary routines and isolates self in room/bed most of the day:

- Providing activities just before or after meal time and where the meal is being served (out of the room);
- Providing in-room volunteer visits, music or videos of choice;
- Encouraging volunteer-type work that begins in the room and needs to be completed outside of the room, or a small group activity in the resident's room, if the resident agrees;

working on failure-free activities, such as simple structured crafts or other activity with a friend; having the resident assist another person;

- Inviting to special events with a trusted peer or family/friend;
- Engaging in activities that give the resident a sense of value (e.g., intergenerational activities that emphasize the resident's oral history knowledge);
- Inviting resident to participate on facility committees;
- Inviting the resident outdoors; and
- Involving in gross motor exercises (e.g., aerobics, light weight training) to increase energy and uplift mood.

For the resident who excessively seeks attention from staff and/or peers: Including in social programs, small group activities, service projects, with opportunities for leadership.

For the resident who lacks awareness of personal safety, such as putting foreign objects in her/his mouth or who is self-destructive and tries to harm self by cutting or hitting self, head banging, or causing other injuries to self:

- Observing closely during activities, taking precautions with materials (e.g., avoiding sharp objects and small items that can be put into the mouth);
- Involving in smaller groups or one-to-one activities that use the hands (e.g., folding towels, putting together PVC tubing);
- Focusing attention on activities that are emotionally soothing, such as listening to music or talking about personal strengths and skills, followed by participation in related activities; and
- Focusing attention on physical activities, such as exercise.

For the resident who has delusional and hallucinatory behavior that is stressful to her/him:

- Focusing the resident on activities that decrease stress and increase awareness of actual surroundings, such as familiar activities and physical activities; offering verbal reassurance, especially in terms of keeping the resident safe; and acknowledging that the resident's experience is real to her/him.

The outcome for the resident, the decrease or elimination of the behavior, either validates the activity intervention or suggests the need for a new approach.

Endnotes

1. Miller, M. E., Peckham, C. W., & Peckham, A. B. (1998). Activities keep me going and going (pp. 217-224). Lebanon, OH: Otterbein Homes.
2. Alzheimer's Association (n.d.). Activity based Alzheimer care: Building a therapeutic program. Training presentation made 1998.
3. Thomas, W.H. (2003). Evolution of Eden. In A. S. Weiner & J. L. Ronch (Eds.), Culture change in long-term care (pp. 146-157). New York: Haworth Press.
4. Bowman, C. S. (2005). Living Life to the Fullest: A match made in OBRA '87. Milwaukee, WI: Action Pact, Inc.

5. Glantz, C.G., & Richman, N. (2001). Leisure activities. In Occupational therapy: Practice skills for physical dysfunction. St Louis: Mosby.

6. Glantz, C.G., & Richman, N. (1996). Evaluation and intervention for leisure activities, ROTE: Role of Occupational Therapy for the Elderly (2nd ed., p. 728). Bethesda, MD.: American Occupational Therapy Association.

7. Glantz, C.G., & Richman, N. (1998). Creative methods, materials and models for training trainers in alzheimer's education (pp. 156-159). Riverwoods, IL: Glantz/Richman Rehabilitation Associates.

8. Hellen, C. (1992). Alzheimer's disease: Activity-focused care (pp. 128-130). Boston, MA: Andover.

9. American Occupatinal Therapy Association. (2002). Occupational therapy practice framework: domain & process. American Journal of Occupational Therapy, 56(6), 616-617. Bethesda, MD: American Occupational Therapy Association.

10. Henderson, A., Cermak, S., Costner, W., Murray, E., Trombly, C., & Tickle-Gegnen, L. (1991). The issue is: Occupational science is multidimensional. American Journal of Occupational Therapy, 45, 370-372, Bethesda, MD: American Occupational Therapy Association.

11. Pedretti, L.W. (1996). Occupational performance: A model for practice in physical dysfunction. In L.W. Pedretti (Ed.), Occupational therapy: Practice skills for physical dysfunction (4th ed., pp. 3-11). St. Louis: Mosby-Year Book

12. Christenson, M.A. (1996). Environmental design, modification, and adaptation, ROTE: Role of occupational therapy for the elderly (2nd ed., pp. 380-408). Bethesda, MD: American Occupational Therapy Association.

13. Coppard, B.M., Higgins, T., & Harvey, K.D. (2004). Working with elders who have orthopedic conditions. In S. Byers-Connon, H.L. Lohman, and R.L. Padilla (Eds.), Occupational therapy with elders: Strategies for the COTA (2nd ed., p. 293). St. Louis, MO: Elservier Mosby.

14. Glantz, C.G., & Richman, N. (1992). Activity programming for the resident with mental illness (pp. 53-76). Riverwoods, IL: Glantz/Richman Rehabilitation Associates.

15. Day, K., & Calkins, M.P. (2002). Design and dementia. In R. B. Bechtel & A. Churchman (Eds.), Handbook of environmental psychology (pp. 374-393). New York: Wiley.

16. Barrick, A.L., Rader, J., Hoeffer, B., & Sloane, P. (2002). Bathing without a battle: Personal care of individuals with dementia (p. 4). New York: Springer.

INVESTIGATIVE PROTOCOL
ACTIVITIES

(Rev).

Objective

To determine if the facility has provided an ongoing program of activities designed to accommodate the individual resident's interests and help enhance her/his physical, mental and psychosocial well-being, according to her/his comprehensive resident assessment.

Use

Use this procedure for each sampled resident to determine through interview, observation and record review whether the facility is in compliance with the regulation.

Procedures

Briefly review the comprehensive assessment and interdisciplinary care plan to guide observations to be made.

1. Observations

Observe during various shifts in order to determine if staff is consistently implementing those portions of the comprehensive plan of care related to activities. Determine if staff takes into account the resident's food preferences and restrictions for activities that involve food, and provide ADL assistance and adaptive equipment as needed during activities programs. For a resident with personal assistive devices such as glasses or hearing aides, determine if these devices are in place, glasses are clean, and assistive devices are functional.

For a resident whose care plan includes group activities, observe if staff informs the resident of the activities program schedule and provide timely transportation, if needed, for the resident to attend in-facility activities and help the resident access transportation to out-of-facility and community activities.

Determine whether the facility provides activities that are compatible with the resident's known interests, needs, abilities and preferences. If the resident is in group activity programs, note if the resident is making attempts to leave, or is expressing displeasure with, or sleeping through, an activity program. If so, determine if staff attempted to identify the reason the resident is attempting to leave, and if they addressed the resident's needs. Determine whether the group activity has been adapted for the resident as needed and whether it is "person appropriate."

Note: If you observe an activity that you believe would be age inappropriate for most residents, investigate further to determine the reason the resident and staff selected this activity. The National Alzheimer's Association has changed from endorsing the idea of "age-appropriate" activities to promoting "person-appropriate" activities. In general, surveyors should not expect to see the facility providing dolls or stuffed animals for most residents, but some residents are attached to these items and should be able to continue having them available if they prefer.

Regarding group activities in common areas, determine if the activities are occurring in rooms that have sufficient space, light, ventilation, equipment and supplies. Sufficient space includes enough space for residents to participate in the activity and space for a resident to enter and leave the room without having to move several other residents. Determine if the room is sufficiently free of extraneous noise, such as environmental noises from mechanical equipment and staff interruptions.

For a resident who is involved in individual activities in her/his room, observe if staff have provided needed assistance, equipment and supplies. Observe if the room has sufficient light and space for the resident to complete the activity.

2. Interviews

Resident/Representative Interview. Interview the resident, family or resident representative as appropriate to identify their involvement in care plan development, defining the approaches and goals that reflect the resident's preferences and choices. Determine:

- What assistance, if any, the facility should be providing to facilitate participation in activities of choice and whether or not the assistance is being provided;
- Whether the resident is participating in chosen activities on a regular basis, and if not, why not;
- Whether the resident is notified of activities opportunities and is offered transportation assistance as needed to the activity location within the facility or access to transportation, where available and feasible, to outside activities;
- Whether the facility tried, to the extent possible, to accommodate the resident's choices regarding her/his schedule, so that service provision (for example, bathing and therapy services) does not routinely conflict with desired activities;
- Whether planned activity programs usually occur as scheduled (instead of being cancelled repeatedly); and
- Whether the resident desires activities that the facility does not provide.

If the resident has expressed any concerns, determine if the resident has discussed these with staff and, if so, what was the staff's response.

Activity Staff Interview

Interview activities staff as necessary to determine:

- The resident's program of activities and related goals;
- What assistance/adaptations they provide in group activities according to the resident's care plan;
- How regularly the resident participates; if not participating, what is the reason(s);
- How they assure the resident is informed of, and transported to, group activities of choice;
- How special dietary needs and restrictions are handled during activities involving food;
- What assistance they provide if the resident participates in any individual (non-group) activities; and
- How they assure the resident has sufficient supplies, lighting, and space for individual activities.

CNA Interview

Interview CNAs as necessary to determine what assistance, if needed, the CNA provides to help the resident participate in desired group and individual activities, specifically:

- Their role in ensuring the resident is out of bed, dressed, and ready to participate in chosen group activities, and in providing transportation if needed;
- Their role in providing any needed ADL assistance to the resident while she/he is participating in group activities;
- Their role in helping the resident to participate in individual activities (if the resident's plan includes these), for example, setup of equipment/supplies, positioning assistance, providing enough lighting and space; and
- How activities are provided for the resident at times when activities staff are not available to provide care planned activities.

Social Services Staff Interview

Interview the social services staff member as necessary to determine how they help facilitate resident participation in desired activities; specifically, how the social services staff member:

- Addresses the resident's psychosocial needs that impact on the resident's ability to participate in desired activities;
- Obtains equipment and/or supplies that the resident needs in order to participate in desired activities (for example, obtaining audio books, helping the resident replace inadequate glasses or a hearing aid); and
- Helps the resident access his/her funds in order to participate in desired activities that require money, such as attending concerts, plays, or restaurant dining events.

Nurse Interview

Interview a nurse who supervises CNAs who work with the resident to determine how nursing staff:

- Assist the resident in participating in activities of choice by:

    - Coordinating schedules for ADLs, medications, and therapies, to the extent possible, to maximize the resident's ability to participate;
    - Making nursing staff available to assist with activities in and out of the facility;
    - If the resident is refusing to participate in activities, how they try to identify and address the reasons; and
    - Coordinate the resident's activities participation when activities staff are not available to provide care planned activities.

3. Record Review

Assessment

Review the RAI, activity documentation/notes, social history, discharge information from a previous setting, and other interdisciplinary documentation that may contain information regarding the resident's activity interests, preferences and needed adaptations.

Compare information obtained by observation of the resident and interviews with staff and the resident/responsible party (as possible), to the information in the resident's record, to help determine if the assessment accurately and comprehensively reflects the resident's status. Determine whether staff have identified:

- Longstanding interests and customary routine, and how the resident's current physical, mental, and psychosocial health status affects her/his choice of activities and her/his ability to participate;
- Specific information about how the resident prefers to participate in activities of interest (for example, if music is an interest, what kinds of music; does the resident play an instrument; does the resident have access to music to which she/he likes to listen; and can the resident participate independently, such as inserting a CD into a player);
- Any significant changes in activity patterns before or after admission;
- The resident's current needs for special adaptations in order to participate in desired activities (e.g., auditory enhancement or equipment to help compensate for physical difficulties such as use of only one hand);
- The resident's needs, if any, for time-limited participation, such as a short attention span or an illness that permits only limited time out of bed;
- The resident's desired daily routine and availability for activities; and
- The resident's choices for group, one-to-one, and self-directed activities.

Comprehensive Care Planning

Review the comprehensive care plan to determine if that portion of the plan related to activities is based upon the goals, interests, and preferences of the resident and reflects the comprehensive assessment. Determine if the resident's care plan:

- Includes participation of the resident (if able) or the resident's representative;
- Considers a continuation of life roles, consistent with resident preferences and functional capacity;
- Encourages and supports the development of new interests, hobbies, and skills;
- Identifies activities in the community, if appropriate;
- Includes needed adaptations that address resident conditions and issues affecting activities participation; and
- Identifies how the facility will provide activities to help the resident reach the goal(s) and who is responsible for implementation (e.g., activity staff, CNAs, dietary staff).

If care plan concerns are noted, interview staff responsible for care planning regarding the rationale for the current plan of care.

Care Plan Revision

Determine if the staff have evaluated the effectiveness of the care plan related to activities and made revisions, if necessary, based upon the following:

- Changes in the resident's abilities, interests, or health;
- A determination that some aspects of the current care plan were unsuccessful (e.g., goals were not being met);
- The resident refuses, resists, or complains about some chosen activities;
- Changes in time of year have made some activities no longer possible (e.g., gardening outside in winter) and other activities have become available; and
- New activity offerings have been added to the facility's available activity choices.

For the resident who refused some or all activities, determine if the facility worked with the resident (or representative, as appropriate) to identify and address underlying reasons and offer alternatives.

Determination of Compliance (Task 6, Appendix P)

Synopsis of Regulation (F248)

This requirement stipulates that the facility's program of activities should accommodate the interests and well-being of each resident. In order to fulfill this requirement, it is necessary for the facility to gain awareness of each resident's activity preferences as well as any current limitations that require adaptation in order to accommodate these preferences.

Criteria for Compliance

The facility is in compliance with this requirement if they:

- Recognized and assessed for preferences, choices, specific conditions, causes and/or problems, needs and behaviors;
- Defined and implemented activities in accordance with resident needs and goals;
- Monitored and evaluated the resident's response; and
- Revised the approaches as appropriate.

If not, cite at F248.

Noncompliance for Tag F248

After completing the Investigative Protocol, analyze the information gained in order to determine whether noncompliance with the regulation exists. Activities (F248) is an outcome-oriented requirement in that compliance is determined separately for each resident sampled. The survey team's review of the facility's activities program is conducted through a review of the individualization of activities to meet each resident's needs and preferences. For each sampled resident for whom activities participation was reviewed, the facility is in compliance if they have provided activities that are individualized to that resident's needs and preferences, and they have provided necessary adaptations to facilitate the resident's participation. Non compliance with F248 may look like, but is not limited to the following:

- The facility does not have an activity program and does not offer any activities to the resident;
- A resident with special needs does not receive adaptations needed to participate in individualized activities;
- Planned activities were not conducted or designed to meet the resident's care plan;

Potential Tags for Additional Investigation

During the investigation of the provision of care and services related to activities, the surveyor may have identified concerns with related outcome, process and/or structure requirements. The surveyor is cautioned to investigate these related requirements before determining whether noncompliance may be present. Some examples of requirements that should be considered include the following (not all inclusive):

- 42 CFR 483.10(e), F164, Privacy and Confidentiality

  ◇ Determine if the facility has accommodated the resident's need for privacy for visiting with family, friends, and others, as desired by the resident.

- 42 CFR 483.10(j)(1) and (2), F172, Access and Visitation Rights

  ◇ Determine if the facility has accommodated the resident's family and/or other visitors (as approved by the resident) to be present with the resident as much as desired, even round-the-clock.

- 42 CFR 483.15(b), F242, Self-Determination and Participation

  ◇ Determine if the facility has provided the resident with choices about aspects of her/his life in the facility that are significant to the resident.

- 42 CFR 483.15(e)(1), F246, Accommodation of Needs

  ◇ Determine if the facility has provided reasonable accommodation to the resident's physical environment (room, bathroom, furniture, etc.) to accommodate the resident's individual needs in relation to the pursuit of individual activities, if any.

- 42 CFR 483.15(f)(2), F249, Qualifications of the Activities Director

  ◇ Determine if a qualified activities director is directing the activities program.

- 42 CFR 483.15(g)(1), F250, Social Services

  ◇ Determine if the facility is providing medically-related social services related to assisting with obtaining supplies/equipment for individual activities (if any), and assisting in meeting the resident's psychosocial needs related to activity choices.

- 43 CFR 483.20(b)(1), F272, Comprehensive Assessment

  ✧ Determine if the facility assessed the resident's activity needs, preferences, and interests specifically enough so that an individualized care plan could be developed.

- 43 CFR 483.20(k)(1), F279, Comprehensive Care Plan

  ✧ Determine if the facility developed specific and individualized activities goals and approaches as part of the comprehensive care plan, unless the resident is independent in providing for her/his activities without facility intervention.

- 43 CFR 483.20(k)(2), F280, Care Plan Revision

  ✧ Determine whether the facility revised the plan of care as needed with input of the resident (or representative, as appropriate).

- 43 CFR 483.30(a), F353, Sufficient Staff

  ✧ Determine if the facility had qualified staff in sufficient numbers to assure the resident was provided activities based upon the comprehensive assessment and care plan.

- 43 CFR 483.70(g), F464, Dining and Activities Rooms

  ✧ Determine if the facility has provided sufficient space to accommodate the activities and the needs of participating residents and that space is well lighted, ventilated, and adequately furnished.

- 43 CFR 483.75(g), F499, Staff Qualifications

  ✧ Determine if the facility has employed sufficient qualified professional staff to assess residents and to develop and implement the activities approaches of their comprehensive care plans.

V. Deficiency of Categorization (Part V, Appendix P)

Deficiencies at F248 are most likely to have psychosocial outcomes. The survey team should compare their findings to the various levels of severity on the Psychosocial Outcome Severity Guide at Appendix P, Part V.

F249 Properly qualified activities program professional

(Rev. 19, Issued: 06-01-06, Effective/Implementation: 06-01-06)

§483.15(f)(2) The activities program must be directed by a qualified professional.

(i) Is a qualified therapeutic recreation specialist or an activities professional who—

(A) Is licensed or registered, if applicable, by the State in which practicing; and

(B) Is eligible for certification as a therapeutic recreation specialist or as an activities professional by a recognized accrediting body on or after October 1, 1990; or

(ii) Has 2 years of experience in a social or recreational program within the last 5 years, 1 of which was full-time in a patient activities program in a health care setting; or

(iii) Is a qualified occupational therapist or occupational therapy assistant; or

(iv) Has completed a training course approved by the State.

§483.15(f)(2)

Intent (F249)

Activities Director

The intent of this regulation is to ensure that the activities program is directed by a qualified professional.

Definitions

"Recognized accrediting body" refers to those organizations that certify, register, or license therapeutic recreation specialists, activity professionals, or occupational therapists.

Activities Director Responsibilities

An activity director is responsible for directing the development, implementation, supervision and ongoing evaluation of the activities program. This includes the completion and/or directing/delegating the completion of the activities component of the comprehensive assessment; and contributing to and/or directing/delegating the contribution to the comprehensive care plan goals and approaches that are individualized to match the skills, abilities, and interests/preferences of each resident. Directing the activity program includes scheduling of activities, both individual and groups, implementing and/or delegating the implementation of the programs, monitoring the response and/or reviewing/evaluating the response to the programs to determine if the activities meet the assessed needs of the resident, and making revisions as necessary.

Note: Review the qualifications of the activities director if there are concerns with the facility's compliance with the activities requirement at §483.15(f)(1), F248, or if there are concerns with the direction of the activity programs.

A person is a qualified professional under this regulatory tag if they meet any one of the qualifications listed under 483.15(f)(2).

Determination of Compliance (Task 6, Appendix P)

Synopsis of Regulation (F249)

This requirement stipulates that the facility's program of activities be directed by a qualified professional.

Criteria for Compliance

The facility is in compliance with this requirement if they:

- Have employed a qualified professional to provide direction in the development and implementation of activities in accordance with resident needs and goals, and the director:

    ✧ Has completed or delegated the completion of the activities component of the comprehensive assessment;
    ✧ Contributed or directed the contribution to the comprehensive care plan of activity goals and approaches that are individualized to match the skills, abilities, and interests/preferences of each resident;
    ✧ Has monitored and evaluated the resident's response to activities and revised the approaches as appropriate; and
    ✧ Has developed, implemented, supervised and evaluated the activities program.

If not, cite at F249.

Noncompliance for F249

Tag F249 is a tag that is absolute, which means the facility must have a qualified activities professional to direct the provision of activities to the residents. Thus, it is cited if the facility is non-compliant with the regulation, whether or not there have been any negative outcomes to residents.

Noncompliance for F249 may include (but is not limited to) one or more of the following, including:

- Lack of a qualified activity director; or
- Lack of providing direction for the provision of an activity program;

V. Deficiency Categorization (Part V, Appendix P)

Once the team has completed its investigation, reviewed the regulatory requirements, and determined that noncompliance exists, the team must determine the severity of each deficiency, based on the resultant effect or potential for harm to the resident. The key elements for severity determination for F249 are as follows:

1. Presence of harm/negative outcome(s) or potential for negative outcomes due to a lack of an activities director or failure of the director to oversee, implement and/or provide activities programming.

   • Lack of the activity director's involvement in coordinating/directing activities; or
   • Lack of a qualified activity director.

2. Degree of harm (actual or potential) related to the noncompliance.

   Identify how the facility practices caused, resulted in, allowed or contributed to the actual or potential for harm:

   • If harm has occurred, determine level of harm; and
   • If harm has not yet occurred, determine the potential for discomfort to occur to the resident.

3. The immediacy of correction required.

   Determine whether the noncompliance requires immediate correction in order to prevent serious injury, harm, impairment, or death to one or more residents.

Severity Level 4 Considerations: Immediate Jeopardy to Resident Health or Safety

Immediate jeopardy is not likely to be issued as it is unlikely that noncompliance with F249 could place a resident or residents into a situation with potential to sustain serious harm, injury or death.

Severity Level 3 Considerations: Actual Harm that is not Immediate Jeopardy

Level 3 indicates noncompliance that results in actual harm, and may include, but is not limited to the resident's inability to maintain and/or reach his/her highest practicable well-being. In order to cite actual harm at this tag, the surveyor must be able to identify a relationship between noncompliance cited at Tag F248 (Activities) and failure of the provision and/or direction of the activity program by the activity director. For Severity Level 3, both of the following must be present:

1. Findings of noncompliance at Severity Level 3 at Tag F248; and
2. There is no activity director; or the facility failed to assure the activity director was responsible for directing the activity program in the assessment, development, implementation and/or revision of an individualized activity program for an individual resident; and/or the activity director failed to assure that the facility's activity program was implemented.

Note: If Severity Level 3 (actual harm that is not immediate jeopardy) has been ruled out based upon the evidence, then evaluate as to whether Level 2 (no actual harm with the potential for more than minimal harm) exists.

Severity Level 2 Considerations: No Actual Harm with Potential for more than Minimal Harm that is not Immediate Jeopardy

Level 2 indicates noncompliance that results in a resident outcome of no more than minimal discomfort and/or has the potential to compromise the resident's ability to maintain or reach his or her highest practicable level of well being. The potential exists for greater harm to occur if interventions are not provided. In order to cite Level 2 at Tag F249, the surveyor must be able to identify a relationship between noncompliance cited at Level 2 at Tag F248 (Activities) and failure of the provision and/or direction of activity program by the activity director. For Severity Level 2 at Tag F249, both of the following must be present:

1. Findings of noncompliance at Severity Level 2 at Tag F248; and
2. There is no activity director; or the facility failed to involve the activity director in the assessment, development, implementation and/or revision of an individualized activity program for an individual resident; and/or the activity director failed to assure that the facility's activity program was implemented.

Severity Level 1 Considerations: No Actual Harm with Potential for Minimal Harm

In order to cite Level 1, no actual harm with potential for minimal harm at this tag, the surveyor must be able to identify that:

There is no activity director and/or the activity director is not qualified, however:

- Tag F248 was not cited;
- The activity systems associated with the responsibilities of the activity director are in place;
- There has been a relatively short duration of time without an activity director; and
- The facility is actively seeking a qualified activity director.

F250 Social services requirements

§483.15(g)(1) The facility must provide medically-related social services to attain or maintain the highest practicable physical, mental, and psychosocial well-being of each resident.

Intent §483.15(g)

To assure that sufficient and appropriate social service are provided to meet the resident's needs.

Interpretive Guidelines §483.15(g)(1)

Regardless of size, all facilities are required to provide for the medically-related social services needs of each resident. This requirement specifies that facilities aggressively identify the need for medically-related social services, and pursue the provision of these services. It is not required that a qualified social worker necessarily provide all of these services. Rather, it is the responsibility of the facility to identify the medically-related social service needs of the resident and assure that the needs are met by the appropriate disciplines.

"Medically-related social services" means services provided by the facility's staff to assist residents in maintaining or improving their ability to manage their everyday physical, mental, and psychosocial needs. These services might include, for example:

- Making arrangements for obtaining needed adaptive equipment, clothing, and personal items;
- Maintaining contact with facility (with resident's permission) to report on changes in health, current goals, discharge planning, and encouragement to participate in care planning;
- Assisting staff to inform residents and those they designate about the resident's health status and health care choices and their ramifications;
- Making referrals and obtaining services from outside entities (e.g., talking books, absentee ballots, community wheelchair transportation);
- Assisting residents with financial and legal matters (e.g., applying for pensions, referrals to lawyers, referrals to funeral homes for preplanning arrangements);
- Discharge planning services (e.g., helping to place a resident on a waiting list for community congregate living, arranging intake for home care services for residents returning home, assisting with transfer arrangements to other facilities);
- Providing or arranging provision of needed counseling services;
- Through the assessment and care planning process, identifying and seeking ways to support resident's individual needs;
- Promoting actions by staff that maintain or enhance each resident's dignity in full recognition of each resident's individuality;
- Assisting residents to determine how they would like to make decisions about their health care, and whether or not they would like anyone else to be involved in those decisions;
- Finding options that most meet the physical and emotional needs of each resident;
- Providing alternatives to drug therapy or restraints by understanding and communicating to staff why residents act as they do, what they are attempting to communicate, and what needs the staff must meet;
- Meeting the needs of residents who are grieving; and
- Finding options which most meet their physical and emotional needs.

Factors with a potentially negative effect on physical, mental, and psychosocial well-being include an unmet need for:

- Dental/denture care;
- Podiatric care;
- Eye care;
- Hearing services;
- Equipment for mobility or assistive eating devices; and
- Need for home-like environment, control, dignity, privacy.

Where needed services are not covered by the Medicaid State plan, nursing facilities are still required to attempt to obtain these services. For example, if a resident requires transportation services that are not covered under a Medicaid state plan, the facility is required to arrange these services. This could be achieved, for example, through obtaining volunteer assistance.

Types of conditions to which the facility should respond with social services by staff or referral include:

- Lack of an effective family/support system;
- Behavioral symptoms;
- If a resident with dementia strikes out at another resident, the facility should evaluate the resident's behavior. For example, a resident may be re-enacting an activity he or she used to perform at the same time everyday. If that resident senses that another is in the way of his re-enactment, the resident may strike out at the resident impeding his or her progress. The facility is responsible for the safety of any potential resident victims while it assesses the circumstances of the residents behavior;
- Presence of a chronic disabling medical or psychological condition (e.g., multiple sclerosis, chronic obstructive pulmonary disease, Alzheimer's disease, schizophrenia);
- Depression;
- Chronic or acute pain;
- Difficulty with personal interaction and socialization skills;
- Presence of legal or financial problems;
- Abuse of alcohol or other drugs;
- Inability to cope with loss of function;
- Need for emotional support;
- Changes in family relationships, living arrangements, and/or resident's condition or functioning; and
- A physical or chemical restraint.

For residents with or who develop mental disorders as defined by the "Diagnostic and Statistical Manual for Mental Disorders (DSM-IV)," see §483.45, F406.

Probes §483.15(g)(1)

For residents selected for a comprehensive or focused review as appropriate:

- How do facility staff implement social services interventions to assist the resident in meeting treatment goals?
- How do staff responsible for social work monitor the resident's progress in improving physical, mental, and psychosocial functioning? Has goal attainment been evaluated and the care plan changed accordingly?
- How does the care plan link goals to psychosocial functioning/well-being?
- Have the staff responsible for social work established and maintained relationships with the resident's family or legal representative?
- [NFs] What attempts does the facility make to access services for Medicaid recipients when those services are not covered by a Medicaid State Plan?

Look for evidence that social services interventions successfully address residents' needs and link social supports, physical care, and physical environment with residents' needs and individuality.

For sampled residents, review MDS, section H.

F251 Social worker qualifications

§483.15(g)(2) and (3)

(2) A facility with more than 120 beds must employ a qualified social worker on a full-time basis.

(3) Qualifications of a social worker. A qualified social worker is an individual with—

(i) A bachelor's degree in social work or a bachelor's degree in a human services field including but not limited to sociology, special education, rehabilitation counseling, and psychology; and

(ii) One year of supervised social work experience in a health care setting working directly with individuals.

Procedures §483.15(g)(2) and (3)

If there are problems with the provision of social services in a facility with over 120 beds, determine if a qualified social worker is employed on a full time basis. See also F250.

F252 Resident's environment

(Rev. 5, Issued: 11-19-04, Effective: 11-19-04, Implementation: 11-19-04)

§483.15(h) Environment

The facility must provide—

§483.15(h)(1) A safe, clean, comfortable, and homelike environment, allowing the resident to use his or her personal belongings to the extent possible;

Interpretive Guidelines §483.15(h)(1)

For "safe" environment, also see Guidelines for §§483.25(h), Accidents and 483.70(a), Life Safety Code.

For Comfortable Environment, see Guidelines for 483.15(h)(5), Adequate and Comfortable Lighting Levels; 483.15(h)(6), Comfortable and Safe Temperature Levels; and 483.15(h)(7), Comfortable Sound Levels.

A determination of "comfortable and homelike" should include, whenever possible, the resident's or representative of the resident's opinion of the living environment.

The absence of a personalized, homelike environment in a resident's room, is not meaningful unless the survey team determines that the absence of personal belongings is a result of facility practices, rather than the result of resident choice or circumstances (e.g., lack of resident funds, lack of family support system, resident's reason for being in the facility, such as short-term rehabilitation).

A "homelike environment" is one that de-emphasizes the institutional character of the setting, to the extent possible, and allows the resident to use those personal belongings that support a homelike environment. A personalized, homelike environment recognizes the individuality and autonomy of the resident, provides an opportunity for self-expression, and encourages links with the past and family members. Use this Tag when the facility fails to allow the resident to personalize his or her individual environment to the extent possible. Use Tag F224, 483.15(c), if the facility fails to have a system in place to prevent the misappropriation of resident's property. For purposes of this requirement, "environment" refers to any environment in the facility that is frequented by residents, including the residents' rooms, bathrooms, hallways, activity areas, and therapy areas.

If the survey team observes that the rooms of residents with dementia do not appear to be homelike, determine if this decision was made in the context of assessment and care planning; i.e., that this environment assists these residents to maintain their highest practicable functioning levels.

If the team observes non-homelike environments for residents with dementia, determine if each of these residents have the same plan of care and the reason why each of these residents have the same plan of care.

By observing the residents' surroundings, what can the survey team learn about their everyday life and interests? Their life prior to residing in the facility? Observe for family photographs, books and magazines, bedspreads, knickknacks, mementos, and furniture that belong to the residents. For residents who have no relatives or friends, and have few assets, determine the extent to which the facility has assisted these residents to make their rooms homelike, if they so desire.

F253 Necessary housekeeping and maintenance services

§483.15(h)(2)

§483.15(h)(2) Housekeeping and maintenance services necessary to maintain a sanitary, orderly, and comfortable interior;

Intent §483.15(h)(2)

The intent of this requirement is to focus on the facility's responsibility to provide effective housekeeping and maintenance services.

Interpretive Guidelines §483.15(h)(2)

"Sanitary" includes, but is not limited to, preventing the spread of disease-causing organisms by keeping resident care equipment clean and properly stored. Resident care equipment includes toothbrushes, dentures, denture cups, glasses and water pitchers, emesis basins, hair brushes and combs, bed pans, urinals, feeding tubes, leg bags and catheter bags, pads, and positioning devices.

For kitchen sanitation, see §483.70(h), Other Environmental Conditions.

For facility-wide sanitary practices affecting the quality of care, see §483.65, Infection Control.

"Orderly" is defined as an uncluttered physical environment that is neat and well-kept.

Procedures §483.15(h)(2)

Balance the resident's need for a homelike environment and the requirements of having a "sanitary" environment in a congregate living situation. For example, a resident may prefer a cluttered room, but does this clutter result in unsanitary or unsafe conditions?

Probes §483.15(h)(2)

Is resident care equipment sanitary?
Is the area orderly?
Is the area uncluttered and in good repair?
Can residents and staff function unimpeded?

F254 Clean bed and bath linens in good condition

§483.15(h)(3)

§483.15(h)(3) Clean bed and bath linens that are in good condition;

Probes §483.15(h)(3)

Are bed linens clean and in good condition? Are there clean towels and wash cloths in good condition available for the resident?

F255 Private closet space for each resident

§483.15(h)(4)

§483.15(h)(4) Private closet space in each resident room, as specified in

§483.70(d)(2)(iv) of this part;

Interpretive Guidelines §483.15(h)(4)

§483.70(d)(2)(iv) states: "The facility must provide each resident with individual closet space in his/her bedroom with clothes racks and shelves accessible to the resident."

Probes §483.15(h)(4)

Are there individual closet spaces with accessible shelves?

Also see F470.

F256 Adequate and comfortable lighting levels

§483.15(h)(5)

§483.15(h)(5) Adequate and comfortable lighting levels in all areas;

Interpretive Guidelines §483.15(h)(5)

"Adequate lighting" is defined as levels of illumination suitable to tasks the resident chooses to perform or the facility staff must perform. For some residents (e.g., those with glaucoma), lower levels of lighting would be more suitable.

"Comfortable" lighting is defined as lighting which minimizes glare and provides maximum resident control, where feasible, over the intensity, location, and direction of illumination so that visually impaired residents can maintain or enhance independent functioning.

Procedures §483.15(h)(5)

Are there adequate and comfortable lighting levels for individual resident and staff work needs?

Consider the illumination available from any source, natural or artificial. For hallways, observe the illumination that is normally present. For resident rooms or for other spaces where residents can control the lighting, turn on the lights and make the rating under these conditions.

F257 Comfortable and safe temperature levels

§483.15(h)(6)

§483.15(h)(6) Comfortable and safe temperature levels. Facilities initially certified after October 1, 1990 must maintain a temperature range of 71–81° F; and

Procedures §483.15(h)(6)

"Comfortable and safe temperature levels" means that the ambient temperature should be in a relatively narrow range that minimizes residents' susceptibility to loss of body heat and risk of hypothermia or susceptibility to respiratory ailments and colds. Although there are no explicit temperature standards for facilities certified on or before October 1, 1990, these facilities still must maintain safe and comfortable temperature levels.

For facilities certified after October 1, 1990, temperatures may exceed the upper range of 81° F for facilities in geographic areas of the country (primarily at the northernmost latitudes) where that temperature is exceeded only during rare, brief unseasonably hot weather. This interpretation would apply in cases where it does not adversely affect resident health and safety, and would enable facilities in areas of the country with relatively cold climates to avoid the expense of installing air conditioning equipment that would only be needed infrequently. Conversely, the temperatures may fall below 71° F for facilities in areas of the country where that temperature is exceeded only during brief episodes of unseasonably cold weather (minimum temperature must still be maintained at a sufficient level to minimize risk of hypothermia and susceptibility to loss of body heat, respiratory ailments and colds).

Measure the air temperature above floor level in resident rooms, dining areas, and common areas. If the temperature is out of the 71–81° F range, then ask staff what actions they take when residents complain of heat or cold, e.g., provide extra fluids during heat waves and extra blankets and sweaters in cold.

F258 Comfortable sound levels

§483.15(h)(7)

§483.15(h)(7) For the maintenance of comfortable sound levels.

Interpretive Guidelines §483.15(h)(7)

"Comfortable" sound levels do not interfere with resident's hearing and enhance privacy when privacy is desired, and encourage interaction when social participation is desired. Of particular concern to comfortable sound levels is the resident's control over unwanted noise.

Procedures §483.15(h)(7)

Determine if the sound levels are comfortable to residents. Do residents and staff have to raise their voices to communicate over background sounds? Are sound levels suitable for the activities occurring in that space during observation?

Consider whether residents have difficulty hearing or making themselves heard because of background sounds (e.g., overuse or excessive volume of intercom, shouting, loud TV, cleaning equipment). Consider if it is difficult for residents to concentrate because of distractions or background noises such as traffic, music, equipment, or staff behavior. Consider the comfort of sound levels based on the needs of the residents participating in a particular activity, e.g., the sound levels may have to be turned up for hard of hearing individuals watching TV or listening to the radio. Consider the effect of noise on the comfort of residents with dementia.

During resident reviews, ask residents if during evenings and at nighttime, sounds are at comfortable levels? (If yes) Have you told staff about it and how have they responded?

F271 Admission orders

§483.20(a) Admission Orders

At the time each resident is admitted, the facility must have physician orders for the resident's immediate care.

Intent §483.20(a)

To ensure the resident receives necessary care and services.

Interpretive Guidelines §483.20(a)

"Physician orders for immediate care" are those written orders facility staff need to provide essential care to the resident, consistent with the resident's mental and physical status upon admission. These orders should, at a minimum, include dietary, drugs (if necessary), and routine care to maintain or improve the resident's functional abilities until staff can conduct a comprehensive assessment and develop an interdisciplinary care plan.

F272 Comprehensive assessments

(Rev. 5, Issued: 11-19-04, Effective: 11-19-04, Implementation: 11-19-04)

§483.20 Resident Assessment

The facility must conduct initially and periodically a comprehensive, accurate, standardized reproducible assessment of each resident's functional capacity.

Intent §483.20

To provide the facility with ongoing assessment information necessary to develop a care plan, to provide the appropriate care and services for each resident, and to modify the care plan and care/services based on the resident's status. The facility is expected to use resident observation and communication as the primary source of information when completing the RAI. In addition to direct observation and communication with the resident, the facility should use a variety of other sources, including communication with licensed and non-licensed staff members on all shifts and may include discussions with the resident's physician, family members, or outside consultants and review of the resident's record.

§483.20(b) Comprehensive Assessments

§483.20(b)(1) Resident Assessment Instrument. A facility must make a comprehensive assessment of a resident's needs, using the RAI specified by the State. The assessment must include at least the following:

(i) Identification and demographic information
(ii) Customary routine
(iii) Cognitive patterns
(iv) Communication
(v) Vision
(vi) Mood and behavior patterns
(vii) Psychological well-being
(viii) Physical functioning and structural problems
(ix) Continence
(x) Disease diagnosis and health conditions
(xi) Dental and nutritional status
(xii) Skin Conditions
(xiii) Activity pursuit
(xiv) Medications
(xv) Special treatments and procedures
(xvi) Discharge potential
(xvii) Documentation of summary information regarding the additional assessment performed through the resident assessment protocols

(xviii) Documentation of participation in assessment

§483.20(b) Intent

To ensure that the RAI is used in conducting comprehensive assessments as part of an ongoing process through which the facility identifies the resident's functional capacity and health status.

§483.20(b) Guidelines

The information required in §483.20(b)(i–xvi) is incorporated into the MDS, which forms the core of each State's approved RAI. Additional assessment information is also gathered using triggered RAPs.

Each facility must use its State-specified RAI (which includes both the MDS and utilization guidelines which include the RAPs) to assess newly admitted residents, conduct an annual re-assessment and assess those residents who experience a significant change in status. The facility is responsible for addressing all needs and strengths of residents regardless of whether the issue is included in the MDS or RAPs. The scope of the RAI does not limit the facility's responsibility to assess and address all care needed by the resident. Furthermore:

(i) Identification and demographic information

"Identification and demographic information" corresponds to MDS v 2.0 sections AA, BB, and A, and refers to information that uniquely identifies each resident and the facility in which he/she resides, date of entry into the facility, and residential history.

(ii) Customary routine

"Customary routine" corresponds to MDS v 2.0 section AC, and refers to information regarding the resident's usual community lifestyle and daily routine in the year prior to the date of entry to the nursing home.

(iii) Cognitive patterns

"Cognitive patterns" (iii) corresponds to MDS v. 2.0 section B. "Cognitive patterns" is defined as the resident's ability to problem solve, decide, remember, and be aware of and respond to safety hazards.

(iv) Communication

"Communication" (iv) corresponds to MDS v. 2.0 section C, and refers to the resident's ability to hear, understand others, make him or herself understood (with assistive devices if they are used).

(v) Vision

"Vision" (v) corresponds to MDS v. 2.0 section D, and I.1.jj, kk, ll, and mm, and refers to the resident's visual acuity, limitations and difficulties, and appliances used to enhance vision.

(vi) Mood and behavior patterns

"Mood and behavior patterns" (vi) corresponds to MDS v. 2.0 section E, and refers to the resident's patterns of mood and behavioral symptoms.

(vii) Psychosocial well-being

"Psychosocial well-being" (vii) corresponds to MDS v. 2.0 sections E1o and p, and F and refers to the resident's positive or negative feelings about him or herself or his/her social relationships.

(viii) Physical functioning and structural problems

"Physical functioning and structural problems" (viii) corresponds to MDS v. 2.0 section G, and refers to the resident's physical functional status, ability to perform activities of daily living, and the resident's need for staff assistance and assistive devices or equipment to maintain or improve functional abilities.

(ix) Continence

"Continence" (ix) corresponds to MDS v. 2.0, section H, and refers to the resident's patterns of bladder and bowel continence (control), pattern of elimination, and appliances used.

(x) Disease diagnosis and health conditions

"Disease diagnoses and health conditions" (x) corresponds to MDS v. 2.0, sections AB.9 and 10, I.1 and 2, and J.

(xi) Dental and nutritional status

"Dental and nutritional status" (xi) corresponds to MDS v. 2.0, sections K1 and L.

"Dental condition status" refers to the condition of the teeth, gums, and other structures of the oral cavity that may affect a resident's nutritional status, communication abilities, or quality of life. The assessment should include the need for, and use of, dentures or other dental appliances.

"Nutritional status" corresponds to MDS v. 2.0, section K2-6.

Nutritional status refers to weight, height, hematologic and biochemical assessments, clinical observations of nutrition, nutritional intake, resident's eating habits and preferences, dietary restrictions, supplements, and use of appliances.

(xii) Skin conditions

"Skin conditions" (xii) corresponds to MDS v. 2.0 sections M, G1a, G6a, H1a, H1b, and P4c, and refers to the resident's development, or risk of development of a pressure sore.

(xiii) Activity pursuit

"Activity pursuit" (xiii) corresponds to MDS v. 2.0 sections N and AC.

"Activity pursuit" refers to the resident's ability and desire to take part in activities which maintain or improve physical, mental, and psychosocial well-being. Activity pursuits refer to any activity outside of activities of daily living (ADLs) which a person pursues in order to obtain a sense of well-being. Also, includes activities which provide benefits in self-esteem, pleasure, comfort, health education, creativity, success, and financial or emotional independence. The assessment should consider the resident's normal everyday routines and lifetime preferences.

(xiv) Medications

"Medications" (xiv) corresponds to MDS v. 2.0, section O, and section U, if completed.

"Medications" refers to all prescription and over-the-counter medications taken by the resident, including dosage, frequency of administration, and recognition of significant side effects that would be most likely to occur in the resident. This information need not appear in the assessment. However, it must be in the resident's clinical record and included in the care plan.

(xv) Special treatments and procedures

"Special treatments and procedures" (xv) corresponds to MDS v. 2.0 sections K5, M5, and P1, and section T, if completed.

"Special treatments and procedures" refers to treatments and procedures that are not part of basic services provided. For example, treatment for pressure sores, naso-gastric feedings, specialized rehabilitation services, respiratory care, or devices and restraints.

(xvi) Discharge potential

"Discharge potential" (xvi) corresponds to MDS v. 2.0 section Q.

"Discharge potential" refers to the facility's expectation of discharging the resident from the facility within the next 3 months.

(xvii) Documentation of summary information regarding the additional assessment performed through the resident assessment protocols

"Documentation of summary information (xvii) regarding the additional assessment performed through the resident assessment protocols (RAPs)" corresponds to MDS v. 2.0 section V, and refers to documentation concerning which RAPs have been triggered, documentation of assessment information in support of clinical decision making relevant to the RAP, documentation regarding where, in the clinical record, information related to the RAP can be found, and for each triggered RAP, whether the identified problem was included in the care plan.

(xviii) Documentation of participation in assessment

"Documentation of participation in the assessment" corresponds to MDS v. 2.0 section R, and refers to documentation of who participated in the assessment process. The assessment process must include direct observation and communication with the resident, as well as communication with licensed and nonlicensed direct care staff members on all shifts.

F273 Frequency of assessments

§483.20(b)(2)

§483.20(b)(2) When required, a facility must conduct a comprehensive assessment of a resident as follows:

(i) Within 14 calendar days after admission, excluding readmissions in which there is no significant change in the resident's physical or mental condition. (For purposes of this section, "readmission" means a return to the facility following a temporary absence for hospitalization for therapeutic leave.)

Intent §483.20(b)(2)

To assess residents in a timely manner.

F274 Frequency of assessments: promptly after a significant change in physical or mental condition

§483.20(b)(2)(ii)

(ii) Within 14 days after the facility determines, or should have determined, that there has been a significant change in the resident's physical or mental condition. (For purposes of this section, a "significant change" means a major decline or improvement in the resident's status that will not normally resolve itself without further intervention by staff or by implementing standard disease-related clinical interventions, that has an impact on more than one area of the resident's health status, and requires interdisciplinary review or revision of the care plan, or both.)

Guidelines §483.20(b)(2)(ii)

The following are the criteria for significant changes:

A significant change reassessment is generally indicated if decline or improvement is consistently noted in 2 or more areas of decline or 2 or more areas of improvement:

Decline:

- Any decline in activities of daily living (ADL) physical functioning where a resident is newly coded as 3, 4, or 8 Extensive Assistance, Total Dependency, activity did not occur (note that even if coding in both columns A and B of an ADL category changes, this is considered 1 ADL change);
- Increase in the number of areas where Behavioral Symptoms are coded as "not easily altered" (e.g., an increase in the use of code 1's for E4B);
- Resident's decision-making changes from 0 or 1, to 2 or 3;
- Resident's incontinence pattern changes from 0 or 1, to 2, 3, or 4, or placement of an indwelling catheter;
- Emergence of sad or anxious mood as a problem that is not easily altered;
- Emergence of an unplanned weight loss problem (5% change in 30 days or 10% change in 180 days);
- Begin to use trunk restraint or a chair that prevents rising for a resident when it was not used before;
- Emergence of a condition/disease in which a resident is judged to be unstable;
- Emergence of a pressure ulcer at Stage II or higher, when no ulcers were previously present at Stage II or higher; or
- Overall deterioration of resident's condition; resident receives more support (e.g., in ADLs or decision making).

Improvement:

- Any improvement in ADL physical functioning where a resident is newly coded as 0, 1, or 2 when previously scored as a 3, 4, or 8;
- Decrease in the number of areas where Behavioral Symptoms or Sad or Anxious Mood are coded as "not easily altered";
- Resident's decision making changes from 2 or 3, to 0 or 1;
- Resident's incontinence pattern changes from 2, 3, or 4, to 0 or 1; or
- Overall improvement of resident's condition; resident receives fewer supports.

§483.20(c) Quality Review Assessment

A facility must assess a resident using the quarterly review instrument specified by the State and approved by CMS not less frequently than once every 3 months.

Intent §483.20(c)

To assure that the resident's assessment is updated on at least a quarterly basis.

- If the resident experiences a significant change in status, the next annual assessment is not due until 366 days after the significant change reassessment has been completed.

F275 Frequency of assessments: at least every 12 months

§483.20(b)(2)(iii)

(iii) Not less than once every 12 months.

Interpretive Guidelines §483.20(b)(2)(iii)

The annual resident assessment must be completed within 366 days after final completion of the most recent comprehensive resident assessment.

Probes §483.20(b)(2)

- Has each resident in the sample been comprehensively assessed using the State-specified RAI within the regulatory time frames (i.e., within 14 days after admission, on significant change in status, and at least annually)?
- Has the facility identified, in a timely manner, those residents who have experienced a change?
- Has the facility reassessed residents using the State-specific RAI who had a significant change in status within 14 days after determining the change was significant.
- Has the facility gathered supplemental assessment information based on triggered RAPs prior to establishing the care plan?
- Does information in the RAI correspond with information obtained during observations of and interviews with the resident, facility staff, and resident's family?

Interpretive Guidelines §483.20(c)

At least each quarter, the facility shall review each resident with respect to those MDS items specified under the State's quarterly review requirement. At a minimum, this would include all items contained in CMS' standard quarterly review form. A Quarterly review assessment must be completed within 92 days of the date at MDS Item R2b of the most recent, clinical assessment (AA8a=1,2,3,4,5 or 10). If the resident has experienced a significant change in status, the next quarterly review is due no later than 3 months after the significant change reassessment.

Probes §483.20(c)

Is the facility assessing and acting, no less than once every 3 months, on the results of resident's functional and cognitive status examinations?

Is the quarterly review of the resident's condition consistent with information in the progress notes, the plan of care, and your resident observations and interviews?

F276 Review of assessments every three months

(Rev. 19, Issued: 06-01-06, Effective/Implementation: 06-01-06)

§483.20(c)

Quarterly Review Assessment

A facility must assess a resident using the quarterly review instrument specified by the State and approved by CMS not less frequently than once every 3 months.

§483.20(c)

Intent:

To assure that the resident's assessment is updated on at least a quarterly basis.

§483.20(c)

Interpretive Guidelines:

At least each quarter, the facility shall review each resident with respect to those MDS items specified under the State's quarterly review requirement. At a minimum, this would include all items contained in CMS' standard quarterly review form. A Quarterly review assessment must be completed within 92 days of the date at MDS Item R2b of the most recent, clinical assessment (AA8a=1,2,3,4,5 or 10). If the resident has experienced a significant change in status, the next quarterly review is due no later than 3 months after the significant change reassessment.

§483.20(c)

Probes:

Is the facility assessing and acting, no less than once every 3 months, on the results of resident's functional and cognitive status examinations?

Is the quarterly review of the resident's condition consistent with information in the progress notes, the plan of care and your resident observations and interviews?

§483.20(d) Use

A facility must maintain all resident assessments completed within the previous 15 months in the resident's active record.

Intent §483.20(d)

Facilities are required to maintain 15 months of assessment data in the resident's active clinical record.

Interpretive Guidelines §483.20(d)

The requirement to maintain 15 months of data in the resident's active clinical record applies regardless of form of storage to all MDS forms, RAP Summary forms, Quarterly Assessment forms, Face Sheet Information and Discharge and Reentry Tracking Forms, and MDS Correction Request Forms (including signed attestation). MDS assessments must be kept in the resident's active clinical record for 15 months following the final completion date, tracking forms for discharge and reentry must be kept for 15 months following the date of the event, Correction Request Forms must be kept for 15 months following the final completion date of the MDS Correction Request form.

The information must be kept in a centralized location, accessible to all professional staff members (including consultants) who need to review the information in order to provide care to the resident.

After the 15-month period, RAI information may be thinned from the clinical record and stored in the medical records department, provided that it is easily retrievable if requested by clinical staff, the State agency, or CMS.

Whether or not the facility's clinical record system is entirely electronic, a hard copy of all MDS forms, including the signatures of the facility staff attesting to the accuracy and completion of the records, must be maintained in the resident's clinical record.

F277 Coordination of assessments with any State programs

§483.20(f) Automated Data Processing Requirement

§483.20(f)(1) Encoding Data. Within 7 days after a facility completes a resident's assessment, a facility must encode the following information for each resident in the facility:

(i) Admission assessment

(ii) Annual assessment updates

(iii) Significant change in status assessments

(iv) Quarterly review assessments

(v) A subset of items upon a resident's transfer, reentry, discharge, and death

(vi) Background (face-sheet) information, if there is no admission assessment

§483.20(f)(2) Transmitting data. Within 7 days after a facility completes a resident's assessment, a facility must be capable of transmitting to the State information for each resident contained in the MDS in a format that conforms to standard record layouts and data dictionaries, and that passes standardized edits defined by CMS and the State.

§483.20(f)(3) Monthly transmittal requirements. A facility must electronically transmit, at least monthly, encoded, accurate, complete MDS data to the State for all assessments conducted during the previous month, including the following:

(i) Admission assessment

(ii) Annual assessment

(iii) Significant change in status assessment

(iv) Significant correction of prior full assessment

(v) Significant correction of prior quarterly assessment

(vi) Quarterly review

(vii) A subset of items upon a resident's transfer, reentry, discharge, and death

(viii) Background (face-sheet) information, for an initial transmission of MDS data on a resident that does not have an admission assessment

§483.20(f)(4) Data format. The facility must transmit data in the format specified by CMS or, for a State which has an alternate RAI approved by CMS, in the format specified by the State and approved by CMS.

Intent §483.20(f)(1-4)

The intent is to enable a facility to better monitor a resident's decline and progress over time. Computer-aided data analysis facilitates a more efficient, comprehensive, and sophisticated review of health data. The primary purpose of maintaining the assessment data is so a facility can monitor resident progress over time. The information should be readily available at all times.

Interpretive Guidelines §483.20(f)(1-4)

"Encoding" means entering MDS information into a computer.

"Transmitting data" refers to electronically sending encoded MDS information, from the facility to the State database, using a modem and communications software.

"Capable of transmitting" means that the facility has encoded and edited according to CMS specifications, the record accurately reflects the resident's overall clinical status as of the assessment reference date, and the record is ready for transmission.

"Passing standard edits" means that the encoded responses to MDS items are consistent and within range, in accordance with CMS specified standards. In general, inconsistent responses are either not plausible or ignore a skip pattern on the MDS. An example of inconsistency would be if one or more MDS items on a list were checked as present, and the "None of the Above" response was also checked for the same list. Out of range responses are invalid responses, such as using a response code of 2 for an MDS item for which the valid responses are zero or 1.

"Monthly Transmittal" means electronically transmitting to the State, an MDS record that passes CMS' standard edits, within 31 days of the final completion date of the record.

"Accurate" means that the encoded MDS data matches the MDS form in the clinical record. Also refer to guidance regarding accuracy at §483.20(g), and the information accurately reflects the resident's status as of the Assessment Reference Date at MDS Item A3a.

"Complete" means that all items required according to the record type, and in accordance with CMS' record specifications and State required edits are in effect at the time the record is completed.

In accordance with the final rule, facilities will be responsible to edit the encoded MDS data to ensure that it meets the standard edit specifications.

We encourage facilities to use software that has a programmed capability to automatically edit MDS records according to CMS' edit specifications.

For §483.20(f)(1)(v), the subset of items required upon a resident's transfer, discharge, and death are contained in the Discharge Tracking form and the items required for reentry are contained in the Reentry Tracking form. Refer to Appendix R for further information about the Discharge Tracking and Reentry Tracking forms.

All nursing homes must computerize MDS information. The facility must edit MDS information using standard CMS-specified edits, revise the information to conform to the edits and to be accurate, and be capable of transmitting that data to the State system within 7 days of:

- Completing a comprehensive assessment (the date at MDS item VB4);
- Completing an assessment that is not comprehensive (the date at MDS item R2b);
- A discharge event (the date at MDS item R4);
- A reentry event (the date at MDS item A4a); or
- Completing a correction request form (the date at MDS item AT6).

Submission must be according to State and Federal time frames. Therefore the facility must:

- Encode the MDS and RAP Summary (where applicable) in machine readable format;
- Edit the MDS and RAP Summary (where applicable) according to edits specified by CMS. Within the 7 day time period specified above for editing, the facility must revise any information on the encoded MDS and RAP Summary (if applicable) that does not

pass CMS-specified edits, revise any otherwise inaccurate information, and make the information ready for submission. The MDS Vendor software used at the facility should have an automated editing process that alerts the user to entries in an MDS record that do not conform with the CMS-specified edits and that prompts the facility to complete revisions within the 7-day editing and revision period. After editing and revision, MDS information and RAP summary information (if applicable) must always accurately reflect the resident's overall clinical status as of the original Assessment Reference date for an assessment or the original event date for a discharge or reentry;

• Print the edited and revised MDS and RAP summary form (where applicable). Discharge or Reentry Tracking form or Correction Request form, and place it in the resident's record. The hard copy of the MDS record must match the record that the facility transmits to the State, and it must accurately reflect the resident's status as of the Assessment Reference date or event date. If a hard copy exists prior to data entry, the facility must correct the hard copy to reflect the changes associated with the editing and revision process.

Electronically submit MDS information to the State MDS database within 31 days of:

• The date the Care Planning Decision process was complete (the date at MDS Item VB4) for comprehensive assessments;
• The date the RN Coordinator certified that the MDS was complete (the date at MDS Item R2b) for assessments that are not comprehensive;
• The date of death or discharge (the date at MDS Item R4) for Discharge Tracking forms;
• The date of reentry (the date at MDS Item A4a) for Reentry Tracking forms; and
• The date of completion of a correction request (the date at MDS Item AT6).

For a discussion of the process that a facility should follow in the event an error is discovered in an MDS record after editing and revision but before it is transmitted to the State, refer to "Correction Policy for MDS Records" in the State Operations Manual, Appendix R, Part IV.

The facility must maintain RAI assessments and Discharge and Reentry Tracking forms, as well as correction information, including Correction Request forms as a part of the resident's clinical record. Whether or not the facility's system is entirely electronic, a hard copy of completed MDS forms, including the signature of the facility staff attesting to the accuracy and completion of the corrected record, must be maintained in the resident's clinical record.

A facility must complete and submit to the State a subset of items when the resident is discharged from the facility (discharge tracking form), or readmitted to the facility (reentry tracking form).

F278 Accuracy of assessments: appropriate participants, registered nurse signature

§483.20(g) Accuracy of Assessment

The assessment must accurately reflect the resident's status.

Intent §483.20(g)

To assure that each resident receives an accurate assessment by staff that are qualified to assess relevant care areas and knowledgeable about the resident's status, needs, strengths, and areas of decline.

Interpretive Guidelines §483.20(g)

"The accuracy of the assessment" means that the appropriate, qualified health professional correctly documents the resident's medical, functional, and psychosocial problems and identifies resident strengths to maintain or improve medical status, functional abilities, and psychosocial status. The initial comprehensive assessment provides baseline data for ongoing assessment of resident progress.

§483.20(h) Coordination

A registered nurse must conduct or coordinate each assessment with the appropriate participation of health professionals.

Intent §483.20(h)

The registered nurse will conduct and/or coordinate the assessment, as appropriate. Whether conducted or coordinated by the registered nurse, he or she is responsible for certifying that the assessment has been completed.

Interpretive Guidelines §483.20(h)

According to the Utilization Guidelines for each State's RAI, the physical, mental, and psychosocial condition of the resident determines the appropriate level of involvement of physicians, nurses, rehabilitation therapists, activities professionals, medical social workers, dietitians, and other professionals, such as developmental disabilities specialists, in assessing the resident, and in correcting resident assessments. Involvement of other disciplines is dependent upon resident status and needs.

Probes §483.20(g)(h)

Have appropriate health professionals assessed the resident? For example, has the resident's nutritional status been assessed by someone who is knowledgeable in nutrition and capable of correctly assessing a resident?

If the resident's medical status, functional abilities, or psychosocial status declined and the decline was not clinically unavoidable, were the appropriate health professionals involved in assessing the resident?

Based on your total review of the resident, is each portion of the assessment accurate?

Are the appropriate certifications in place, including the RN Coordinator's certification of completion of an assessment or Correction Request form, and the certification of individual assessors of the accuracy and completion of the portion(s) of the assessment, tracking form or face sheet they completed or corrected. On an assessment or correction request, the RN Assessment Coordinator is responsible for certifying overall completion once all individual assessors have completed and signed their portion(s) of the MDS forms. When MDS forms are completed directly on the facility's computer, (e.g., no paper form has been manually completed), the RN Coordinator signs and dates the computer generated hard copy after reviewing it for completeness, including the signatures of all individual assessors. Backdating a completion date is not acceptable.

§483.20(i) Certification

(1) A registered nurse must sign and certify that the assessment is completed.

(2) Each individual who completes a portion of the assessment must sign and certify the accuracy of that portion of the assessment.

Interpretive Guidelines §483.20(i)

Whether the MDS forms are manually completed, or computer generated following data entry, each individual assessor is responsible for certifying the accuracy of responses on the forms relative to the resident's condition and discharge or reentry status. Manually completed forms are signed and dated by each individual assessor the day they complete their portion(s) of the MDS record. When MDS forms are completed directly on the facility's computer (e.g., no paper form has been manually completed), then each individual assessor signs and dates a computer generated hard copy, after they review it for accuracy of the portion(s) they completed. Backdating completion dates is not acceptable.

§483.20(j) Penalty for Falsification

(1) Under Medicare and Medicaid, an individual who willfully and knowingly—

(i) Certifies a material and false statement in a resident assessment is subject to a civil money penalty of not more than $1,000 for each assessment; or

(ii) Causes another individual to certify a material and false statement in a resident assessment is subject to a civil money penalty of not more than $5,000 for each assessment.

(2) Clinical disagreement does not constitute a material and false statement.

Interpretive Guidelines §483.20(j)

MDS information serves as the clinical basis for care planning and delivery. With the introduction of additional uses of MDS information such as for payment rate setting and quality monitoring, MDS information as it is reported impacts a nursing home's payment rate and standing in terms of the quality monitoring process. A pattern within a nursing home of clinical documentation or of MDS assessment or reporting practices that result in higher RUG scores, untriggering RAP(s), or unflagging QI(s), where the information does not accurately reflect the resident's status, may be indicative of payment fraud or avoidance of the quality monitoring process. Such practices may include but are not limited to a pattern or high prevalence of the following:

- Submitting MDS Assessments (including any reason(s) for assessment, routine or non-routine); Discharge or Reentry Tracking forms, where the information does not accurately reflect the resident's status as of the Assessment Reference date, or the Discharge or Reentry date, as applicable;
- Submitting correction(s) to information in the State MDS database where the corrected information does not accurately reflect the resident's status as of the original Assessment Reference date, or the original Discharge or Reentry date, as applicable, or where the record it claims to correct does not appear to have been in error;
- Submitting Significant Correction Assessments where the assessment it claims to correct does not appear to have been in error;
- Submitting Significant Change in Status Assessments where the criteria for significant change in the resident's status do not appear to be met; Delaying or withholding MDS Assessments (including any reason(s) for assessment, routine or non-routine), Discharge or Reentry Tracking information, or correction(s) to information in the State MDS database.

When such patterns or practices are noticed, they should be reported by the State Agency to the proper authority.

F279 Comprehensive care plans

(Rev. 5, Issued: 11-19-04, Effective: 11-19-04, Implementation: 11-19-04)

§483.20(d) A facility must use the results of the assessment to develop, review, and revise the resident's comprehensive plan of care.

§483.20(k) Comprehensive Care Plans

(1) The facility must develop a comprehensive care plan for each resident that includes measurable objectives and timetables to meet a resident's medical, nursing, and mental and psychosocial needs that are identified in the comprehensive assessment. The care plan must describe the following:

(i) The services that are to be furnished to attain or maintain the resident's highest practicable physical, mental, and psychosocial well-being as required under §483.25; and

(ii) Any services that would otherwise be required under §483.25 but are not provided due to the resident's exercise of rights under §483.10, including the right to refuse treatment under §483.10(b)(4).

Interpretive Guidelines §483.20(k)

An interdisciplinary team, in conjunction with the resident, resident's family, surrogate, or representative, as appropriate, should develop quantifiable objectives for the highest level of functioning the resident may be expected to attain, based on the comprehensive assessment. The interdisciplinary team should show evidence in the RAP summary or clinical record of the following:

- The resident's status in triggered RAP areas;
- The facility's rationale for deciding whether to proceed with care planning; and
- Evidence that the facility considered the development of care planning interventions for all RAPs triggered by the MDS.

The care plan must reflect intermediate steps for each outcome objective if identification of those steps will enhance the resident's ability to meet his/her objectives. Facility staff will use these objectives to monitor resident progress. Facilities may, for some residents, need to prioritize their care plan interventions. This should be noted in the clinical record or on the plan of care.

The requirements reflect the facility's responsibilities to provide necessary care and services to attain or maintain the highest practicable physical, mental, and psychosocial well-being, in accordance with the comprehensive assessment and plan of care. However, in some cases, a resident may wish to refuse certain services or treatments that professional staff believe may be indicated to assist the resident in reaching his or her highest practicable level of well-being. Desires of the resident should be documented in the clinical record (see guidelines at §483.10(b)(4) for additional guidance concerning refusal of treatment).

Probes §483.20(k)(1)

Does the care plan address the needs, strengths, and preferences identified in the comprehensive resident assessment?

Is the care plan oriented toward preventing avoidable declines in functioning or functional levels? How does the care plan attempt to manage risk factors? Does the care plan build on resident strengths?

Does the care plan reflect standards of current professional practice?

Do treatment objectives have measurable outcomes?

Corroborate information regarding the resident's goals and wishes for treatment in the plan of care by interviewing residents, especially those identified as refusing treatment.

Determine whether the facility has provided adequate information to the resident so that the resident was able to make an informed choice regarding treatment.

If the resident has refused treatment, does the care plan reflect the facility's efforts to find alternative means to address the problem?

For implementation of care plan, see §483.20(k)(3).

F280 Comprehensive care plan requirements

(Rev. 5, Issued: 11-19-04, Effective: 11-19-04, Implementation: 11-19-04)

§483.10(d)(3) — The resident has the right to — unless adjudged incompetent or otherwise found to be incapacitated under the laws of the State — participate in planning care and treatment or changes in care and treatment.

Interpretive Guidelines §483.10(d)(3)

"Participates in planning care and treatment" means that the resident is afforded the opportunity to select from alternative treatments. This applies both to initial decisions about care and treatment and to decisions about changes in care and treatment. The resident's right to participate in care planning and to refuse treatment are covered in §§483.20(d)(2) and 483.10(b)(4).

A resident whose ability to make decisions about care and treatment is impaired, or a resident who has been formally declared incompetent by a court, should, to the extent practicable, be kept informed and be consulted on personal preferences.

Whenever there appears to be a conflict between a resident's right and the resident's health or safety, determine if the facility attempted to accommodate both the exercise of the resident's rights and the resident's health, including exploration of care alternatives through a thorough care planning process in which the resident may participate.

Procedures §483.10(d)(3)

Look for evidence that the resident was afforded the right to participate in care planning or was consulted about care and treatment changes (e.g., ask residents or their representatives during interviews).

§483.20(k)(2)

§483.20(k)(2) A comprehensive care plan must be—

(i) Developed within 7 days after the completion of the comprehensive assessment;

(ii) Prepared by an interdisciplinary team, that includes the attending physician, a registered nurse with responsibility for the resident, and other appropriate staff in disciplines as determined by the resident's needs, and, to the extent practicable, the participation of the resident, the resident's family, or the resident's legal representative; and

(iii) Periodically reviewed and revised by a team of qualified persons after each assessment.

Interpretive Guidelines §483.20(k)(2)

As used in this requirement, "Interdisciplinary" means that professional disciplines, as appropriate, will work together to provide the greatest benefit to the resident. It does not mean that every goal must have an interdisciplinary approach. The mechanics of how the interdisciplinary team meets its responsibilities in developing an interdisciplinary care plan (e.g., a face-to-face meeting, teleconference, written communication) is at the discretion of the facility.

The physician must participate as part of the interdisciplinary team, and may arrange with the facility for alternative methods, other than attendance at care planning conferences, of providing his/her input, such as one-on-one discussions and conference calls.

The resident's right to participate in choosing treatment options, decisions in care planning, and the right to refuse treatment are addressed at §483.20(k)(2)(ii) and 483.10(b)(4), respectively, and include the right to accept or refuse treatment. The facility has a responsibility to assist residents to participate, e.g., helping residents, and families, legal surrogates, or representatives understand the assessment and care planning process; when feasible, holding care planning meetings at the time of day when a resident is functioning best; planning enough time for information exchange and decision making; encouraging a resident's advocate to attend (e.g., family member, friend) if desired by a resident.

The resident has the right to refuse specific treatments and to select among treatment options before the care plan is instituted. (See §483.20(k)(2)(ii) and 483.10(b)(4).) The facility should encourage residents, legal surrogates, and representatives to participate in care planning, including attending care planning conferences if they so desire.

While Federal regulations affirm the resident's right to participate in care planning and to refuse treatment, the regulations do not create the right for a resident, legal surrogate, or representative to demand that the facility use specific medical intervention or treatment that the facility deems inappropriate. Statutory requirements hold the facility ultimately accountable for the resident's care and safety, including clinical decisions.

Probes §483.20(k)(2)

1. Was interdisciplinary expertise utilized to develop a plan to improve the resident's functional abilities?

   a. For example, did an occupational therapist design needed adaptive equipment or a speech therapist provide techniques to improve swallowing ability?

   b. Do the dietitian and speech therapist determine, for example, the optimum textures and consistency for the resident's food that provide both a nutritionally adequate diet and effectively use oropharyngeal capabilities of the resident?

   c. Is there evidence of physician involvement in development of the care plan (e.g., presence at care plan meetings, conversations with team members concerning the care plan, conference calls)?

2. In what ways do staff involve residents and families, surrogates, and/or representatives in care planning?

3. Do staff make an effort to schedule care plan meetings at the best time of the day for residents and their families?

4. Ask the ombudsman if he/she has been involved in a care planning meeting as a resident advocate. If yes, ask how the process worked.

5. Do facility staff attempt to make the process understandable to the resident/family?

6. Ask residents whether they have brought questions or concerns about their care to the attention of facility's staff. If so, what happened as a result?

Interpretive Guidelines §483.20(k)(2)(iii)

See §483.75(g)(2)(iii) for "Qualified Person."

Probes §483.20(k)(2)(iii)

Is the care plan evaluated and revised as the resident's status changes?

F281 Services must meet professional standards of quality

§483.20(k)(3)

(3) The services provided or arranged by the facility must—

(i) Meet professional standards of quality and;

Intent §483.20(k)(3)(i)

The intent of this regulation is to assure that services being provided meet professional standards of quality (in accordance with the definition provided below) and are provided by appropriate qualified persons (e.g., licensed, certified).

Interpretive Guidelines §483.20(k)(3)(i)

"Professional standards of quality" means services that are provided according to accepted standards of clinical practice. Standards may apply to care provided by a particular clinical discipline or in a specific clinical situation or setting. Standards regarding quality care practices may be published by a professional organization, licensing board, accreditation body, or other regulatory agency. Recommended practices to achieve desired resident outcomes may also be found in clinical literature. Possible reference sources for standards of practice include:

- Current manuals or textbooks on nursing, social work, physical therapy, etc.
- Standards published by professional organizations such as the American Dietetic Association, American Medical Association, American Medical Directors Association, American Nurses Association, National Association of Activity Professionals, National Association of Social Work, etc.
- Clinical practice guidelines published by the Agency of Health Care Policy and Research
- Current professional journal articles

If a negative resident outcome is determined to be related to the facility's failure to meet professional standards, and the team determines a deficiency has occurred, it should be cited under the appropriate quality of care or other relevant requirement.

Probes §483.20(k)(3)

Question only those practices which have a negative outcome or have a potential negative outcome. Ask the facility to produce references upon which the practice is based.

- Do nurses notify physicians, as appropriate, and show evidence of discussions of acute medical problems?
- Are residents with acute conditions who require intensive monitoring and hospital-level treatments that the facility is unable to provide, promptly hospitalized?
- Are there errors in the techniques of medication administration? (Cite actual medication errors at §483.25(m).)
- Is there evidence of assessment and care planning sufficient to meet the needs of newly admitted residents, prior to completion of the first comprehensive assessment and comprehensive care plan?
- Are physicians' orders carried out, unless otherwise indicated by an advanced directive?

F282 Services to be provided by qualified persons in accordance with each resident's written plan of care

§483.20(k)(3)(ii) Be provided by qualified persons in accordance with each resident's written plan of care.

Interpretive Guidelines §483.20(k)(3)(ii)

If you find problems with quality of care, quality of life, or resident rights, are these problems attributable to the qualifications of the facility staff, or lack of, inadequate, or incorrect implementation of the care plan?

Probes §483.20(k)(3)(ii)

- Can direct care-giving staff describe the care, services, and expected outcomes of the care they provide; do they have a general knowledge of the care and services being provided by other therapists; do they have an understanding of the expected outcomes of this care, and understand the relationship of these expected outcomes to the care they provide?

F283 Discharge summary: recapitulation of the resident's stay

§483.20(l) Discharge Summary

When the facility anticipates discharge, a resident must have a discharge summary that includes:

(1) A recapitulation of the resident's stay;

(2) A final summary of the resident's status to include items in paragraph (b)(2) of this section, at the time of the discharge that is available for release to authorized persons and agencies, with the consent of the resident or legal representative; and

Intent §483.20(l)

To ensure appropriate discharge planning and communication of necessary information to the continuing care provider.

Interpretive Guidelines §483.20(l)

"Anticipates" means that the discharge was not an emergency discharge (e.g., hospitalization for an acute condition) or due to the resident's death.

"Adjust to his or her living environment" means that the post-discharge plan, as appropriate, should describe the resident's and family's preferences for care, how the resident and family will access these services, and how care should be coordinated if continuing treatment involves multiple caregivers. It should identify specific resident needs after discharge such as personal care, sterile dressings, and physical therapy, as well as describe resident/caregiver education needs and ability to meet care needs after discharge.

F284 A post-discharge plan of care developed with participation

§483.20(l)(3) A post-discharge plan of care that is developed with the participation of the resident and his or her family, which will assist the resident to adjust to his or her new living environment.

Interpretive Guidelines §483.20(l)(3)

A post-discharge plan of care for an anticipated discharge applies to a resident whom the facility discharges to a private residence, to another NF or SNF, or to another type of residential facility such as a board and care home or an intermediate care facility for individuals with mental retardation. Resident protection concerning transfer and discharge are found at §483.12. A "post-discharge plan of care" means the discharge planning process which includes: assessing continuing care needs and developing a plan designed to ensure the individual's needs will be met after discharge from the facility into the community.

Probes §483.20(l)

- Does the discharge summary have information pertinent to continuing care for the resident?
- Is there evidence of discharge planning in the records of discharged residents who had an anticipated discharge or those residents to be discharged shortly (e.g., in the next 7–14 days)?
- Do discharge plans address necessary post-discharge care?
- Has the facility aided the resident and his/her family in locating and coordinating post-discharge services?
- What types of pre-discharge preparation and education has the facility provided the resident and his/her family?

F285 Preadmission screening for mentally ill and mentally retarded persons

(Rev. 5, Issued: 11-19-04, Effective: 11-19-04, Implementation: 11-19-04)

§483.20(e) Coordination

A facility must coordinate assessments with the preadmission screening and resident review program under Medicaid in part 483, subpart C to the maximum extent practicable to avoid duplicative testing and effort.

Interpretive Guidelines §483.20(e)

With respect to the responsibilities under the Pre-Admission Screening and Resident Review (PASRR) program, the State is responsible for conducting the screens, preparing the PASRR report, and providing or arranging the specialized services that are needed as a result of conducting the screens. The State is required to provide a copy of the PASRR report to the facility. This report must list the specialized services that the individual requires and that are the responsibility of the State to provide. All other needed services are the responsibility of the facility to provide.

§483.20(m) Preadmission Screening for Mentally Ill Individuals and Individuals with Mental Retardation.

§483.20(m)(1) A nursing facility must not admit, on or after January 1, 1989, any new residents with:

(i) Mental illness as defined in paragraph (m)(2)(i) of this section, unless the State mental health authority has determined, based on an independent physical and mental evaluation performed by a person or entity other than the State mental health authority, prior to admission;

(A) That, because of the physical and mental condition of the individual, the individual requires the level of services provided by a nursing facility; and

(B) If the individual requires such level of services, whether the individual requires specialized services for mental retardation.

(ii) Mental retardation, as defined in paragraph (m)(2)(ii) of this section, unless the State mental retardation or developmental disability authority has determined prior to admission—

(A) That, because of the physical and mental condition of the individual, the individual requires the level of services provided by a nursing facility; and

(B) If the individual requires such level of services, whether the individual requires specialized services for mental retardation.

§483.20(m)(2) Definitions. For purposes of this section:

(i) An individual is considered to have "mental illness" if the individual has a serious mental illness defined at 483.102(b)(1).

(ii) An individual is considered to be "mentally retarded" if the individual is mentally retarded as defined in 483.102(b)(3) or is a person with a related condition as described in 42 CFR 1009.

Intent §483.20(m)

To ensure that individuals with mental illness and mental retardation receive the care and services they need in the most appropriate setting.

"Specialized services" are those services the State is required to provide or arrange for that raise the intensity of services to the level needed by the resident. That is, specialized services are an "add-on" to NF services—they are of a higher intensity and frequency than specialized rehabilitation services, which are provided by the NF.

The statute mandates preadmission screening for all individuals with mental illness (MI) or mental retardation (MR) who apply to NFs, regardless of the applicant's source of payment, except as provided below. (See §1919(b)(3)(F).) Residents readmitted and individuals who initially apply to a nursing facility directly following a discharge from an acute care stay are exempt if:

- They are certified by a physician prior to admission to require a nursing facility stay of less than 30 days; and
- They require care at the nursing facility for the same condition for which they were hospitalized.

The State is responsible for providing specialized services to residents with MI/MR residing in Medicaid-certified facilities. The facility is required to provide all other care and services appropriate to the resident's condition. Therefore, if a facility has residents with MI/MR, do not survey for specialized services, but survey for all other requirements, including resident rights, quality of life, and quality of care.

If the resident's PAS report indicates that he or she needs specialized services but the resident is not receiving them, notify the Medicaid agency. NF services ordinarily are not of the intensity to meet the needs of residents with MI or MR.

Probes §483.20(m)

If sampled residents have MI or MR, did the State Mental Health or Mental Retardation Authority determine:

- Whether the residents needed the services of a NF?
- Whether the residents need specialized services for their MR or MI?

§483.25 Quality of Care   Tags 309 – 354

§483.25(a) Activities of Daily Living
§483.25(b) Vision and Hearing
§483.25(c) Pressure Sores
§483.25(d) Urinary Incontinence
§483.25(e) Range of Motion
§483.25(f) Mental and Psychosocial Functioning
§483.25(g) Naso-Gastric Tubes
§483.25(h) Accidents
§483.25(i) Nutrition
§483.25(j) Hydration
§483.25(k) Special Needs
§483.25(l) Unnecessary Drugs
§483.25(m) Medication Errors
§483.25(n) Influenza and Pneumococcal Immunizations

F309 Quality of care

(Rev. 4, Issued: 11-12-04, Effective: 11-12-04, Implementation: 11-12-04)

§483.25 Quality of Care

Each resident must receive and the facility must provide the necessary care and services to attain or maintain the highest practicable physical, mental, and psychosocial well-being, in accordance with the comprehensive assessment and plan of care.

Use F309 for quality of care deficiencies not covered by §483.25(a)-(m).

Intent §483.25

The facility must ensure that the resident obtains optimal improvement or does not deteriorate within the limits of a resident's right to refuse treatment, and within the limits of recognized pathology and the normal aging process.

Definitions §483.25

- "Highest practicable" is defined as the highest level of functioning and well-being possible, limited only by the individual's presenting functional status and potential for improvement or reduced rate of functional decline. Highest practicable is determined through the comprehensive resident assessment by competently and thoroughly addressing the physical, mental, or psychosocial needs of the individual.
- "Skin Ulcer/Wound"

NOTE: Skin ulcer definitions are included to clarify clinical terms related to skin ulcers. At the time of the assessment and diagnosis, the clinician is expected to document the clinical basis (e.g., underlying condition contributing to the ulceration, ulcer edges and wound bed, location, shape, condition of surrounding tissues) which permit differentiating the ulcer type, especially if the ulcer has characteristics consistent with a pressure ulcer, but is determined not to be one.

- ✧ "Arterial Ulcer" is ulceration that occurs as the result of arterial occlusive disease when non-pressure related disruption or blockage of the arterial blood flow to an area causes tissue necrosis.

  Inadequate blood supply to the extremity may initially present as intermittent claudication. Arterial/Ischemic ulcers may be present in individuals with moderate to severe peripheral vascular disease, generalized arteriosclerosis, inflammatory or autoimmune disorders (such as arteritis), or significant vascular disease elsewhere (e.g., stroke or heart attack). The arterial ulcer is characteristically painful, usually occurs in the distal portion of the lower extremity and may be over the ankle or bony areas of the foot (e.g., top of the foot or toe, outside edge of the foot). The wound bed is frequently dry and pale with minimal or no exudate. The affected foot may exhibit: diminished or absent pedal pulse, coolness to touch, decreased pain when hanging down (dependent) or increased pain when elevated, blanching upon elevation, delayed capillary fill time, hair loss on top of the foot and toes, toenail thickening.

- ✧ "Diabetic neuropathic ulcer" requires that the resident be diagnosed with diabetes mellitus and have peripheral neuropathy. The diabetic ulcer characteristically occurs on the foot, e.g., at mid-foot, at the ball of the foot over the metatarsal heads, or on the top of toes with Charcot deformity.
- ✧ "Pressure ulcer." See Guidance at 42 CFR 483.25(c)-F314.
- ✧ "Venous insufficiency ulcer" (previously known as "stasis ulcer") is an open lesion of the skin and subcutaneous tissue of the lower leg, usually occurring in the pretibial area of the lower leg or above the medial ankle. Venous ulcers are reported to be the most common vascular ulceration and may be difficult to heal, may occur off and on for several years, and may occur after relatively minor trauma. The ulcer may have a moist, granulating wound bed, may be superficial, and may have minimal to copious serous drainage unless the wound is infected. The resident may experience pain which may be increased when the foot is in a dependent position, such as when a resident is seated with her or his feet on the floor. Recent literature implicates venous hypertension as a causative factor. Earlier, the ulceration was believed to be due to the pooling of blood in the veins.

  Venous hypertension may be caused by one (or a combination of) factor(s) including: loss of (or compromised) valve function in the vein, partial or complete obstruction of the vein (e.g., deep vein thrombosis, obesity, malignancy), and/or failure of the calf muscle to pump the blood (e.g., paralysis, decreased activity). Venous insufficiency may result in edema and induration, dilated superficial veins, cellulitis in the lower third of the leg or dermatitis (typically characterized by change in skin pigmentation). The pigmentation may appear as darkening skin, tan, or purple areas in light-skinned residents and dark purple, black, or dark brown areas in dark-skinned residents.

Interpretive Guidelines §483.25

Use F309 when the survey team determines there are quality of care deficiencies not covered by §§483.25(a)-(m). "Highest practicable" is defined as the highest level of functioning and well-being possible, limited only by the individual's presenting functional status and potential for improvement or reduced rate of functional decline. Highest practicable is determined through the comprehensive resident assessment by competently and thoroughly addressing the physical, mental, or psychosocial needs of the individual.

The facility must ensure that the resident obtains optimal improvement or does not deteriorate within the limits of a resident's right to refuse treatment, and within the limits of recognized pathology and the normal aging process.

In any instance in which there has been a lack of improvement or a decline, the survey team must determine if the occurrence was unavoidable or avoidable. A determination of unavoidable decline or failure to reach highest practicable well-being may be made only if all of the following are present:

- An accurate and complete assessment (see §483.20);
- A care plan which is implemented consistently and based on information from the assessment;
- Evaluation of the results of the interventions and revising the interventions as necessary.

Determine if the facility is providing the necessary care and services based on the findings of the RAI. If services and care are being provided, determine if the facility is evaluating the outcome to the resident and changing the interventions if needed. This should be done in accordance with the resident's customary daily routine. Use Tag F309 to cite quality of care deficiencies that are not explicit in the quality of care regulations.

Procedures §483.25

Assess a facility's compliance with these requirements by determining if the services noted in the plan of care, based on a comprehensive and accurate functional assessment of the resident's strengths, weaknesses, risk factors for deterioration, and potential for improvement, is continually and aggressively implemented and updated by the facility staff. In looking at assessments, use both the MDS and RAPs information, any other pertinent assessments, and resulting care plans.

If the resident has been in the facility for less than 14 days (before completion of all the RAI is required), determine if the facility is conducting ongoing assessment and care planning, and, if appropriate, care and services are being provided.

If quality of care problems are noted in areas of nurse aide responsibility, review nurse aide competency requirements at §483.75(e).

F310 Activities of daily living

§483.25(a) Activities of Daily Living (ADLs)

Based on the comprehensive assessment of a resident, the facility must ensure that

Intent §483.25(a)

The intent of this regulation is that the facility must ensure that a resident's abilities in ADLs do not deteriorate unless the deterioration was unavoidable.

§483.25(a)(1) A resident's abilities in activities of daily living do not diminish unless circumstances of the individual's clinical condition demonstrate that diminution was unavoidable. This includes the resident's ability to—

(i) Bathe, dress, and groom;

(ii) Transfer and ambulate;

(iii) Toilet;

(iv) Eat; and

(v) Use speech, language, or other functional communication systems.

Interpretive Guidelines §483.25(a)

The mere presence of a clinical diagnosis, in itself, justify a decline in a resident's ability to perform ADLs. Conditions which may demonstrate unavoidable diminution in ADLs include:

- The natural progression of the resident's disease;
- Deterioration of the resident's physical condition associated with the onset of a physical or mental disability while receiving care to restore or maintain functional abilities; and
- The resident's or his/her surrogate's or representative's refusal of care and treatment to restore or maintain functional abilities after aggressive efforts by the facility to counsel and/or offer alternatives to the resident, surrogate, or representative. Refusal of such care and treatment should be documented in the clinical record. Determine which interventions were identified on the care plan and/or could be in place to minimize or decrease complications. Note also that depression is a potential cause of excess disability and, where appropriate, therapeutic interventions should be initiated.

Appropriate treatment and services includes all care provided to residents by employees, contractors, or volunteers of the facility to maximize the individual's functional abilities. This includes pain relief and control, especially when it is causing a decline or a decrease in the quality of life of the resident.

If the survey team identifies a pattern of deterioration in ADLs, i.e., a number of residents have deteriorated in more than one ADL or a number of residents have deteriorated in only one ADL (one in bathing, one in eating, one in toileting) and it is determined there is deficient practice, cite at F310.

For evaluating a resident's ADLs and determining whether a resident's abilities have declined, improved, or stayed the same within the last twelve months, use the following definitions as specified in the State's RAI:

1. Independent — No help or staff oversight; or staff help/oversight provided only 1 or 2 times during prior 7 days.

2. Supervision — Oversight encouragement or cuing provided 3 or more times during the last 7 days, or supervision plus physical assistance provided only 1 or 2 times during the last 7 days.

3. Limited Assistance — Resident highly involved in activity, received physical help in guided maneuvering of limbs, and/or other non-weight bearing assistance 3 or more times; or more help provided only 1 or 2 times over 7-day period.

4. Extensive Assistance — While resident performed part of activity, over prior 7-day period, help of following type(s) was provided 3 or more times;

   a. Weight-bearing support; or

   b. Full staff performance during part (but not all) of week.

5. Total Dependence — Full staff performance of activity over entire 7-day period.

§483.25(a)(1)(i) Bathing, Dressing, Grooming

Interpretive Guidelines §483.25(a)(1)(i)

This corresponds to MDS section E; version 2.0, section G, when specified for use by the State.

"Bathing" means how resident takes full-body bath, sponge bath, and transfers in/out of tub/shower. Exclude washing of back and hair.

"Dressing" means how resident puts on, fastens, and takes off all items of clothing, including donning/removing prosthesis.

"Grooming" means how resident maintains personal hygiene, including preparatory activities; combing hair; brushing teeth; shaving; applying make-up; and washing/drying face, hands and perineum. Exclude baths and showers.

BATHING, DRESSING, GROOMING

Procedures §483.25(a)(1)(i)

For each sampled resident selected for the comprehensive review or the focused review, as appropriate, determine:

1. Whether the resident's ability to bathe, dress, and/or groom has changed since admission, or over the past 12 months;

2. Whether the resident's ability to bathe, dress, and groom has improved, declined, or stayed the same;

3. Whether any deterioration or lack of improvement was avoidable or unavoidable by:

4. Identifying if resident triggers RAPs for ADL functional/rehabilitation potential.

   a. What risk factors for decline of bathing, dressing, and/or grooming abilities did the facility identify?

   b. What care did the resident receive to address unique needs to maintain his/her bathing, dressing, and/or grooming abilities (e.g., resident needs a button hook to button his shirt; staff teaches the resident how to use it; staff provides resident with dementia with cues that allow him/her to dress him or herself)?

   c. Were individual objectives of the plan of care periodically evaluated, and if the objectives were not met, were alternative approaches developed to encourage maintenance of bathing, dressing, and/or grooming abilities (e.g., resident now unable to button dress, even with encouragement; will ask family if we may use velcro in place of buttons so resident can continue to dress herself)?

Probes §483.25(a)(1)(i)

If the resident's abilities in bathing, dressing, and grooming have been maintained, what evidence is there that the resident could have improved if appropriate treatment and services were provided:

- Identify relevant sections of the MDS and consider whether assessment triggers the RAPs and the RAPs were followed.
- Are there physical and psychosocial deficits that could affect improvement in functional abilities?
- Was the care plan driven by resident strengths identified in the comprehensive assessment?
- Was the care plan consistently implemented?
- What changes were made in treatment if the resident failed to progress or when initial rehabilitation goals were achieved, but additional progress might have been possible?

TRANSFER AND AMBULATION

§483.25(a)(1)(ii)

Interpretive Guidelines §483.25(a)(1)(ii)

This corresponds to MDS section E; MDS 2.0 section G when specified for use by the State.

"Transfer" means how resident moves between surfaces — to/from: bed, chair, wheelchair, standing position. (Exclude to/from bath/toilet.)

"Ambulation" means how resident moves between locations in his/her room and adjacent corridor on same floor. If in wheelchair, self-sufficiency once in chair.

Procedures §483.25(a)(1)(ii)

Determine for each resident selected for a comprehensive review, or a focused review as appropriate, whether the resident's ability to transfer and ambulate has declined, improved, or stayed the same and whether any deterioration or decline in function was avoidable or unavoidable.

Probes §483.25(a)(1)(ii)

If the resident's transferring and ambulating abilities have declined, what evidence is there that the decline was unavoidable:

- What risk factors for decline of transferring or ambulating abilities did the facility identify (e.g., necrotic area of foot ulcer becoming larger, postural hypotension)?
- What care did the resident receive to address risk factors and unique needs to maintain transferring or ambulating abilities (e.g., a transfer board is provided to maintain ability to transfer from bed to wheelchair and staff teaches the resident how to use it)?
- What evidence is there that sufficient staff time and assistance are provided to maintain transferring and ambulating abilities?
- Has resident been involved in activities that enhance mobility skills?
- Were individual objectives of the plan of care periodically evaluated, and if goals were not met, were alternative approaches developed to encourage maintenance of transferring and ambulation abilities (e.g., resident remains unsteady when using a cane, returns to walker, with staff encouraging the walker's consistent use)?
- Identify if resident triggers RAPs for ADL functional/rehabilitation potential, psychosocial well-being, or mood state and the RAPs are followed.

If the resident's abilities in transferring and ambulating have been maintained, is there evidence that the resident could have improved if appropriate treatment and services were provided?

- Are there physical and psychosocial deficits that could affect improvement in functional abilities?

- Was the care plan driven by resident strengths identified in the comprehensive assessment?
- Was the care plan consistently implemented? What changes were made in treatment if the resident failed to progress or when initial rehabilitation goals were achieved, but additional progress seemed possible?

TOILETING

§483.25(a)(1)(ii)

Interpretive Guidelines §483.25(a)(1)(iii)

This corresponds to MDS sections E; MDS 2.0 sections G and H when specified for use by the State.

"Toilet use" means how the resident uses the toilet room (or commode, bedpan, urinal); transfers on/off the toilet, cleanses self, changes pad, manages ostomy or catheter, adjusts clothes.

Procedures §483.25(a)(1)(iii)

Determine for each resident selected for a comprehensive review, or focused review as appropriate, whether the resident's ability to use the toilet has improved, declined, or stayed the same and whether any deterioration or decline in improvement was avoidable or unavoidable.

Probes §483.25(a)(1)(iii)

If the resident's toilet use abilities have declined, what evidence is there that the decline was unavoidable.

- What risk factors for the decline of toilet use abilities did the facility identify (e.g., severe arthritis in hands makes use of toilet paper difficult)?
- What care did resident receive to address risk factors and unique needs to maintain toilet use abilities (e.g., assistive devices to maintain ability to use the toilet such as using a removable elevated toilet seat or wall grab bar to facilitate rising from seated position to standing position)?
- Is there sufficient staff time and assistance provided to maintain toilet use abilities (e.g., allowing residents enough time to use the toilet independently or with limited assistance)?
- Were individual objectives of the plan of care periodically evaluated, and if objectives were not met, were alternative approaches developed to encourage maintaining toilet use abilities (e.g., if resident has not increased sitting stability, seek occupational therapy consult to determine the need for therapy to increase sitting balance, ability to transfer safely and manipulate clothing during the toileting process. For residents with dementia, remind periodically to use the toilet)?
- Identify if resident triggers RAPs for urinary incontinence, and ADL functional/rehabilitation potential and the RAPs were used to assess causal factors for decline or potential for decline or lack of improvement.

If the resident's toilet use abilities have been maintained, what evidence is there that the resident could have improved if appropriate treatment and services were provided?

- Are there physical and psychosocial deficits that could affect improvement in functional abilities?
- Was the care plan driven by resident strengths identified in the comprehensive assessment?
- Was the care plan consistently implemented? What changes were made to treatment if the resident failed to progress or when initial rehabilitation goals were achieved, but additional progress seemed possible?
- Identify if resident triggers RAPs for mood state and psychosocial well-being.

EATING

§483.25(a)(1)(iv)

Interpretive Guidelines §483.25(a)(1)(iv)

This corresponds to MDS sections E, L1 and MI; MDS 2.0, sections G and K when specified for use by the State.

"Eating" means how resident ingests and drinks (regardless of self-feeding skill).

Procedures §483.25(a)(1)(iv)

Determine for each resident selected for a comprehensive review, or focused review, as appropriate, whether the resident's ability to eat or eating skills have improved, declined, or stayed the same and whether any deterioration or lack of improvement was avoidable or unavoidable.

If the resident's eating abilities have declined, is there any evidence that the decline was unavoidable?

1. What risk factors for decline of eating skills did the facility identify?

   a. A decrease in the ability to chew and swallow food;

   b. Deficit in neurological and muscular status necessary for moving food onto a utensil and into the mouth;

   c. Oral health status affecting eating ability;

   d. Depression or confused mental state.

2. What care did the resident receive to address risk factors and unique needs to maintain eating abilities?

   a. Assistive devices to improve resident's grasp or coordination;

b. Seating arrangements to improve sociability;

c. Seating in a calm, quiet setting for residents with dementia.

3. Is there sufficient staff time and assistance provided to maintain eating abilities (e.g., allowing residents enough time to eat independently or with limited assistance)?

4. Identify if resident triggers RAPs for ADL functional/rehabilitation potential, feeding tubes, and dehydration/fluid maintenance, and the RAPs were used to assess causal reasons for decline, potential for decline, or lack of improvement.

5. Were individual objectives of the plan of care periodically evaluated, and if the objectives were not met, were alternative approaches developed to encourage maintaining eating abilities?

Probes §483.25(a)(1)(iv)

If the resident's eating abilities have been maintained, what evidence is there that the resident could have improved if appropriate treatment and services were provided:

- Are there physical and psychosocial deficits that could affect improvement in functional abilities?
- Was the care plan driven by resident strengths identified in the comprehensive assessment?
- Was the care plan consistently implemented? What changes are made to treatment if the resident failed to progress or when initial rehabilitation goals were achieved, but additional progress seemed possible?

USE OF SPEECH, LANGUAGE, OR OTHER FUNCTIONAL COMMUNICATION SYSTEMS

§483.25(a)(1)(v)

Interpretive Guidelines §483.25(a)(1)(v)

This corresponds to MDS, section C; MDS 2.0 sections B and C when specified for use by the State.

"Speech, language or other functional communication systems" is defined as the ability to effectively communicate requests, needs, opinions, and urgent problems; to express emotion; to listen to others; and to participate in social conversation whether in speech, writing, gesture, or a combination of these (e.g., a communication board or electronic augmentative communication device).

Procedures §483.25(a)(1)(v)

Determine for each resident selected for a comprehensive review, or focused review, as appropriate, if resident's ability to communicate has declined, improved, or stayed the same and whether any deterioration or lack of improvement was avoidable or unavoidable.

Identify if resident triggers RAPs for communication, psychosocial well-being, mood state, and visual function, and if the RAPs were used to assess causal factors for decline, potential for decline, or lack of improvement.

Probes §483.25(a)(1)(v)

If the resident's communication abilities have diminished, is there any evidence that the decline was unavoidable:

- What risk factors for decline of communication abilities did the facility identify and how did they address them (e.g., dysarthria, poor-fitting dentures, few visitors, poor relationships with staff, Alzheimer's disease)?
- Has the resident received audiologic and vision evaluation? If not, did the resident refuse such services? (See also §483.10(b)(4).)
- What unique resident needs and risk factors did the facility identify (e.g., does the resident have specific difficulties in transmitting messages, comprehending messages, and/or using a variety of communication skills such as questions and commands; does the resident receive evaluation and training in the use of assistive devices to increase and/or maintain writing skills)?
- What care does the resident receive to improve communication abilities (e.g., nurse aides communicate in writing with deaf residents or residents with severe hearing problems; practice exercises with residents receiving speech-language pathology services; increase number of resident's communication opportunities; non-verbal means of communication; review of the effect of medications on communication ability)?
- Is there sufficient staff time and assistance provided to maintain communication abilities?
- Were individual objectives of the plan of care periodically evaluated, and if the objectives were not met, were alternative approaches developed to encourage maintenance of communication abilities (e.g., if drill-oriented therapy is frustrating the resident, a less didactic approach should be attempted)?

If the resident's speech, language, and other communication abilities have been maintained, what evidence is there that the resident could have improved if appropriate treatment and services were provided:

- Are there physical and psychosocial deficits that could affect improvement in functional abilities?
- Was the care plan driven by resident strengths identified in the comprehensive assessment?
- Was the care plan consistently implemented?

• What changes were made to treatment if the resident failed to progress or when initial rehabilitation goals were achieved, but additional progress seemed possible?

F311 Appropriate treatment and services to resident

§483.25(a)(2)

(2) A resident is given the appropriate treatment and services to maintain or improve his or her abilities specified in paragraph (a)(1) of this section; and

Intent §483.25(a)(2)

The intent of this regulation is to stress that the facility is responsible for providing maintenance and restorative programs that will not only maintain, but improve, as indicated by the resident's comprehensive assessment to achieve and maintain the highest practicable outcome.

Procedures §483.25(a)(2)

Use the survey procedures and probes at §483.25(a)(1)(i) through (v) to assist in making this determination

F312 Resident unable to carry out ADLs gets necessary services

§483.25(a)(3)

(3) A resident who is unable to carry out activities of daily living receives the necessary services to maintain good nutrition, grooming, and personal and oral hygiene.

Intent §483.25(a)(3)

The intent of this regulation is that the resident receives the care and services needed because he/she is unable to do their own ADL care independently.

Interpretive Guidelines §483.25(a)(3)

This corresponds to MDS section L; MDS 2.0 section K when specified by the State.

"Unable to carry out ADLs" means those residents who need extensive or total assistance with maintenance of nutrition, grooming, and personal and oral hygiene, receive this assistance from the facility.

Methods for maintenance of good nutrition may include hand feeding of foods served on dishes; tube feedings provided through naso-gastric, gastrostomy, or other external tubes; or total parenteral nutrition provided through a central intravenous line.

"Grooming" — See §483.25(a)(1)(i) for definition.

"Personal hygiene" — Those activities described in dressing and bathing as defined in §483.25(a)(1)(i).

"Oral hygiene" means maintaining the mouth in a clean and intact condition and treating oral pathology such as ulcers of the mucosa. Services to maintain oral hygiene may include brushing the teeth, cleaning dentures, cleaning the mouth and tongue either by assisting the resident with a mouth wash or by manual cleaning with a gauze sponge, and application of medication as prescribed.

Procedures §483.25(a)(3)

For residents selected for a comprehensive review, or focused review, as appropriate, who are unable to carry out these ADLs without extensive assistance, determine if poor nutritional status, poor grooming, or lack of effective personal and oral hygiene exist. To what extent are these negative outcomes attributable to the lack of receiving necessary services?

Identify if residents trigger RAPs for nutritional status, ADL functional/rehabilitation potential, behavior problems, and dental care. Consider whether the RAPs were used to assess causal factors for decline, potential for decline, or lack of improvement. Determine if the facility proceeded properly with care planning and delivery of care for these residents.

F313 Vision and hearing

§483.25(b) Vision and Hearing

To ensure that residents receive proper treatment and assistive devices to maintain vision and hearing abilities, the facility must, if necessary, assist the resident—

1. In making appointments, and

2. By arranging for transportation to and from the office of a practitioner specializing in the treatment of vision or hearing impairment or the office of a professional specializing in the provision of vision or hearing assistive devices.

Intent §483.25(b)

The intent of this regulation is to require a facility to assist residents in gaining access to vision and hearing services by making appointments and arranging for transportation, and assistance with the use of any devices needed to maintain vision and hearing.

Interpretive Guidelines §483.25(b)

This corresponds to MDS, sections C and O; MDS 2.0 sections C, D, and P when specified for use by the State.

Assistive devices to maintain vision include glasses, contact lenses, and magnifying glasses. Assistive devices to maintain hearing include hearing aids.

This requirement does not mean that the facility must provide refractions, glasses, contact lenses, conduct comprehensive audiological evaluations (although screening is a part of the required assessment in §483.20(b)), or provide hearing aids.

The facility's responsibility is to assist residents and their families in locating and utilizing any available resources (e.g., Medicare or Medicaid program payment, local health organizations offering items and services which are available free to the community) for the provision of the services the resident needs. This includes making appointments and arranging transportation to obtain needed services.

Probes §483.25(b)

- Identify if resident triggers RAPs for visual function, and communication. Consider whether the RAPs were used to assess causal factors for decline, potential for decline, or lack of improvement.
- If the resident needs, and/or requests and does not have vision and/or hearing assistive devices, what has the facility done to assist the resident in making appointments and obtaining transportation to obtain these services?
- If the resident has assistive devices but is not using them, why not (e.g., are repairs or batteries needed)?

F314 Pressure sores

(Rev. 4, Issued: 11-12-04, Effective: 11-12-04, Implementation: 11-12-04)

§483.25(c) Pressure Sores

Based on the comprehensive Assessment of a resident, the facility must ensure that—

(1) A resident who enters the facility without pressure sores does not develop pressure sores unless the individual's clinical condition demonstrates that they were unavoidable; and

(2) A resident having pressure sores receives necessary treatment and services to promote healing, prevent infection, and prevent new sores from developing.

Intent (F314) 42 CFR 483.25(c)

The intent of this requirement is that the resident does not develop pressure ulcers unless clinically unavoidable and that the facility provides care and services to:

- Promote the prevention of pressure ulcer development;
- Promote the healing of pressure ulcers that are present (including prevention of infection to the extent possible); and
- Prevent development of additional pressure ulcers.

NOTE: Although the regulatory language refers to pressure sores, the nomenclature widely accepted presently refers to pressure ulcers, and the guidance provided in this document will refer to pressure ulcers.

DEFINITIONS

Definitions are provided to clarify clinical terms related to pressure ulcers and their evaluation and treatment.

- "Pressure Ulcer" — A pressure ulcer is any lesion caused by unrelieved pressure that results in damage to the underlying tissue(s).[1] Although friction and shear are not primary causes of pressure ulcers, friction and shear are important contributing factors to the development of pressure ulcers.
- "Avoidable/Unavoidable" Pressure Ulcers

  ✧ "Avoidable" means that the resident developed a pressure ulcer and that the facility did not do one or more of the following: evaluate the resident's clinical condition and pressure ulcer risk factors; define and implement interventions that are consistent with resident needs, resident goals, and recognized standards of practice; monitor and evaluate the impact of the interventions; or revise the interventions as appropriate.
  ✧ "Unavoidable" means that the resident developed a pressure ulcer even though the facility had evaluated the resident's clinical condition and pressure ulcer risk factors; defined and implemented interventions that are consistent with resident needs, goals, and recognized standards of practice; monitored and evaluated the impact of the interventions; and revised the approaches as appropriate.

- "Cleansing/Irrigation"

  ✧ "Cleansing" refers to the use of an appropriate device and solution to clean the surface of the wound bed and to remove the looser foreign debris or contaminants in order to decrease microbial growth.[2]
  ✧ "Irrigation" refers to a type of mechanical debridement, which uses an appropriate solution delivered under pressure to the wound bed to vigorously attempt to remove debris from the wound bed.[3]

- "Colonized/Infected" Wound[4, 5]

❖ "Colonized" refers to the presence of bacteria on the surface or in the tissue of a wound without the signs and symptoms of an infection.

❖ "Infected" refers to the presence of micro-organisms in sufficient quantity to overwhelm the defenses of viable tissues and produce the signs and symptoms of infection.

• "Debridement" — Debridement is the removal of devitalized/necrotic tissue and foreign matter from a wound to improve or facilitate the healing process.[6, 7, 8] Various debridement methods include:

❖ "Autolytic debridement" refers to the use of moisture retentive dressings to cover a wound and allow devitalized tissue to self-digest by the action of enzymes present in the wound fluids.

❖ "Enzymatic (chemical) debridement" refers to the topical application of substances e.g., enzymes to break down devitalized tissue.

❖ "Mechanical debridement" refers to the removal of foreign material and devitalized or contaminated tissue from a wound by physical rather than by chemical or autolytic means.

❖ "Sharp or surgical debridement" refers to removal of foreign material or devitalized tissue by a surgical instrument.

❖ "Maggot debridement therapy (MDT)" or medicinal maggots refers to a type of sterile intentional biological larval or biosurgical debridement that uses disinfected (sterile) maggots to clean wounds by dissolving the dead and infected tissue and by killing bacteria.[9]

• "Eschar/Slough"

❖ "Eschar" is described as thick, leathery, frequently black or brown in color, necrotic (dead) or devitalized tissue that has lost its usual physical properties and biological activity. Eschar may be loose or firmly adhered to the wound.

❖ "Slough" is necrotic/avascular tissue in the process of separating from the viable portions of the body and is usually light colored, soft, moist, and stringy (at times).

• "Exudate"

❖ "Exudate" is any fluid that has been forced out of the tissues or its capillaries because of inflammation or injury. It may contain serum, cellular debris, bacteria, and leukocytes.

❖ "Purulent exudate/drainage/discharge" is any product of inflammation that contains pus (e.g., leukocytes, bacteria, and liquefied necrotic debris).

❖ "Serous drainage or exudate" is watery, clear, or slightly yellow/tan/pink fluid that has separated from the blood and presents as drainage.

• "Friction/Shearing"

- ✧ "Friction" is the mechanical force exerted on skin that is dragged across any surface.
- ✧ "Shearing" is the interaction of both gravity and friction against the surface of the skin. Friction is always present when shear force is present.[10] Shear occurs when layers of skin rub against each other or when the skin remains stationary and the underlying tissue moves and stretches and angulates or tears the underlying capillaries and blood vessels causing tissue damage.

- • "Granulation Tissue"

  - ✧ "Granulation tissue" is the pink-red moist tissue that fills an open wound, when it starts to heal. It contains new blood vessels, collagen, fibroblasts, and inflammatory cells.

- • "Tunnel/Sinus Tract/Undermining"—Tunnel and sinus tract are often used interchangeably.

  - ✧ "Tunneling" is a passageway of tissue destruction under the skin surface that has an opening at the skin level from the edge of the wound.
  - ✧ A "sinus tract" is a cavity or channel underlying a wound that involves an area larger than the visible surface of the wound.
  - ✧ "Undermining" is the destruction of tissue or ulceration extending under the skin edges (margins) so that the pressure ulcer is larger at its base than at the skin surface. Undermining often develops from shearing forces and is differentiated from tunneling by the larger extent of the wound edge involved in undermining and the absence of a channel or tract extending from the pressure ulcer under the adjacent intact skin.

OVERVIEW

A pressure ulcer can occur wherever pressure has impaired circulation to the tissue. Critical steps in pressure ulcer prevention and healing include: identifying the individual resident at risk for developing pressure ulcers; identifying and evaluating the risk factors and changes in the resident's condition; identifying and evaluating factors that can be removed or modified; implementing individualized interventions to attempt to stabilize, reduce, or remove underlying risk factors; monitoring the impact of the interventions; and modifying the interventions as appropriate. It is important to recognize and evaluate each resident's risk factors and to identify and evaluate all areas at risk of constant pressure.

A complete assessment is essential to an effective pressure ulcer prevention and treatment program. A comprehensive individual evaluation helps the facility to:

- • Identify the resident at risk of developing pressure ulcers, the level and nature of risk(s); and
- • Identify the presence of pressure ulcers.

This information allows the facility to develop and implement a comprehensive care plan that reflects each resident's identified needs.

The care process should include efforts to stabilize, reduce, or remove underlying risk factors; to monitor the impact of the interventions; and to modify the interventions as appropriate.

The facility should have a system/procedure to assure: assessments are timely and appropriate; interventions are implemented, monitored, and revised as appropriate; and changes in condition are recognized, evaluated, reported to the practitioner, and addressed. The quality assessment and assurance committee may help the facility evaluate existing strategies to reduce the development and progression of pressure ulcers, monitor the incidence and prevalence of pressure ulcers within the facility, and ensure that facility policies and procedures are consistent with current standards of practice.

Research into appropriate practices for the prevention, management, and treatment of pressure ulcers, continues to evolve. As such, there are many recognized clinical resources regarding the prevention and management of pressure ulcers (including wound care and complications such as infections and pain). Some of these resources include:

- The Clinical Practice Guidelines from the Agency for Healthcare Research and Quality (AHRQ) www.ahrq.gov (Guideline No. 15: Treatment of Pressure Ulcers and Guideline No. 3: Pressure Ulcers in Adults: Prediction and Prevention) (AHRQ was previously known as the Agency for Health Care Policy and Research [AHCPR]);
- The National Pressure Ulcer Advisory Panel (NPUAP) www.npuap.org;
- The American Medical Directors Association (AMDA) www.amda.com (Clinical Practice Guidelines: Pressure Ulcers, 1996 and Pressure Ulcer Therapy Companion, 1999);
- The Quality Improvement Organizations, Medicare Quality Improvement Community Initiatives site at www.medqic.org;
- The Wound, Ostomy, and Continence Nurses Society (WOCN) www.wocn.org; and
- The American Geriatrics Society guideline "The Management of Persistent Pain in Older Persons", www.healthinaging.org.

NOTE: References to non-CMS sources or sites on the Internet are provided as a service and do not constitute or imply endorsement of these organizations or their programs by CMS or the U.S. Department of Health and Human Services. CMS is not responsible for the content of pages found at these sites. URL addresses were current as of the date of this publication.

PREVENTION OF PRESSURE ULCERS

42 CFR 483.25 (c) requires that a resident who is admitted without a pressure ulcer doesn't develop a pressure ulcer unless clinically unavoidable, and that a resident who has an ulcer receives care and services to promote healing and to prevent additional ulcers.

The first step in prevention is the identification of the resident at risk of developing pressure ulcers. This is followed by implementation of appropriate individualized interventions and monitoring for the effectiveness of the interventions.

ASSESSMENT

An admission evaluation helps identify the resident at risk of developing a pressure ulcer, and the resident with existing pressure ulcer(s) or areas of skin that are at risk for breakdown. Because a resident at risk can develop a pressure ulcer within 2 to 6 hours of the onset of pressure,[11] the at-risk resident needs to be identified and have interventions implemented promptly to attempt to prevent pressure ulcers. The admission evaluation helps define those initial care approaches.

In addition, the admission evaluation may identify pre-existing signs (such as a purple or very dark area that is surrounded by profound redness, edema, or induration)[12] suggesting that deep tissue damage has already occurred and additional deep tissue loss may occur.

This deep tissue damage could lead to the appearance of an unavoidable Stage III or IV pressure ulcer or progression of a Stage I pressure ulcer to an ulcer with eschar or exudate within days after admission. Some situations, which may have contributed to this tissue damage, include pressure resulting from immobility during hospitalization or surgical procedures, during prolonged ambulance transport, or while waiting to be discovered or assisted after a debilitating event, such as a fall or a cerebral vascular accident.

Some evidence suggests that because it may be harder to identify erythema in an older adult with darkly pigmented skin, older individuals with darkly pigmented skin may be more at risk for developing pressure ulcers.[13-16] It may be necessary, therefore, in a darker skinned individual to focus more on other evidence of pressure ulcer development, such as bogginess, induration, coolness, or increased warmth, as well as signs of skin discoloration.

Multiple factors, including pressure intensity, pressure duration, and tissue tolerance, significantly affect the potential for the development and healing of pressure ulcers. An individual may also have various intrinsic risks due to aging, for example: decreased subcutaneous tissue and lean muscle mass, decreased skin elasticity, and impaired circulation or innervation.

The comprehensive assessment, which includes the Resident Assessment Instrument (RAI), evaluates the resident's intrinsic risks, the resident's skin condition, other factors (including causal factors) which place the resident at risk for developing pressure ulcers and/or experiencing delayed healing, and the nature of the pressure to which the resident may be subjected. The assessment should identify which risk factors can be removed or modified.

The assessment also helps identify the resident who has multi-system organ failure or an end-of-life condition or who is refusing care and treatment. If the resident is refusing care, an evaluation of the basis for the refusal, and the identification and evaluation of potential alternatives is indicated.

This comprehensive assessment should address those factors that have been identified as having an impact on the development, treatment, and/or healing of pressure ulcers, including, at a minimum: risk factors, pressure points, under-nutrition and hydration deficits, and moisture and the impact of moisture on skin. Each of these factors is discussed in additional detail in the following sections.

Risk Factors

Many studies and professional documents identify risk factors that increase a resident's susceptibility to develop or to not heal pressure ulcers.[17-19] Examples of these risk factors include, but are not limited to:

- Impaired/decreased mobility and decreased functional ability;
- Co-morbid conditions, such as end stage renal disease, thyroid disease, or diabetes mellitus;
- Drugs such as steroids that may affect wound healing;
- Impaired diffuse or localized blood flow, for example, generalized atherosclerosis or lower extremity arterial insufficiency;
- Resident refusal of some aspects of care and treatment;
- Cognitive impairment;
- Exposure of skin to urinary and fecal incontinence;
- Under-nutrition, malnutrition, and hydration deficits; and
- A healed ulcer. The history of a healed pressure ulcer and its stage [if known] is important, since areas of healed Stage III or IV pressure ulcers are more likely to have recurrent breakdown.

Some residents have many risk factors for developing pressure ulcers, such as diabetic neuropathy, frailty, cognitive impairment, and under-nutrition. Not all factors are fully modifiable and some potentially modifiable factors (e.g., under-nutrition) may not be corrected immediately, despite prompt intervention, while other factors such as pressure may be modified promptly. It may be necessary to stabilize, when possible, the underlying causes (e.g., control blood sugars or ensure adequate food and fluid intake).

Although the requirements do not mandate any specific assessment tool, other than the RAI, validated instruments are available to assess risk for developing pressure ulcers. Research has shown that a significant number of pressure ulcers develop within the first four weeks after admission to a long-term care facility.[20] Therefore, many clinicians recommend using a standardized pressure ulcer risk assessment tool to assess a resident's pressure ulcer risks upon admission, weekly for the first four weeks after admission for each resident at risk, then quarterly, or whenever there is a change in cognition or functional ability.[21, 22] A resident's risk may increase due to an acute illness or condition change (e.g., upper respiratory infection, pneumonia, or exacerbation of underlying congestive heart failure) and may require additional evaluation.

Regardless of any resident's total risk score, the clinicians responsible for the resident's care should review each risk factor and potential cause(s) individually[23] to: a) Identify those that increase the potential for the resident to develop pressure ulcers; b) Decide whether and to what extent the factor(s) can be modified, stabilized, removed, etc., and c) Determine whether targeted management protocols need to be implemented. In other words, an overall risk score indicating the resident is not at high risk of developing pressure ulcers does not mean that existing risk factors or causes should be considered less important or addressed less vigorously than those factors or causes in the resident whose overall score indicates he or she is at a higher risk of developing a pressure ulcer.

Pressure Points and Tissue Tolerance

Assessment of a resident's skin condition helps define prevention strategies. The skin assessment should include an evaluation of the skin integrity and tissue tolerance (ability of the skin and its supporting structures to endure the effects of pressure without adverse effects) after pressure to that area has been reduced or redistributed.

Tissue closest to the bone may be the first tissue to undergo necrosis. Pressure ulcers are usually located over a bony prominence, such as the sacrum, heel, the greater trochanter, ischial tuberosity, fibular head, scapula, and ankle (malleolus).

An at-risk resident who sits too long on a static surface may be more prone to get ischial ulceration. Slouching in a chair may predispose an at-risk resident to pressure ulcers of the spine, scapula, or elbow (elbow ulceration is often related to arm rests or lap boards). Friction and shearing are also important factors in tissue ischemia, necrosis, and pressure ulcer formation.

Pressure ulcers may develop at other sites where pressure has impaired the circulation to the tissue, such as pressure from positioning or use of medical devices. For example, pressure ulcers may develop from pressure on an earlobe related to positioning of the head; pressure or friction on areas (e.g., nares, urinary meatus, extremities) caused by tubes, casts, orthoses, braces, cervical collars, or other medical devices; pressure on the labia or scrotum related to positioning (e.g., against a pommel type cushion); pressure on the foot related to ill-fitting shoes causing blistering; or pressure on legs, arms, and fingers due to contractures or deformity resulting from rheumatoid arthritis, etc.

While pressure ulcers on the sacrum remain the most common location, pressure ulcers on the heel are occurring more frequently,[24] are difficult to assess and heal, and require early identification of skin compromise over the heel.

It is, therefore, important for clinical staff to regularly conduct thorough skin assessments on each resident who is at risk for developing pressure ulcers.

Under-Nutrition and Hydration Deficits

Adequate nutrition and hydration are essential for overall functioning. Nutrition provides vital energy and building blocks for all of the body's structures and processes. Any organ or body system may require additional energy or structural materials for repair or function. The skin is the body's largest organ system. It may affect, and be affected by, other body processes and organs. Skin condition reflects overall body function; skin breakdown may be the most visible evidence of a general catabolic state.

Weight reflects a balance between intake and utilization of energy. Significant unintended weight loss may indicate under-nutrition or worsening health status. Weight stability (in the absence of fluid excess or loss) is a useful indicator of overall caloric balance. Severely impaired organs (heart, lungs, kidneys, liver, etc.) may be unable to use nutrients effectively. A resident with a pressure ulcer who continues to lose weight either needs additional caloric intake or correction (where possible) of conditions that are creating a hypermetabolic state. Continuing weight loss and failure of a pressure ulcer to heal despite reasonable efforts to improve caloric and nutrient intake may indicate the resident is in multi-system failure or an end-stage or end-of-life condition warranting an additional assessment of the resident's overall condition.

Before instituting a nutritional care plan, it helps to summarize resident specific evidence, including: severity of nutritional compromise, rate of weight loss or appetite decline, probable causes, the individual's prognosis and projected clinical course, and the resident's wishes and goals. Because there are no wound-specific nutritional measures, the interdisciplinary team should develop nutritional goals for the whole person. Unless contraindicated, nutritional goals for a resident with nutritional compromise who has a pressure ulcer or is at risk of developing pressure ulcers should include protein intake of approximately 1.2–1.5 gm/kg body weight daily (higher end of the range for those with larger, more extensive, or multiple wounds). A simple multivitamin is appropriate, but unless the resident has a specific vitamin or mineral deficiency, supplementation with additional vitamins or minerals may not be indicated.

NOTE: Although some laboratory tests may help clinicians evaluate nutritional issues in a resident with pressure ulcers, no laboratory test is specific or sensitive enough to warrant serial/repeated testing. Serum albumin, pre-albumin and cholesterol may be useful to help establish overall prognosis; however, they may not correlate well with clinical observation of nutritional status.[25, 26] At his or her discretion, a practitioner may order test(s) that provide useful additional information or help with management of treatable conditions.

Water is essential to maintain adequate body functions. As a major component of blood, water dissolves vitamins, minerals, glucose, amino acids, etc.; transports nutrients into cells; removes waste from the cells; and helps maintain circulating blood volume as well as fluid and electrolyte balance. It is critical that each resident at risk for hydration deficit or imbalance, including the resident with a pressure ulcer or at risk of developing an ulcer, be identified and that hydration needs be addressed.

(The surveyor should refer to the Guidance at 42 CFR 483.25 (i), F325, Nutrition, and 483.25(j), F327 Hydration for investigation of potential non-compliance with the nutrition and hydration requirements. A low albumin level combined with the facility's lack of supplementation, for example, is not sufficient to cite a pressure ulcer deficiency.)

Moisture and Its Impact

Both urine and feces contain substances that may irritate the epidermis and may make the skin more susceptible to breakdown. Some studies have found that fecal incontinence may pose a greater threat to skin integrity,[27] most likely due to bile acids and enzymes in the feces. Irritation or maceration resulting from prolonged exposure to urine and feces may hasten skin breakdown, and moisture may make skin more susceptible to damage from friction and shear during repositioning.

It may be difficult to differentiate dermatitis related to incontinence from partial thickness skin loss (pressure ulcer). This differentiation should be based on the clinical evidence and review of presenting risk factors. A Stage I pressure ulcer usually presents as a localized area of erythema or skin discoloration, while perineal dermatitis may appear as a more diffuse area of erythema or discoloration where the urine or stool has come into contact with the skin. The dermatitis may occur in the area where the incontinence brief or underpad has been used. Also, the dermatitis/rash more typically presents as intense erythema, scaling, itching, papules, weeping, and eruptions.[28]

INTERVENTIONS

The comprehensive assessment should provide the basis for defining approaches to address residents at risk of developing or already having a pressure ulcer. A determination that a resident is at high risk to develop a pressure ulcer has significant implications for preventive and treatment strategies, but does not by itself indicate that development of a pressure ulcer was unavoidable. Effective prevention and treatment are based upon consistently providing routine and individualized interventions.

In the context of the resident's choices, clinical condition, and physician input, the resident's plan of care should establish relevant goals and approaches to stabilize or improve co-morbidities, such as attempts to minimize clinically significant blood sugar fluctuations and other interventions aimed at limiting the effects of risk factors associated with pressure ulcers. Alternatively, facility staff and practitioners should document clinically valid reasons why such interventions were not appropriate or feasible. Repeated hospitalizations or emergency room visits within a 6-month period may indicate overall decline or instability.

Resident Choice

In order for a resident to exercise his or her right appropriately to make informed choices about care and treatment or to refuse treatment, the facility and the resident (or the resident's legal representative) must discuss the resident's condition, treatment options, expected outcomes, and consequences of refusing treatment. The facility is expected to address the resident's concerns and offer relevant alternatives, if the resident has refused specific treatments. (See Resident Rights at 42 CFR 483.10(b)(3) and (4), F154, and F155.)

Advance Directive

A resident at the end of life, in terminal stages of an illness or having multiple system failures may have written directions for his or her treatment goals (or a decision has been made by the resident's surrogate or representative, in accordance with state law).

If a resident has a valid Advance Directive, the facility's care must reflect a resident's wishes as expressed in the Directive, in accordance with state law. However, the presence of an Advance Directive does not absolve the facility from giving supportive and other pertinent care that is not prohibited by the Advance Directive. If the facility has implemented individualized approaches for end-of-life care in accordance with the resident's wishes, and has implemented appropriate efforts to try to stabilize the resident's condition (or indicated why the condition cannot or should not be stabilized) and to provide care to prevent or treat the pressure ulcer (including pertinent, routine, lesser aggressive approaches, such as, cleaning, turning, repositioning), then the development, continuation, or progression of a pressure ulcer may be consistent with regulatory requirements.

NOTE: The presence of a "Do Not Resuscitate" (DNR) order is not sufficient to indicate the resident is declining other appropriate treatment and services. It only indicates that the resident should not be resuscitated if respirations and/or cardiac function cease.

Based upon the assessment and the resident's clinical condition, choices, and identified needs, basic or routine care should include interventions to: a) Redistribute pressure (such as repositioning, protecting heels, etc); b) Minimize exposure to moisture and keep skin clean, especially of fecal contamination; c) Provide appropriate, pressure-redistributing, support surfaces; d) Provide non-irritating surfaces; and e) Maintain or improve nutrition and hydration status, where feasible. Adverse drug reactions related to the resident's drug regimen may worsen risk factors for development of pressure ulcers or for non-healing pressure ulcers (for example, by causing lethargy or anorexia or creating/increasing confusion) and should be identified and addressed. These interventions should be incorporated into the plan of care and revised as the condition of the resident indicates.

Repositioning

Repositioning is a common, effective intervention for an individual with a pressure ulcer or who is at risk of developing one.[29, 30] Assessment of a resident's skin integrity after pressure has been reduced or redistributed should guide the development and implementation of repositioning plans. Such plans should be addressed in the comprehensive plan of care consistent with the resident's need and goals. Repositioning is critical for a resident who is immobile or dependent upon staff for repositioning. The care plan for a resident at risk of friction or shearing during repositioning may require the use of lifting devices for repositioning. Positioning the resident on an existing pressure ulcer should be avoided since it puts additional pressure on tissue that is already compromised and may impede healing.

Surveyors should consider the following repositioning issues:

- A resident who can change positions independently may need supportive devices to facilitate position changes. The resident also may need instruction about why repositioning is important and how to do it, encouragement to change positions regularly, and monitoring of frequency of repositioning.
- The care plan for a resident who is reclining and is dependent on staff for repositioning should address position changes to maintain the resident's skin integrity. This may include repositioning at least every 2 hours or more frequently depending upon the resident's condition and tolerance of the tissue load (pressure). Depending on the individualized assessment, more frequent repositioning may be warranted for individuals who are at higher risk for pressure ulcer development or who show evidence (e.g., Stage I pressure ulcers) that repositioning at 2-hour intervals is inadequate. With rare exception (e.g., both sacral and ischial pressure ulcers are present) the resident should not be placed directly on the greater trochanter for more than momentary placement. Elevating the head of the bed or the back of a reclining chair to or above a 30 degree angle creates pressure comparable to that exerted while sitting, and requires the same considerations regarding repositioning as those for a dependent resident who is seated.
- Many clinicians recommend a position change "off loading" hourly for dependent residents who are sitting or who are in a bed or a reclining chair with the head of the bed or back of the chair raised 30 degrees or more.[31] Based upon an assessment including evidence of tissue tolerance while sitting (checking for Stage I ulcers as noted above), the res-

ident may not tolerate sitting in a chair in the same position for 1 hour at a time and may require a more frequent position change.

- Postural alignment, weight distribution, sitting balance and stability, and pressure redistribution should all be considered when positioning a resident in a chair.[32] A teachable resident should be taught to shift his/her weight approximately every 15 minutes while sitting in a chair.
- Wheelchairs are often used for transporting residents, but they may severely limit repositioning options and increase the risk of pressure ulcer development. Therefore, wheelchairs with sling seats may not be optimal for prolonged sitting during activities or meals, etc. However, available modifications to the seating can provide a more stable surface and provide better pressure reduction.
- There isn't evidence that momentary pressure relief followed by return to the same position (that is a "microshift" of five or 10 degrees or a 10–15 second lift from a seated position) is beneficial. This approach does not allow sufficient capillary refill and tissue perfusion for a resident at risk of developing pressure ulcers. Ongoing monitoring of the resident's skin integrity and tissue tolerance is critical to prevent development or deterioration of pressure ulcers.

Support Surfaces and Pressure Redistribution

Pressure redistribution refers to the function or ability to distribute a load over a surface or contact area. Redistribution results in shifting pressure from one area to another and requires attention to all affected areas. Pressure redistribution has incorporated the concepts of both pressure reduction (reduction of interface pressure, not necessarily below capillary closure pressure) and pressure relief (reduction of interface pressure below capillary closure pressure).

Appropriate support surfaces or devices should be chosen by matching a device's potential therapeutic benefit with the resident's specific situation; for example, multiple ulcers, limited turning surfaces, ability to maintain position. The effectiveness of pressure redistribution devices (e.g., 4-inch convoluted foam pads, gels, air fluidized mattresses, and low loss air mattresses) is based on their potential to address the individual resident's risk, the resident's response to the product, and the characteristics and condition of the product. For example, an overinflated overlay product, or one that "bottoms out" (completely compressing the overlay, when, for example, the caregiver can feel less than one inch between the resident and support material) is unlikely to effectively reduce the pressure risk. These products are more likely to reduce pressure effectively if they are used in accord with the manufacturer's instructions. The effectiveness of each product used needs to be evaluated on an ongoing basis. Surveyors should consider the following pressure redistribution issues:

- Static pressure redistribution devices (e.g., solid foam, convoluted foam, gel mattress) may be indicated when a resident is at risk for pressure ulcer development or delayed healing. A specialized pressure redistribution cushion or surface, for example, might be used to extend the time a resident is sitting in a chair; however, the cushion does not eliminate the necessity for periodic repositioning.
- Dynamic pressure reduction surfaces may be helpful when: 1) The resident cannot assume a variety of positions without bearing weight on a pressure ulcer, 2) The resident com-

pletely compresses a static device that has retained its original integrity, or 3) The pressure ulcer is not healing as expected, and it is determined that pressure may be contributing to the delay in healing.

- Because the heels and elbows have relatively little surface area, it is difficult to redistribute pressure on these two surfaces. Therefore, it is important to pay particular attention to reducing the pressure on these areas for the resident at risk in accord with resident's overall goals and condition. Pillows used to support the entire lower leg may effectively raise the heel from contact with the bed, but use of the pillows needs to take into account the resident's other conditions. The use of donut-type cushions is not recommended by the clinicians.
- A resident with severe flexion contractures also may require special attention to effectively reduce pressure on bony prominences or prevent breakdown from skin-to-skin contact.

Some products serve mainly to provide comfort and reduce friction and shearing forces, e.g., sheepskin, heel and elbow protectors. Although these products are not effective at redistributing pressure, they (in addition to pillows, foam wedges, or other measures) may be employed to prevent bony prominences from rubbing together.

MONITORING

At least daily, staff should remain alert to potential changes in the skin condition and should evaluate and document identified changes. For example, a resident's complaint about pain or burning at a site where there has been pressure or a nursing assistant's observation during the resident's bath that there is a change in skin condition should be reported so that the resident may be evaluated further.

After completing a thorough evaluation, the interdisciplinary team should develop a relevant care plan to include prevention and management interventions with measurable goals. Many clinicians recommend evaluating skin condition (e.g., skin color, moisture, temperature, integrity, and turgor) at least weekly, or more often if indicated, such as when the resident is using a medical device that may cause pressure.

The resident should be monitored for condition changes that might increase the risk for breakdown and the defined interventions should be implemented and monitored for effectiveness.

ASSESSMENT AND TREATMENT OF PRESSURE ULCER(S)

It is important that each existing pressure ulcer be identified, whether present on admission or developed after admission, and that factors that influenced its development, the potential for development of additional ulcers or for the deterioration of the pressure ulcer(s) be recognized, assessed, and addressed (see discussion under Prevention regarding overall assessment and interventions). Any new pressure ulcer suggests a need to reevaluate the adequacy of the plan for preventing pressure ulcers.

When assessing the ulcer itself, it is important to:

- Differentiate the type of ulcer (pressure-related versus non-pressure-related) because interventions may vary depending on the specific type of ulcer;

- Determine the ulcer's stage;
- Describe and monitor the ulcer's characteristics;
- Monitor the progress toward healing and for potential complications;
- Determine if infection is present;
- Assess, treat, and monitor pain, if present; and
- Monitor dressings and treatments.

TYPES OF ULCERS

Three of the more common types of ulcers are pressure, vascular insufficiency/ischemia (venous stasis and arterial ischemic ulcers), and neuropathic. See Guidance to Surveyors at 42 CFR 483.25 (F309) for definition and description of ulcer types other than pressure ulcers.

At the time of the assessment, clinicians (physicians, advance practice nurses, physician assistants, and certified wound care specialists, etc.) should document the clinical basis (for example, type of skin injury/ulcer, location, shape, ulcer edges and wound bed, condition of surrounding tissues) for any determination that an ulcer is not pressure-related, especially if the injury/ulcer has characteristics consistent with a pressure ulcer, but is determined not to be one.

ULCER CHARACTERISTICS

It is important that the facility have a system in place to assure that the protocols for daily monitoring and for periodic documentation of measurements, terminology, frequency of assessment, and documentation are implemented consistently throughout the facility.

When a pressure ulcer is present, daily monitoring, (with accompanying documentation, when a complication or change is identified), should include:

- An evaluation of the ulcer, if no dressing is present;
- An evaluation of the status of the dressing, if present (whether it is intact and whether drainage, if present, is or is not leaking);
- The status of the area surrounding the ulcer (that can be observed without removing the dressing);
- The presence of possible complications, such as signs of increasing area of ulceration or soft tissue infection (for example: increased redness or swelling around the wound or increased drainage from the wound); and
- Whether pain, if present, is being adequately controlled.

The amount of observation possible will depend upon the type of dressing that is used, since some dressings are meant to remain in place for several days, according to manufacturers' guidelines.

With each dressing change or at least weekly (and more often when indicated by wound complications or changes in wound characteristics), an evaluation of the pressure ulcer wound should be documented. At a minimum, documentation should include the date observed and:

- Location and staging;
- Size (perpendicular measurements of the greatest extent of length and width of the ulceration); depth; and the presence, location, and extent of any undermining or tunneling/sinus tract;
- Exudate, if present: type (such as purulent/serous), color, odor, and approximate amount;
- Pain, if present: nature and frequency (e.g., whether episodic or continuous);
- Wound bed: Color and type of tissue/character including evidence of healing (e.g., granulation tissue), or necrosis (slough or eschar); and
- Description of wound edges and surrounding tissue (e.g., rolled edges, redness, hardness/induration, maceration) as appropriate.

Photographs may be used to support this documentation, if the facility has developed a protocol consistent with accepted standards[33] (e.g., frequency, consistent distance from the wound, type of equipment used, means to assure digital images are accurate and not modified, inclusion of the resident identification/ulcer location/dates/etc. within the photographic image, and parameters for comparison).

STAGES OF PRESSURE ULCERS

The staging system is one method of summarizing certain characteristics of pressure ulcers, including the extent of tissue damage. This is the system used within the RAI.

Stage I pressure ulcers may be difficult to identify because they are not readily visible and they present with greater variability. Advanced technology (not commonly available in nursing homes) has shown that a Stage I pressure ulcer may have minimal to substantial tissue damage in layers beneath the skin's surface, even when there is no visible surface penetration. The Stage I indicators identified below will generally persist or be evident after the pressure on the area has been removed for 30–45 minutes.

The definitions for the stages of pressure ulcers identified below, are from the NPUAP and used with permission.[34]

- "Stage I" — An observable, pressure-related alteration of intact skin, whose indicators as compared to an adjacent or opposite area on the body may include changes in one or more of the following parameters:

  - ✧ Skin temperature (warmth or coolness);
  - ✧ Tissue consistency (firm or boggy);
  - ✧ Sensation (pain, itching); and/or
  - ✧ A defined area of persistent redness in lightly pigmented skin, whereas in darker skin tones, the ulcer may appear with persistent red, blue, or purple hues.

- "Stage II" — Partial thickness skin loss involving epidermis, dermis, or both. The ulcer is superficial and presents clinically as an abrasion, blister, or shallow crater.
- "Stage III" — Full thickness skin loss involving damage to, or necrosis of, subcutaneous tissue that may extend down to, but not through, underlying fascia. The ulcer presents clinically as a deep crater with or without undermining of adjacent tissue.

- "Stage IV" — Full thickness skin loss with extensive destruction, tissue necrosis, or damage to muscle, bone, or supporting structures (e.g., tendon, joint capsule). Undermining and sinus tracts also may be associated with Stage IV pressure ulcers.

NOTE: If eschar and necrotic tissue are covering and preventing adequate staging of a pressure ulcer, the RAI User's Manual Version 2 instructs the assessor to code the pressure ulcer as a Stage IV. These instructions must be followed for MDS coding purposes until they are revised. Although the AHCPR and NPUAP system for staging pressure ulcers indicates that the presence of eschar precludes accurate staging of the ulcer, the facility must use the RAI directions in order to code the MDS, but not necessarily to render treatment.

THE HEALING PRESSURE ULCER

Ongoing evaluation and research have indicated that pressure ulcers do not heal in a reverse sequence, that is, the body does not replace the types and layers of tissue (e.g., muscle, fat and dermis) that were lost during the pressure ulcer development.

There are different types of clinical documentation to describe the progression of the healing pressure ulcer(s). The regulation at 42 CFR 483.20(b)(1), F272, requires that facilities use the Resident Assessment Instrument (RAI), which includes direction to describe the healing of the pressure ulcer(s) for coding purposes for the MDS: The RAI User's Manual Version 2.0, instructs staff to identify the stages of pressure ulcer(s) by describing depth in reverse order from deepest to lesser stages to describe the healing or improvement of a pressure ulcer (e.g., a Stage IV becomes a Stage III and so forth). This has been referred to as "reverse staging" or "back staging."

Some clinicians utilize validated instruments to describe the healing of a pressure ulcer. Although such instruments are appropriate for making treatment decisions, they may not be utilized for coding the MDS. Until the MDS is revised, the present coding system (reverse staging) must be used for completion of the RAI.

Clinicians may use the National Pressure Ulcer Advisory Panel — Pressure Ulcer Scale for Healing (NPUAP-PUSH) tool. The NPUAP always refers to a healed pressure ulcer as a healed ulcer at the deepest stage of its development (e.g., a healed Stage IV or a healing Stage IV). The NPUAP cautions that the tool does not represent a comprehensive pressure ulcer assessment, and other factors may need to be considered when selecting pressure ulcer treatment options.

Since surveyors may encounter clinician's notes in which the NPUAP-PUSH tool is used as part of the facility's documentation protocol, the following description of the tool is provided. The NPUAP-PUSH tool documents pressure ulcer healing consistent with the healing process, describes a healing pressure ulcer in terms of three ulcer characteristics, and assigns a numeric value to the characteristics: length (cm) × width (cm), exudate amount, and type of tissue (closed with epithelium; new pink, shiny epithelial tissue; clean, pink or beefy red, shiny, moist granulation tissue; slough tissue; or necrotic, eschar tissue).

The 1994 AHCPR Guidelines and current literature[35] indicate that a clean pressure ulcer with adequate blood supply and innervation should show evidence of stabilization or some healing within 2–4 weeks. Evidence accumulating since 1962 indicates that management of wound exudate coupled with a clean, moist wound environment allows a chronic wound (e.g., pressure ulcer) to lay down healthy granulating tissue more efficiently.[36, 37]

If a pressure ulcer fails to show some evidence of progress toward healing within 2–4 weeks, the pressure ulcer (including potential complications) and the resident's overall clinical condition should be reassessed. Re-evaluation of the treatment plan including determining whether to continue or modify the current interventions is also indicated. Results may vary depending on the resident's condition and interventions/treatments used. The complexity of the resident's condition may limit responsiveness to treatment or tolerance for certain treatment modalities. The clinicians, if deciding to retain the current regimen, should document the rationale for continuing the present treatment (for example, why some, or all, of the plan's interventions remain relevant despite little or no apparent healing).

Pressure ulcers may progress or may be associated with complications such as infection of the soft tissues around the wound (cellulitis), infection of the bone (osteomyelitis), infection of a joint (septic arthritis), abscess, spread of bacteria into the bloodstream (bacteremia/septicemia), chronic infection, or development of a sinus tract. Sometimes these complications may occur despite apparent improvement in the pressure ulcer itself. The physician's involvement is integral whenever significant changes in the nature of the wound or overall resident condition are identified.

INFECTIONS RELATED TO PRESSURE ULCERS

Current literature reports that all Stage II, III, and IV pressure ulcers are colonized with bacteria but may not be infected. Identification, diagnosis, and treatment of infection, when present, are critical to healing a pressure ulcer.[38] The infection occurs when the bacteria have invaded the tissue surrounding or within the pressure ulcer.

As with any infection, classic signs and symptoms of infection may include purulent exudate, peri-wound warmth, swelling, induration or erythema (erythema may not be readily determined in individuals with dark skin pigmentation), increasing pain or tenderness around the site, or delayed wound healing. These classic signs may not be as evident in someone with a granulating, chronic wound or an immuno-compromised or aged resident. Some infections may present primarily with pain or delayed healing without other typical clinical signs of infection.[39] Clinicians have developed some tools, which may facilitate identifying and assessing an infection[40, 41] and documenting progress toward healing.

Wounds may be classified as infected if the signs and symptoms of infection are present and/or a wound culture (obtained in accord with accepted standards, such as sterile tissue aspirate, a "quantitative surface swab" using the Levine technique or semi-quantitative swab) contains 100,000 (10^5) or greater micro-organisms per gram of tissue. A superficial swab may show the presence of bacteria, but is not a reliable method to identify infection.

Findings such as an elevated white blood cell count, bacteremia, sepsis, or fever may signal an infection related to a pressure ulcer area or a co-existing infection from a different source.

PAIN

The assessment and treatment of a resident's pain are integral components of pressure ulcer prevention and management. "The goal of pain management in the pressure ulcer patient is to eliminate the cause of pain, to provide analgesia, or both."[42] Pain that interferes with movement and/or affects mood may contribute to immobility and contribute to the potential for developing a pressure ulcer or for delayed healing or non-healing of an already existing ulcer.

It may be difficult to assess the degree of pain in a resident who is cognitively impaired. Some strategies and tools exist to help determine the presence and characteristics of pain (e.g., nature, intensity, and frequency).[43, 44] Recent research suggests that a resident with a Stage IV pressure ulcer can feel as much pain as those with a Stage I or II ulcer.[45] The relationship of pain to the pressure ulcer healing process is not yet clear. Pain is an individual perception and response and an individual's report of pain is a generally valid indicator of pain. One resident may experience pain of varying intensity and frequency (e.g., continually or periodically) or episodically in association with treatments (e.g., debridement, dressing changes) or movement or infection, while another resident may not have or report pain.

DRESSINGS AND TREATMENTS

Research has found that chronic wounds such as pressure ulcers heal differently from acute wounds, primarily because of differing biochemical and cellular characteristics. Current clinical practice indicates that Stage III and Stage IV ulcers should be covered. Determination of the need for a dressing for a Stage I or Stage II ulcer is based upon the individual practitioner's clinical judgment and facility protocols based upon current clinical standards of practice. No particular dressing promotes healing of all pressure ulcers within an ulcer classification.[46]

For those pressure ulcers with significant exudate, management of the exudate is critical for healing. A balance is needed to assure that the wound is moist enough to support healing but not too moist to interfere with healing.[47] Since excess wound exudate generally impairs wound healing, selecting an appropriate absorptive dressing is an important part of managing chronic wound exudate.

Product selection should be based upon the relevance of the specific product to the identified pressure ulcer(s) characteristics, the treatment goals, and the manufacturer's recommendations for use. Current literature does not indicate significant advantages of any single specific product over another, but does confirm that not all products are appropriate for all pressure ulcers. Wound characteristics should be assessed throughout the healing process to assure that the treatments and dressings being used are appropriate to the nature of the wound.

Present literature suggests that pressure ulcer dressing protocols may use clean technique rather than sterile, but that appropriate sterile technique may be needed for those wounds that recently have been surgically debrided or repaired.[48]

Debridement of non-viable tissue is frequently performed to reduce the amount of wound debris or non-viable tissue and to reduce the risk of sepsis. A variety of debridement methods (e.g., mechanical, sharp or surgical, enzymatic, autolytic, MDT) are available. Removal of necrotic tissue should enhance wound healing. Ongoing monitoring (and timely intervention in case of change in the character of the wound) is critical for areas with eschar and those areas that have been debrided.[49] Many clinicians believe that stable, dry, adherent, and intact eschar on the foot/heel should not be debrided, unless signs and symptoms of local infection or instability are detected.[50]

Some facilities may use "wet to dry gauze dressings" or irrigation with chemical solutions to remove slough. The use of wet-to-dry dressings or irrigations may be appropriate in limited circumstances, but repeated use may damage healthy granulation tissue in healing ulcers and may lead to excessive bleeding and increased resident pain.

A facility should be able to show that its treatment protocols are based upon current standards of practice and are in accord with the facility's policies and procedures as developed with the medical director's review and approval.

ENDNOTES

(For more information on the references below, visit the CMS Sharing Innovations in Quality website: www.cms.hhs.gov/medicaid/survey-cert/siqhome.asp)

1. Cuddigan, J., Ayello, E.A., Sussman, C., & Baranoski, S. (Eds.). (2001). Pressure Ulcers in America: Prevalence, Incidence, and Implications for the Future. National Pressure Ulcer Advisory Panel Monograph (pp. 181). Reston, VA: NPUAP.

2. Gardner, S.E. & Frantz, R.A. (2003). Wound Bioburden. In Baranoski, S. & Ayello, E.A. (Eds.), Wound Care Essentials: Practice Principles. Philadelphia, PA: Lippincott, Williams, & Wilkins.

3. Ayello, E.A. & Cuddigan, J.E. (2004). Debridement: Controlling the Necrotic/Cellular Burden. Advances in Skin and Wound Care, 17(2), 66–75.

4. Bergstrom, N., Bennett, M.A., Carlson, C.E., et al. (1994). Treatment of Pressure Ulcers in Adults (Publication 95-0652). Clinical Practice Guideline, 15, Rockville, MD: U.S. Department of Health and Human Services, Agency for Health Care Policy and Research.

5. Thompson, P.D. & Smith, D.J. (1994). What is Infection? American Journal of Surgery, 167, 7–11.

6. Ayello, E.A., Baranoski, S., Kerstein, M.D., & Cuddigan, J. (2003). Wound Debridement. In Baranoski. S. & Ayello, E.A. (Eds.) Wound Care Essentials: Practice Principles. Philadelphia, PA: Lippincott Williams & Wilkins.

7. Bergstrom, N., et al. (1994). Clinical Practice Guideline, 15.

8. Ayello & Cuddigan. (2004). Advances in Skin and Wound Care, 66–75.

9. Sherman, R.A. (1998). Maggot Debridement in Modem Medicine. Infections in Medicine, 15(9), 651–656.

10. Piper, B. (2000). Mechanical Forces: Pressure, Shear, and Friction. In Bryant, R.A. (Ed.) Acute and Chronic Wounds. Nursing Management (2nd ed., pp. 221–264). St. Louis, MO: Mosby.

11. Kosiak, M. (1961). Etiology of Decubitus Ulcers. Archives of Physical Medicine and Rehabilitation, 42, 19–29.

12. Frequently Asked Questions: Pressure Ulcer Staging and Assessment, Question 202 (2000, July 28). Retrieved July 1, 2004 from http://www.npuap.org/archive/stagingdefinition.htm.

13. Lyder, C., Yu, C., Emerling, J., Empleo-Frazier, O., Mangat, R., Stevenson, D. & McKay, J. (1999). Evaluating the Predictive Validity of the Braden Scale for Pressure Ulcer Risk in Blacks and Latino/Hispanic Elders. Applied Nursing Research, 12, 60–68.

14. Lyder, C. (2003). Pressure Ulcer Prevention and Management. Journal of the American Medical Association, 289, 223–226.

15. Fuhrer, M., Garber, S., Rintola, D., Clearman, R., Hart, K. (1993). Pressure Ulcers in Community-resident persons with spinal cord injury: Prevalence and Risk Factors. Archives of Physical Medicine Rehabilitation, 74, 1172–1177.

16. Cuddigan, Ayello, Sussman, & Baranoski S. (Eds.). (2001). NPUAP Monograph, 153.

17. Ayello, E.A., Braden, B. (May-June 2002). How and Why to do Pressure Ulcer Risk Assessment. Advances in Skin and Wound Care, 15(3), 125–32.

18. Bergstrom, N. & Braden, B.A. (1992). A Prospective Study of Pressure Sore Risk Among Institutionalized Elderly. Journal of the American Geriatric Society, 40(8), 747–758.

19. Gosnell, S.J. (1973). An Assessment Tool to Identify Pressure Sores. Nursing Research, 22(1), 55–59.

20. Bergstrom, N., Braden, B., Kemp, M., Champagne, M., Ruby, E. (1998). Predicting Pressure Ulcer Risk: A Multistate Study of the Predictive Validity of the Braden Scale. Nursing Research, 47(5), 261–269.

21. Bergstrom, N. & Braden, B.A. (1992). Journal of the American Geriatric Society, 747–758.

22. Braden, B. (2001). Risk Assessment in Pressure Ulcer Prevention. In Krasner, D.L., Rodeheaver, G.T., Sibbeald, R.G. (Eds.) Chronic Wound Care: A Clinical Source Book for Healthcare Professionals (3rd ed., pp. 641<nd.651). Wayne, PA: HMP Communications Pub.

23. Ayello, E.A., Baranoski, S., Lyder, C.H., Cuddigan, J. (2003). Pressure Ulcers. In Baranoski, S. & Ayello, E.A. (Eds.) Wound Care Essentials: Practice Principles (pp. 245). Philadelphia, PA: Lippincott Williams & Wilkins.

24. Cuddigan, J., Ayello, E.A., Sussman, C., & Baranoski, S. (Eds.). (2001). NPUAP Monograph, 27 & 168.

25. Ferguson, R., O'Connor, P., Crabtree, B., Batchelor, A., Mitchell, J., Coppola, D. (1993). Serum Albumin and Pre-albumin as Predictors of Hospitalized Elderly Nursing Home Patients. Journal of the American Geriatric Society, 41, 545–549.

26. Covinsky, K.E., Covinsky, K.H., Palmer, R.M., & Sehgal, A.R. (2002). Serum Albumin Concentration and Clinical Assessments of Nutritional Status in Hospitalized Older People: Different Sides of Different Coins? Journal of the American Geriatric Society, 50, 631–637.

27. Maklebust, J. & Sieggreen, M. (2001). Pressure Ulcers: Guidelines for Prevention and Management (3rd ed., pp. 49). Springhouse, PA: Springhouse.

28. Lyder, C. (1997). Perineal Dermatitis in the Elderly: A Critical Review of the Literature. Journal of Gerontological Nursing, 23(12), 5–10.

29. Bergstrom N., et al. (1994). Clinical Practice Guideline, 15.

30. Agency for Health Care Policy and Research (AHCPR). (1992). Pressure Ulcers in Adults: Prediction and Prevention (Publication 92-0050). Clinical Practice Guideline, 3.

31. Wound Ostomy Continence Nurses Society. (2003). Guidelines for Prevention and Management of Pressure Ulcers (pp. 12). Glenview, IL: Author.

32. Kloth, L.C. & McCulloch, J.M. (Eds.) (2002). Prevention and Treatment of Pressure Ulcer. Wound Healing: Alternatives in Management (3rd ed., pp. 434–438). Philadelphia: FA Davis Company.

33. Jones, V., Bale, S., & Harding, K. (2003). Acute and Chronic Wound Healing. In Baranoski, S. & Ayello, E.A. (Eds.), Wound Care Essentials: Practice Principles (pp. 72–73). Philadelphia, PA: Lippincott Williams & Wilkins.

34. Cuddigan, J., Ayello, E.A., Sussman, C., & Baranoski, S. (Eds.) (2001). NPUAP Monograph,181.

35. Morrison, M.J. (Ed.). (2001). The Prevention and Treatment of Pressure Ulcers. London: Mosby.

36. Bullen, E.C., Longaker, M.T., Updike, D.L., Benton, R., Ladin, D., Hou, Z., & Howard, E.W. (1996). Tissue inhibitor of metalloproteinases-1 is decreased and activated gelatinases are increased in chronic wounds. Journal of Investigative Dermatology, 106(2), 335–341.

37. Ayello, E.A. & Cuddigan, J. (2003). Jump start the healing process. Nursing Made Incredibly Easy! 1(2), 18–26.

38. Bergstrom N., et al. (1994). Clinical Practice Guideline, 15.

39. Gardner, S.E., Frantz, R.A., & Doebbeling, B.N. (2001). The Validity of the Clinical Signs and Symptoms Used to Identify Localized Chronic Wound Infection. Wound Repair and Regeneration, 9, 178–186.

40. Gardner, S.E. & Frantz, R.A. (2001). A Tool to Assess Clinical Signs and Symptoms of Localized Chronic Wound Infection: Development and Reliability. Ostomy/Wound Management, 47(1), 40–47.

41. Cutting, K.F. & Harding, K.G. (1994). Criteria for Identifying Wound Infection. Journal of Wound Care, 3(4), 198–201.

42. Bergstrom, N., et al. (1994). Clinical Practice Guideline, 15.

43. American Geriatric Society. (2002). American Geriatric Society Guideline: The Management of Persistent Pain in Older Persons. Journal of American Geriatric Society, 50(6), S205–S224.

44. Gomez, S., Osborn, C., Watkins, T. & Hegstrom, S. (2002). Caregivers team up to manage chronic pain. Provider, 28(4), 51–58.

45. Dallam, L.E., Barkauskas, C., Ayello, E.A., & Baranoski, S. (2003). Pain Management and Wounds. In Baranoski, S. & Ayello, E.A. (Eds.). Wound Care Essentials: Practice Principles (pp. 223–224). Philadelphia, PA: Lippincott Williams & Wilkins.

46. Ayello, E.A., Baranoski, S., Lyder, C.H., & Cuddigan, J. (2003). Pressure Ulcers. In Baranoski, S. & Ayello, E.A. Wound Care Essentials: Practice Principles (pp. 257). Philadelphia, PA: Lippincott Williams & Wilkins.

47. Schultz, G.S., Sibbald, R.G., Falanga, V., Ayello, E.A., Dowsett, C., Harding, K., Romanelli, M., Stacey, M.C., Teot, L., Vanscheidt, W. (2003). Wound Bed Preparation: A systematic Approach to Wound Management. Wound Repair Regeneration, 11, 1–28.

48. Association for Professionals in Infection Control and Epidemiology, Inc. (March/April 2001). Position Statement: Clean vs. Sterile: Management of Chronic Wounds. Retrieved July 6, 2004 from www.apic.org resource center.

49. Black, J.M., & Black, S.B. (2003). Complex Wounds. In Baranoski, S. & Ayello, E.A. (Eds.). Wound Care Essentials: Practice Principles (pp. 372). Philadelphia, PA: Lippincott Williams & Wilkins.

50. Bergstrom N., et al. (1994). Clinical Practice Guideline, 15.

INVESTIGATIVE PROTOCOL

PRESSURE ULCER

Objectives

- To determine if the identified pressure ulcer(s) is avoidable or unavoidable; and
- To determine the adequacy of the facility's interventions and efforts to prevent and treat pressure ulcers.

Use

Use this protocol for a sampled resident having—or at risk of developing—a pressure ulcer.

If the resident has an ulcer, determine if it was identified as non-pressure related, e.g., vascular insufficiency or a neuropathic ulcer. If record review, staff and/or physician interview, and observation (unless the dressing protocol precludes observing the wound) support the conclusion that the ulcer is not pressure related, do not proceed with this protocol unless the resident is at risk for developing, or also has, pressure ulcers. Evaluate care and services regarding non-pressure related ulcers at F309, Quality of Care.

Procedures

Briefly review the assessment, care plan, and orders to identify facility interventions and to guide observations to be made. For a newly admitted resident either at risk or with a pressure ulcer, the staff is expected to assess and provide appropriate care from the day of admission. Corroborate observations by interview and record review.

1. Observation

Observe whether staff consistently implements the care plan over time and across various shifts. During observations of the interventions, note and/or follow up on deviations from the care plan as well as potential negative outcomes, including but not limited to the following:

- Erythema or color changes on areas such as the sacrum, buttocks, trochanters, posterior thigh, popliteal area, or heels when moved off an area:

    ✧ If erythema or color change are noted, return approximately $1/2$–$3/4$ hours later to determine if the changes or other Stage I characteristics persist;
    ✧ If the changes persist and exhibit tenderness, hardness, or alteration in temperature from surrounding skin, ask staff how they determine repositioning schedules and how they evaluate and address a potential Stage I pressure ulcer;

- Previously unidentified open areas;
- Whether the positioning avoids pressure on an existing pressure ulcer(s);
- Measures taken to prevent or reduce the potential for shearing or friction during transfers, elevation, and repositioning; and
- Whether pressure-redistributing devices for the bed and/or chair, such as gel-type surfaces or overlays are in place, working, and used according to the manufacturer's recommendations.

Observation of Existing Ulcer/Wound Care

If a dressing change is scheduled during the survey, observe the wound care to determine if the record reflects the current status of the ulcer(s) and note:

- Characteristics of the wound and surrounding tissues such as presence of granulation tissue, the Stage, presence of exudates, necrotic tissue such as eschar or slough, or evidence of erythema or swelling around the wound;
- The form or type of debridement, if used;
- Whether treatment and infection control practices reflect current standards of practice; and
- Based on location, steps taken to cleanse and protect the wound from likely contamination by urine or fecal incontinence.

If unable to observe the dressing change due to the dressing protocol, observe the area surrounding the ulcer(s). For ulcers with dressings that are not scheduled to be changed, the surveyor may request that the dressing be removed to observe the wound and surrounding area if other information suggests a possible treatment or assessment problem.

If the resident expresses (or appears to be in) pain related to the ulcer or treatment, determine if the facility:

- Assessed for pain related to the ulcer, addressed and monitored interventions for effectiveness; and/or
- Assessed and took preemptive measures for pain related to dressing changes or other treatments, such as debridement/irrigations, and monitored for effectiveness.

2. Resident/Staff Interviews

Interview the resident, family, or responsible party to the degree possible to identify:

- Involvement in care plan, choices, goals, and if interventions reflect preferences;
- Awareness of approaches, such as pressure redistribution devices or equipment, turning/repositioning, weight shifting to prevent or address pressure ulcer(s);
- Presence of pain, if any, and how it is managed;
- If treatment(s) was refused, whether counseling on alternatives, consequences, and/or other interventions was offered; and
- Awareness of current or history of an ulcer(s). For the resident who has or has had a pressure ulcer, identify, as possible, whether acute illness, weight loss, or other condition changes occurred prior to developing the ulcer.

Interview staff on various shifts to determine:

- Knowledge of prevention and treatment, including facility-specific guidelines/protocols and specific interventions for the resident;
- If nursing assistants know what, when, and to whom to report changes in skin condition; and
- Who monitors for the implementation of the care plan, changes in the skin, the development of pressure ulcers, and the frequency of review and evaluation of an ulcer.

3. Record Review

Assessment

Review the RAI and other documents such as physician orders, progress notes, nurses' notes, pharmacy or dietary notes regarding the assessment of the resident's overall condition, risk factors, and presence of a pressure ulcer(s) to determine if the facility identified the resident at risk and evaluated the factors placing the resident at risk:

- For a resident who was admitted with an ulcer or who developed one within 1 to 2 days, review the admission documentation regarding the wound site and characteristics at the time of admission, the possibility of underlying tissue damage because of immobility or illness prior to admission, skin condition on or within a day of admission, history of impaired nutrition, and history of previous pressure ulcers; and
- For a resident who subsequently developed or has an existing pressure ulcer, review documentation regarding the wound site, characteristics, progress and complications including reassessment if there were no signs of progression towards healing within 2 to 4 weeks.

In considering the appropriateness of a facility's response to the presence, progression, or deterioration of a pressure ulcer, take into account the resident's condition, complications, time needed to determine the effectiveness of a treatment, and the facility's efforts, where possible, to remove, modify, or stabilize the risk factors and underlying causal factors.

Care Plan

For the resident at risk for developing or who has a pressure ulcer, determine if the facility developed an individualized care plan that addresses prevention, care, and treatment of any existing pressure ulcers, including specific interventions, measurable objectives, and approximate time frames.

If the facility's care of a specific resident refers to a treatment protocol that contains details of the treatment regimen, the care plan should refer to that protocol. The care plan should clarify any major deviations from, or revisions to, that protocol in a specific resident.

A specific care plan intervention for risk of pressure ulcers is not needed if other components of the care plan address related risks adequately. For example, the risk of skin breakdown posed by fecal/urinary incontinence might be addressed in that part of the care plan that deals with incontinence management.

If the resident refuses or resists staff interventions to reduce risk or treat existing pressure ulcers, determine if the care plan reflects efforts to seek alternatives to address the needs identified in the assessment.

Revision of the Care Plan

Determine if the staff have been monitoring the resident's response to interventions for prevention and/or treatment and have evaluated and revised the care plan based on the resident's response, outcomes, and needs. Review the record and interview staff for information and/or evidence that:

- Continuing the current approaches meets the resident's needs, if the resident has experienced recurring pressure ulcers or lack of progression toward healing and staff did not revise the care plan; and
- The care plan was revised to modify the prevention strategies and to address the presence and treatment of a newly developed pressure ulcer, for the resident who acquired a new ulcer.

4. Interviews with Health Care Practitioners and Professionals

If the interventions defined or care provided appear not to be consistent with recognized standards of practice, interview one or more health care practitioners and professionals as necessary (e.g., physician, charge nurse, director of nursing) who, by virtue of training and knowledge of the resident, should be able to provide information about the causes, treatment, and evaluation of the resident's condition or problem. Depending on the issue, ask about:

- How it was determined that chosen interventions were appropriate;
- Risks identified for which there were no interventions;
- Changes in condition that may justify additional or different interventions; or
- How they validated the effectiveness of current interventions.

If the attending physician is unavailable, interview the medical director, as appropriate.

DETERMINATION OF COMPLIANCE (Task 6, Appendix P)

Synopsis of Regulation (F314)

The pressure ulcer requirement has two aspects. The first aspect requires the facility to prevent the development of pressure ulcer(s) in a resident who is admitted without pressure ulcer(s), unless the development is clinically unavoidable. The second aspect requires the facility to provide necessary treatment and services to promote healing, prevent infection, and prevent new ulcers from developing. A facility may have non-compliance in either or both aspects of this requirement.

Criteria for Compliance

- Compliance with 42 CFR 483.25(c)(1), F314, Pressure Sore

  ◇ For a resident who developed a pressure ulcer after admission, the facility is in compliance with this requirement, if staff have:

  - Recognized and assessed factors placing the resident at risk for developing a pressure ulcer, including specific conditions, causes and/or problems, needs, and behaviors;
  - Defined and implemented interventions for pressure ulcer prevention in accordance with resident needs, goals, and recognized standards of practice;
  - Monitored and evaluated the resident's response to preventive efforts; and
  - Revised the approaches as appropriate.

If not, the development of the pressure ulcer is avoidable, cite at F314.

- Compliance with 42 CFR 483.25(c)(2), F314, Pressure Sore

  ✧ For a resident who was admitted with a pressure ulcer, who has a pressure ulcer that is not healing, or who is at risk of developing subsequent pressure ulcers, the facility is in compliance with this requirement if they:

    - Recognized and assessed factors placing the resident at risk of developing a new pressure ulcer or experiencing non-healing or delayed healing of a current pressure ulcer, including specific conditions, causes and/or problems, needs, and behaviors;
    - Defined and implemented interventions for pressure ulcer prevention and treatment in accordance with resident needs, goals, and recognized standards of practice;
    - Addressed the potential for infection;
    - Monitored and evaluated the resident's response to preventive efforts and treatment interventions; and
    - Revised the approaches as appropriate.

If not, cite at F314.

Non-compliance for F314

After completing the Investigative Protocol, analyze the data in order to determine whether or not non-compliance with the regulation exists. Non-compliance for F314 may include (but is not limited to) one or more of the following, including failure to:

- Accurately or consistently assess a resident's skin integrity on admission and as indicated thereafter;
- Identify a resident at risk of developing a pressure ulcer(s);
- Identify and address risk factors for developing a pressure ulcer, or explain adequately why they could not or should not do so;
- Implement preventive interventions in accord with the resident's need and current standards of practice;
- Provide clinical justification for the unavoidable development or non-healing/delayed healing or deterioration of a pressure ulcer;
- Provide appropriate interventions, care, and treatment to an existing pressure ulcer to minimize infections and to promote healing;
- Implement interventions for existing wounds;
- Notify the physician of the resident's condition or changes in the resident's wound(s);
- Adequately implement pertinent infection management practices in relation to wound care; and
- Identify or know how to apply relevant policies and procedures for pressure ulcer prevention and treatment.

Potential Tags for Additional Investigation

During the investigation of F314, the surveyor may have determined that concerns may also be present with related outcome, process and/or structure requirements. The surveyor is cautioned to investigate these related requirements before determining whether non-compliance may be present. Some examples of related requirements that should be considered include the following:

- 42 CFR 483.10(b)(11)(i)(B)&(C), F157, Notification of Changes

  ✧ Determine if staff notified the physician of significant changes in the resident's condition or failure of the treatment plan to prevent or heal pressure ulcers; or the resident's representative (if known) of significant changes in the resident's condition in relation to the development of a pressure ulcer or a change in the progression of healing of an existing pressure ulcer.

- 42 CFR 483.20(b)(1), F272, Comprehensive Assessments

  ✧ Determine if the facility comprehensively assessed the resident's skin condition, including existing pressure ulcers, and resident-specific risk factors (including potential causative factors) for the development of a pressure ulcer or non-healing of the ulcer.

- 42 CFR 483.20(k)(1), F279, Comprehensive Care Plans

  ✧ Determine if the facility developed a care plan that was consistent with the resident's specific conditions, risks, needs, behaviors, and preferences and current standards of practice and included measurable objectives and timetables, specific interventions/services to prevent the development of pressure ulcers and/or to treat existing pressures ulcers.

- 42 CFR 483.20(k)(2)(iii), F280, Comprehensive Care Plan Revision

  ✧ Determine if the care plan was periodically reviewed and revised as necessary to prevent the development of pressure ulcers and to promote the healing of existing pressure ulcers.

- 42 CFR 483.20(k)(3)(i), F281, Services Provided Meet Professional Standards

  ✧ Determine if pressure ulcer care was provided in accordance with accepted professional standards.

- 42 CFR 483.25, F309, Quality of Care

  ✧ Determine if staff identified and implemented appropriate measures for the management of pain as indicated as related to pressure ulcers and pressure ulcer treatment.

- 42 CFR 482.30(a), F353, Sufficient Staff

✧ Determine if the facility had qualified staff in sufficient numbers to assure the resident was provided necessary care and services, based upon the comprehensive assessment and care plan, to prevent or treat pressure ulcers.

- 42 CFR 483.40(a)(1), F385, Physician Supervision

  ✧ Determine if the physician has assessed and developed a treatment regimen relevant to preventing or healing a pressure ulcer and responded appropriately to the notice of changes in condition.

- 42 CFR 483.75(i)(2), F501, Medical Director

  ✧ Determine whether the medical director assisted the facility in the development and implementation of policies and procedures for pressure ulcer prevention and treatment, and that these are based on current standards of practice; and whether the medical director interacts with the physician supervising the care of the resident if requested by the facility to intervene on behalf of the resident with a pressure ulcer(s).

V. DEFICIENCY CATEGORIZATION (Part V, Appendix P)

Once the team has completed its investigation, analyzed the data, reviewed the regulatory requirement, and identified the deficient practices that demonstrate that the facility failed to provide care and treatment to prevent or treat pressure ulcers and that non-compliance exists, the team must determine the severity of the deficient practice(s) and the resultant harm or potential for harm to the resident. The key elements for severity determination for F314 are as follows:

1. Presence of harm/negative outcome(s) or potential for negative outcomes because of lack of appropriate treatment and care. Actual or potential harm/negative outcome for F314 may include but is not limited to:

- Potential for development of, occurrence, or recurrence of (an) avoidable pressure ulcer(s);
- Complications such as sepsis or pain related to the presence of avoidable pressure ulcer(s); and/or
- Pressure ulcers that fail to improve as anticipated or develop complications such as sepsis or pain because of the lack of appropriate treatment and care.

2. Degree of harm (actual or potential) related to the non-compliance

Identify how the facility practices caused, resulted in, allowed, or contributed to the actual or potential for harm:

- If harm has occurred, determine if the harm is at the level of serious injury, impairment, death, compromise, or discomfort; and
- If harm has not yet occurred, determine how likely is the potential for serious injury, impairment, death, compromise, or discomfort to occur to the resident.

3. The immediacy of correction required

Determine whether the non-compliance requires immediate correction in order to prevent serious injury, harm, impairment, or death to one or more residents.

The survey team must evaluate the harm or potential for harm based upon the following levels of severity for tag F314. First, the team must rule out whether Severity Level 4, Immediate Jeopardy to a resident's health or safety exists by evaluating the deficient practice in relation to immediacy, culpability, and severity. (Follow the guidance in Appendix Q.)

Severity Level 4 Considerations: Immediate Jeopardy to Resident Health or Safety

Immediate Jeopardy is a situation in which the facility's non-compliance:

- With one or more requirements of participation has caused/resulted in, or is likely to cause, serious injury, harm, impairment, or death to a resident; and
- Requires immediate correction as the facility either created the situation or allowed the situation to continue by failing to implement preventative or corrective measures.

Examples of possible avoidable negative outcomes may include:

- Development of avoidable Stage IV pressure ulcer(s): As a result of the facility's non-compliance, permanent tissue damage (whether or not healing occurs) has compromised the resident, increasing the potential for serious complications including osteomyelitis and sepsis.
- Admitted with a Stage IV pressure ulcer(s) that has shown no signs of healing or shows signs of deterioration: As a result of the facility's non-compliance, a Stage IV pressure ulcer has shown signs of deterioration or a failure to progress towards healing with an increased potential for serious complications including osteomyelits and sepsis.
- Stage III or IV pressure ulcers with associated soft tissue or systemic infection: As a result of the facility's failure to assess or treat a resident with an infectious complication of a pressure ulcer. (See discussion in guidelines and definitions that distinguishes colonization from infection.)
- Extensive failure in multiple areas of pressure ulcer care: As a result of the facility's extensive non-compliance in multiple areas of pressure ulcer care, the resident developed recurrent and/or multiple, avoidable Stage III or Stage IV pressure ulcer(s).

NOTE: If immediate jeopardy has been ruled out based upon the evidence, then evaluate whether actual harm that is not immediate jeopardy exists at Severity Level 3.

Severity Level 3 Considerations: Actual Harm That Is Not Immediate Jeopardy

Level 3 indicates non-compliance that results in actual harm, and can include but may not be limited to clinical compromise, decline, or the resident's ability to maintain and/or reach his/her highest practicable well-being.

Examples of avoidable negative outcomes may include but are not limited to:

- The development of avoidable Stage III pressure ulcer(s): As a result of the facility's non-compliance, Stage III pressure ulcers occurred, which are open wounds in which damage has occurred into the subcutaneous level and may be painful.
- The development of recurrent or multiple avoidable Stage II pressure ulcer(s): As a result of the facility's non-compliance, the resident developed multiple and/or recurrent avoidable Stage II ulcers.
- Failure to implement the comprehensive care plan for a resident who has a pressure ulcer: As a result of a facility's failure to implement a portion of an existing plan related to pressure ulcer care, such as failure to provide for pressure redistribution, or inappropriate treatment/dressing changes, a wound increased in size or failed to progress towards healing as anticipated, or the resident experienced untreated pain.

NOTE: If Severity Level 3 (actual harm that is not immediate jeopardy) has been ruled out based upon the evidence, then evaluate as to whether Level 2 (no actual harm with the potential for more than minimal harm) exists.

Severity Level 2 Considerations: No Actual Harm with Potential for More Than Minimal Harm That Is Not Immediate Jeopardy

Level 2 indicates non-compliance that results in a resident outcome of no more than minimal discomfort and/or has the potential to compromise the resident's ability to maintain or reach his or her highest practicable level of well-being. The potential exists for greater harm to occur if interventions are not provided.

Examples of avoidable negative outcomes may include but are not limited to:

- The development of a single avoidable Stage II pressure ulcer that is receiving appropriate treatment: As a result of the facility's non-compliance, a resident developed an avoidable Stage II pressure ulcer.
- The development of an avoidable Stage I pressure ulcer: As a result of the facility's non-compliance, a resident developed an avoidable Stage I pressure ulcer.
- Failure to implement an element of the care plan for a resident who has a pressure ulcer however, there has been no evidence of decline or failure to heal.
- Failure to recognize or address the potential for developing a pressure ulcer: As a result of the facility's non-compliance, staff failed to identify the risks, develop a plan of care, and/or consistently implement a plan that has been developed to prevent pressure ulcers.

Severity Level 1: No Actual Harm with Potential for Minimal Harm

The failure of the facility to provide appropriate care and services to prevent pressure ulcers or heal existing pressure ulcers is more than minimal harm. Therefore, Severity Level 1 doesn't apply for this regulatory requirement.

F315 Urinary incontinence

§483.25(d) Urinary Incontinence

(Rev. 8, Issued: 06-28-05, Effective: 06-28-05, Implementation: 06-28-05)

Based on the resident's comprehensive assessment, the facility must ensure that—

§483.25(d) (1) A resident who enters the facility without an indwelling catheter is not catheterized unless the resident's clinical condition demonstrates that catheterization was necessary; and

§483.25(d) (2) A resident who is incontinent of bladder receives appropriate treatment and services to prevent urinary tract infections and to restore as much normal bladder function as possible.

Intent (F315) 42 CFR 483.25 (d) (1) and (2) Urinary Incontinence and Catheters

The intent of this requirement is to ensure that:

- Each resident who is incontinent of urine is identified, assessed, and provided appropriate treatment and services to achieve or maintain as much normal urinary function as possible;
- An indwelling catheter is not used unless there is valid medical justification;
- An indwelling catheter for which continuing use is not medically justified is discontinued as soon as clinically warranted;
- Services are provided to restore or improve normal bladder function to the extent possible, after the removal of the catheter; and
- A resident, with or without a catheter, receives the appropriate care and services to prevent infections to the extent possible.

DEFINITIONS

Definitions are provided to clarify clinical terms related to evaluation and treatment of urinary incontinence and catheter use.

- "Bacteremia" is the presence of bacteria in the bloodstream.
- "Bacteriuria" is defined as the presence of bacteria in the urine.
- "Urinary Incontinence" is the involuntary loss or leakage of urine. There are several types of urinary incontinence, and the individual resident may experience more than one type at a time. Some of the more common types include:

  ✧ "Functional Incontinence" refers to loss of urine that occurs in residents whose urinary tract function is sufficiently intact that they should be able to maintain continence, but who cannot remain continent because of external factors (e.g., inability to utilize the toilet facilities in time);
  ✧ "Mixed Incontinence" is the combination of stress incontinence and urge incontinence;
  ✧ "Overflow Incontinence" is associated with leakage of small amounts of urine when the bladder has reached its maximum capacity and has become distended;
  ✧ "Stress Incontinence" (outlet incompetence) is associated with impaired urethral closure (malfunction of the urethral sphincter) which allows small amounts of urine leak-

age when intra-abdominal pressure on the bladder is increased by sneezing, coughing, laughing, lifting, standing from a sitting position, climbing stairs, etc.;

⋄ "Transient Incontinence" refers to temporary episodes of urinary incontinence that are reversible once the cause(s) of the episode(s) is (are) identified and treated; and

⋄ "Urge Incontinence" (overactive bladder) is associated with detrusor muscle overactivity (excessive contraction of the smooth muscle in the wall of the urinary bladder resulting in a sudden, strong urge (also known as urgency) to expel moderate to large amounts of urine before the bladder is full).

- "Urinary Retention" is the inability to completely empty the urinary bladder by micturition.
- "Urinary Tract Infection" (UTI) is a clinically detectable condition associated with invasion by disease-causing microorganisms of some part of the urinary tract, including the urethra (urethritis), bladder (cystitis), ureters (ureteritis), and/or kidney (pyelonephritis). An infection of the urethra or bladder is classified as a lower tract UTI and infection involving the ureter or kidney is classified as an upper tract UTI.
- "Urosepsis" refers to the systemic inflammatory response to infection (sepsis) that appears to originate from a urinary tract source. It may present with symptoms such as fever, hypotension, reduced urine output, or acute change in mental status.

OVERVIEW

Urinary incontinence is not normal. Although aging affects the urinary tract and increases the potential for urinary incontinence, urinary incontinence is not a normal part of aging. In the younger person, urinary incontinence may result from a single cause. In the older individual, urinary incontinence generally involves psychological, physiological, pharmacological, and/or pathological factors or co-morbid conditions (e.g., later stages of dementia, diabetes, prostatectomy, medical conditions involving dysfunction of the central nervous system, urinary tract infections, etc.). Because urinary incontinence is a symptom of a condition and may be reversible, it is important to understand the causes and to address incontinence to the extent possible. If the underlying condition is not reversible, it is important to treat or manage the incontinence to try to reduce complications.

Many older adults are incontinent of urine prior to admission to a nursing home. Urinary incontinence and related loss of independence are prominent reasons for a nursing home admission. Articles[1] and data currently available, including CMS data (e.g., MDS Active Resident Information Report (Item H1b) at www.cms.hhs.gov/states/mdsreports), indicate that more than 50% of the nursing home population experience some degree of urinary incontinence. Whether the resident is incontinent of urine on admission or develops incontinence after admission, the steps of assessment, monitoring, reviewing, and revising approaches to care (as needed) are essential to managing urinary incontinence and to restoring as much normal bladder function as possible.

Various conditions or situations may aggravate the severity of urinary incontinence in nursing home residents. In addition, urinary incontinence may be associated with changes in skin integrity, skin irritation or breakdown, urinary tract infections, falls and fractures, sleep disturbances, and psychosocial complications including social withdrawal, embarrassment, loss of dignity, feelings of isolation, and interference with participation in activities.

Various factors common to elderly individuals may increase the risk of infection including: underlying diseases (e.g., diabetes mellitus), medications that affect immune responses to infection (e.g., steroids and chemotherapy, history of multiple antibiotic usage), conditions that cause incontinence, and indwelling urinary catheters.

The urinary tract is a common source of bacteremia in nursing home residents. UTI is one of the most common infections occurring in nursing homes and is often related to an indwelling urinary catheter. Without a valid clinical rationale for an indwelling catheter, its use is not an acceptable approach to manage urinary incontinence. Although UTIs can result from the resident's own flora, they may also be the result of microorganisms transmitted by staff when handling the urinary catheter drainage system and/or providing incontinence care. Hand washing remains one of the most effective infection control tools available.

Resources

It is important for the facility to have in place systems/procedures to assure: assessments are timely and appropriate; interventions are defined, implemented, monitored, and revised as appropriate in accordance with current standards of practice; and changes in condition are recognized, evaluated, reported to the practitioner, and addressed. The medical director and the quality assessment and assurance committee may help the facility evaluate existing strategies for identifying and managing incontinence, catheter use, and UTIs, and ensure that facility policies and procedures are consistent with current standards of practice.

Research into appropriate practices to prevent, manage, and treat urinary incontinence, urinary catheterization, and UTI continues to evolve. Many recognized clinical resources on the prevention and management of urinary incontinence, infection, and urinary catheterization exist. Some of these resources include:

- The American Medical Directors Association (AMDA) at www.amda.com (Clinical Practice Guidelines: Clinical Practice Guidelines, 1996);
- The Quality Improvement Organizations, Medicare Quality Improvement Community Initiatives at www.medqic.org;
- The CMS Sharing Innovations in Quality website at www.cms.hhs.gov/medicaid/survey-cert/siqhome.asp;
- Association for Professionals in Infection Control and Epidemiology (APIC) at www.apic.org;
- Centers for Disease Control at www.cdc.gov;
- The Annals of Long Term Care publications at www.mmhc.com;
- American Foundation for Urologic Disease, Inc. at www.afud.org; and
- The American Geriatrics Society at www.americangeriatrics.org.

NOTE: References to non-CMS sources or sites on the internet are provided as a service and do not constitute or imply endorsement of these organizations or their programs by CMS or the U. S. Department of Health and Human Services. CMS is not responsible for the content of pages found at these sites. URL addresses were current as of the date of this publication.

Resident Choice

In the course of developing and implementing care plan interventions for treatment and services related to achieving the highest practicable level of urinary continence, preventing and treating urinary tract infections, and avoiding the use of indwelling catheters without medical justification, it is important to involve the resident and/or her or his surrogate in care decisions and to consider whether the resident has an advance directive in place.

In order for a resident to exercise his or her right appropriately to make informed choices about care and treatment or to refuse treatment, the facility and the resident (or the resident's legal representative) must discuss the resident's condition, treatment options, expected outcomes, and consequences of refusing treatment. The facility should address the resident's concerns and offer relevant alternatives, if the resident has refused specific treatments. (See Resident Rights 483.10(b) (3) and (4) (F154 and F155).)

Advance Directive. A resident who is at the end of life or in terminal stages of an illness or who has multiple organ system failures may have written directions for his or her treatment goals (or a decision has been made by the resident's surrogate or representative, in accordance with State law).

Although a facility's care must reflect a resident's wishes as expressed in the Directive, in accordance with State law, the presence of an Advance Directive does not absolve the facility from giving supportive and other pertinent care that is not prohibited by the Advance Directive. The presence of a "Do Not Resuscitate" (DNR) order does not indicate that the resident is declining appropriate treatment and services. It only indicates that the resident should not be resuscitated if respirations and/or cardiac function cease.

If the facility has implemented individualized approaches for end-of-life care in accordance with the resident's wishes, and has implemented appropriate efforts to try to stabilize the resident's condition (or indicated why the condition cannot or should not be stabilized), and has provided care based on the assessed needs of the resident, then the development, continuation, or progression of urinary incontinence; the insertion and prolonged use of an indwelling urinary catheter; or the development of infection or skin-related complications from urine or an indwelling catheter may be consistent with regulatory requirements.

URINARY INCONTINENCE

42 CFR 483.25 (d) (2) Urinary Incontinence requires that a resident who is incontinent of bladder receives appropriate treatment and services to prevent urinary tract infections and to restore as much normal bladder function as possible.

Urinary incontinence generally involves a number of transitory or chronic progressive factors that affect the bladder and/or the urethral sphincter. Any condition, medication, or factor that affects lower urinary tract function, bladder capacity, urination, or the ability to toilet can predispose residents to urinary incontinence and may contribute to incomplete bladder emptying.

The first steps toward assuring that a resident receives appropriate treatment and services to restore as much bladder function as possible or to treat and manage the incontinence are to identify the resident already experiencing some level of incontinence or at risk of developing urinary incontinence and to complete an accurate, thorough assessment of factors that may predispose the resident to having urinary incontinence. This is followed by implementing appropriate, individualized interventions that address the incontinence, including the resident's capabilities and underlying factors that can be removed, modified, or stabilized, and by monitoring the effectiveness of the interventions and modifying them, as appropriate. The practitioner, may at his or her option, refer residents to various practitioners who specialize in diagnosing and treating conditions that affect urinary function.

Assessment

Factors contributing to urinary incontinence sometimes may be resolved after a careful examination and review of history. In addition, for a resident who is incontinent of urine, determining the type of urinary incontinence can allow staff to provide more individualized programming or interventions to enhance the resident's quality of life and functional status. A resident should be evaluated at admission and whenever there is a change in cognition, physical ability, or urinary tract function. This evaluation is to include identification of individuals with reversible and irreversible (e.g., bladder tumors and spinal cord disease) causes of incontinence. If the resident has urinary incontinence that has already been investigated, documented, and determined to be irreversible or not significantly improvable, additional studies may be of limited value, unless there has been advancement in available treatments.

Documentation of assessment information may be found throughout the medical record, such as in an admission assessment, hospital records, history and physical, and the Resident Assessment Instrument (RAI). The location of RAI assessment information is identified on the Resident Assessment Protocol (RAP) summary form. It is important that staff, when completing the comprehensive assessment, consider the following:

- Prior history of urinary incontinence, including onset, duration and characteristics, precipitants of urinary incontinence, associated symptoms (e.g., dysuria, polyuria, hesitancy), and previous treatment and/or management, including the response to the interventions and the occurrence of persistent or recurrent UTI;
- Voiding patterns (such as frequency, volume, nighttime or daytime, quality of stream) and, for those already experiencing urinary incontinence, voiding patterns over several days;
- Medication review, particularly those that might affect continence, such as medications with anticholinergic properties (may cause urinary retention and possible overflow incontinence), sedative/hypnotics (may cause sedation leading to functional incontinence), diuretics (may cause urgency, frequency, overflow incontinence), narcotics, alpha-adrenergic agonists (may cause urinary retention in men) or antagonists (may cause stress incontinence in women), calcium channel blockers (may cause urinary retention);[2]

- Patterns of fluid intake, such as amounts, time of day, alterations and potential complications, such as decreased or increased urine output;
- Use of urinary tract stimulants or irritants (e.g., frequent caffeine intake);[3]
- Pelvic and rectal examination to identify physical features that may directly affect urinary incontinence, such as prolapsed uterus or bladder, prostate enlargement, significant constipation or fecal impaction, use of a urinary catheter, atrophic vaginitis, distended bladder, or bladder spasms;
- Functional and cognitive capabilities that could enhance urinary continence and limitations that could adversely affect continence, such as impaired cognitive function or dementia, impaired immobility, decreased manual dexterity, the need for task segmentation, decreased upper and lower extremity muscle strength, decreased vision, pain with movement;
- Type and frequency of physical assistance necessary to assist the resident to access the toilet, commode, urinal, etc. and the types of prompting needed to encourage urination;
- Pertinent diagnoses such as congestive heart failure, stroke, diabetes mellitus, obesity, and neurological disorders (e.g., multiple sclerosis, Parkinson's Disease, or tumors that could affect the urinary tract or its function);
- Identification of and/or potential of developing complications such as skin irritation or breakdown;
- Tests or studies indicated to identify the type(s) of urinary incontinence (e.g., post-void residual(s) for residents who have, or are at risk of, urinary retention; results of any urine culture if the resident has clinically significant systemic or urinary symptoms), or evaluations assessing the resident's readiness for bladder rehabilitation programs; and
- Environmental factors and assistive devices that may restrict or facilitate a resident's ability to access the toilet (e.g., grab bars, raised or low toilet seats, inadequate lighting, distance to toilet or bedside commodes, availability of urinals, use of bed rails or restraints, or fear of falling).

Types of Urinary Incontinence

Identifying the nature of the incontinence is a key aspect of the assessment and helps identify the appropriate program/interventions to address incontinence.

- Urge Incontinence is characterized by abrupt urgency, frequency, and nocturia (part of the overactive bladder diagnosis). It may be age-related or have neurological causes (e.g., stroke, diabetes mellitus, Parkinson's Disease, multiple sclerosis) or other causes such as bladder infection, urethral irritation, etc. The resident can feel the need to void, but is unable to inhibit voiding long enough to reach and sit on the commode. It is the most common cause of urinary incontinence in elderly persons.
- Stress Incontinence is the loss of a small amount of urine with physical activity such as coughing, sneezing, laughing, walking stairs, or lifting. Urine leakage results from an increase in intra-abdominal pressure on a bladder that is not over distended and is not the result of detrusor contractions. It is the second most common type of urinary incontinence in older women.

- Mixed Incontinence is the combination of urge incontinence and stress incontinence. Many elderly persons (especially women) will experience symptoms of both urge and stress called mixed incontinence.

- Overflow Incontinence occurs when the bladder is distended from urine retention. Symptoms of overflow incontinence may include: weak stream, hesitancy, or intermittency; dysuria; nocturia; frequency; incomplete voiding; frequent or constant dribbling. Urine retention may result from outlet obstruction (e.g., benign prostatic hypertrophy (BPH), prostate cancer, and urethral stricture), hypotonic bladder (detrusor under activity), or both. Hypotonic bladder may be caused by outlet obstruction, impaired or absent contractility of the bladder (neurogenic bladder), or other causes. Neurogenic bladder may also result from neurological conditions such as diabetes mellitus, spinal cord injury, or pelvic nerve damage from surgery or radiation therapy. In overflow incontinence, post void residual (PVR) volume (the amount of urine remaining in the bladder within 5 to 10 minutes following urination) exceeds 200 milliliters (ml). Normal PVR is usually 50 ml. or less. A PVR of 150 to 200 may suggest a need for retesting to determine if this finding is clinically significant. Overflow incontinence may mimic urge or stress incontinence but is less common than either of those.

- Functional Incontinence refers to incontinence that is secondary to factors other than inherently abnormal urinary tract function. It may be related to physical weakness or poor mobility/dexterity (e.g., due to poor eyesight, arthritis, deconditioning, stroke, contracture), cognitive problems (e.g., confusion, dementia, unwillingness to toilet), various medications (e.g., anti-cholinergics, diuretics), or environmental impediments (e.g., excessive distance of the resident from the toilet facilities, poor lighting, low chairs that are difficult to get out of, physical restraints and toilets that are difficult to access). Refer to 42 CFR 483.15(e) (1) for issues regarding unmet environmental needs (e.g., handicap toilet, lighting, assistive devices).

NOTE: Treating the physiological causes of incontinence, without attending to functional components that may have an impact on the resident's continence, may fail to solve the incontinence problem.

- Transient Incontinence refers to temporary or occasional incontinence that may be related to a variety of causes, for example: delirium, infection, atrophic urethritis or vaginitis, some pharmaceuticals (such as sedatives/hypnotics, diuretics, anti-cholinergic agents), increased urine production, restricted mobility, or fecal impaction. The incontinence is transient because it is related to a potentially improvable or reversible cause.

Interventions

It is important that the facility follow the care process (accurate assessment, care planning, consistent implementation and monitoring of the care plan with evaluation of the effectiveness of the interventions, and revision, as appropriate). Recording and evaluating specific information (such as frequency and times of incontinence and toileting and response to specific interventions) is important for determining progress, changes, or decline.

A number of factors may contribute to the decline or lack of improvement in urinary continence, for example: underlying medical conditions, an inaccurate assessment of the resident's
type of incontinence (or lack of knowledge about the resident's voiding patterns) may contribute to inappropriate interventions or unnecessary use of an indwelling catheter. Facility practices that may promote achieving the highest practicable level of functioning, may prevent or
minimize a decline or lack of improvement in degree of continence include providing treatment and services to address factors that are potentially modifiable, such as:

- Managing pain and/or providing adaptive equipment to improve function for residents suffering from arthritis, contractures, neurological impairments, etc;
- Removing or improving environmental impediments that affect the resident's level of continence (e.g., improved lighting, use of a bedside commode or reducing the distance to the
  toilet);
- Treating underlying conditions that have a potentially negative impact on the degree of
  continence (e.g., delirium causing urinary incontinence related to acute confusion);
- Possibly adjusting medications affecting continence (e.g., medication cessation, dose reduction, selection of an alternate medication, change in time of administration); and
- Implementing a fluid and/or bowel management program to meet the assessed needs.

Options for managing urinary incontinence in nursing home residents include primarily behavioral programs and medication therapy. Other measures and supportive devices used in the
management of urinary incontinence and/or urinary retention may include intermittent catheterization; pelvic organ support devices (pessaries); the use of incontinence products, garments,
and an external collection system for men and women; and environmental accommodation and/
or modification.

Behavioral Programs — Interventions involving the use of behavioral programs are among the
least invasive approaches to address urinary incontinence and have no known adverse complications. Behavior programs involve efforts to modify the resident's behavior and/or environment.
Critical aspects of a successful behavioral program include education of the caregiver and the
resident, availability of the staff, and the consistent implementation of the interventions.

NOTE: It is important for the comprehensive assessment to identify the essential skills the resident must possess to be successful with specific interventions being attempted. These skills include the resident's ability to: comprehend and follow through on education and instructions;
identify urinary urge sensation; learn to inhibit or control the urge to void until reaching a toilet; contract the pelvic floor muscle (Kegel exercises) to lessen urgency and/or urinary leakage;
and/or respond to prompts to void.[4] Voiding records help detect urinary patterns or intervals between incontinence episodes and facilitate planning care to avoid or reduce the frequency of
episodes.

Programs that require the resident's cooperation and motivation in order for learning and practice to occur include the following:

- "Bladder Rehabilitation/Bladder Retraining" is a behavioral technique that requires the resident to resist or inhibit the sensation of urgency (the strong desire to urinate), to postpone
  or delay voiding, and to urinate according to a timetable rather than to the urge to void.

Depending upon the resident's successful ability to control the urge to void, the intervals between voiding may be increased progressively. Bladder training generally consists of education, scheduled voiding with systematic delay of voiding, and positive reinforcement. This program is difficult to implement in cognitively impaired residents and may not be successful in frail, elderly, or dependent residents. The resident who may be appropriate for a bladder rehabilitation (retraining) program is usually fairly independent in activities of daily living, has occasional incontinence, is aware of the need to urinate (void), may wear incontinence products for episodic urine leakage, and has a goal to maintain his/her highest level of continence and decrease urine leakage. Successful bladder retraining usually takes at least several weeks. Residents who are assessed with urge or mixed incontinence and are cognitively intact may be candidates for bladder retraining; and

- "Pelvic Floor Muscle Rehabilitation," also called Kegel and pelvic floor muscle exercise, is performed to strengthen the voluntary periuretheral and perivaginal muscles that contribute to the closing force of the urethra and the support of the pelvic organs. These exercises are helpful in dealing with urge and stress incontinence. Pelvic floor muscle exercises (PFME) strengthen the muscular components of urethral supports and are the cornerstone of noninvasive treatment of stress urinary incontinence. PFME requires residents who are able and willing to participate and the implementation of careful instructions and monitoring provided by the facility. Poor resident adherence to the exercises may occur even with close monitoring.

Programs that are dependent on staff involvement and assistance, as opposed to resident function, include the following:

- "Prompted Voiding" is a behavioral technique appropriate for use with dependent or more cognitively impaired residents. Prompted voiding techniques have been shown to reduce urinary incontinence episodes up to 40% for elderly incontinent nursing home residents, regardless of their type of urinary incontinence or cognitive deficit—provided that they at least are able to say their name or reliably point to one of two objects.[5] Prompted voiding has three components: regular monitoring with encouragement to report continence status, prompting to toilet on a scheduled basis, and praise and positive feedback when the resident is continent and attempts to toilet. These methods require training, motivation, and continued effort by the resident and caregivers to ensure continued success. Prompted voiding focuses on teaching the resident, who is incontinent, to recognize bladder fullness or the need to void, to ask for help, or to respond when prompted to toilet.

Residents who are assessed with urge or mixed incontinence and are cognitively impaired may be candidates for prompted voiding. As the resident's cognition changes, the facility should consider other factors, such as mobility, when deciding to conduct a voiding trial to determine feasibility of an ongoing toileting program; and

- "Habit Training/Scheduled Voiding" is a behavioral technique that calls for scheduled toileting at regular intervals on a planned basis to match the resident's voiding habits. Unlike bladder retraining, there is no systematic effort to encourage the resident to delay voiding and resist urges. Habit training includes timed voiding with the interval based on the resident's usual voiding schedule or pattern. Scheduled voiding is timed voiding, usually every three to four hours while awake. Residents who cannot self-toilet may be candidates for habit training or scheduled voiding programs.

Intermittent Catheterization — Sterile insertion and removal of a catheter through the urethra every 3–6 hours for bladder drainage may be appropriate for the management of acute or chronic urinary retention. See additional discussion below in "Catheterization".

Medication Therapy — Medications are often used to treat specific types of incontinence, including stress incontinence and those categories associated with an overactive bladder, which may involve symptoms including urge incontinence, urinary urgency, frequency, and nocturia. The current literature identifies classifications and names of medications used for various types of incontinence. When using medications, potentially problematic anti-cholinergic and other side effects must be recognized. The use of medication therapy to treat urinary incontinence may not be appropriate for some residents because of potential adverse interactions with their other medications or other co-morbid conditions. Therefore, it is important to weigh the risks and benefits before prescribing medications for continence management and to monitor for both effectiveness and side effects. As with all approaches attempting to improve control or management of incontinence, the education and discussion with the resident (or the resident's surrogate) regarding the benefits and risks of pharmacologic therapies is important.

Pessary — A pessary is an intra-vaginal device used to treat pelvic muscle relaxation or prolapse of pelvic organs. Women whose urine retention or urinary incontinence is exacerbated by bladder or uterine prolapse may benefit from placement of a pessary. Female residents may be admitted to the nursing home with a pessary device. The assessment should note whether the resident has a pessary in place or has had a history of successful pessary use. If a pessary is to be used, it is important to develop a plan of care for ongoing management and for the prevention of and monitoring for complications.

Absorbent Products, Toileting Devices, and External Collection Devices — Absorbent incontinence products include perineal pads or panty liners for slight leakage, undergarments and protective underwear for moderate to heavy leakage, guards and drip collection pouches for men, and products (called adult briefs) for moderate or heavy loss. Absorbent products can be a useful, rational way to manage incontinence; however, every absorbent product has a saturation point. Factors contributing to the selection of the type of product to be used should include the severity of incontinence, gender, fit, and ease of use.

Advantages of using absorbent products to manage urinary incontinence include the ability to contain urine (some may wick the urine away from the skin), provide protection for clothing, and preserve the resident's dignity and comfort.

NOTE: Although many residents have used absorbent products prior to admission to the nursing home and the use of absorbent products may be appropriate, absorbent products should not be used as the primary long-term approach to continence management until the resident has been appropriately evaluated and other alternative approaches have been considered.

The potential disadvantages of absorbent products are the impact on the resident's dignity, cost, the association with skin breakdown and irritation, and the amount of time needed to check and change them.[6]

It is important that residents using various toileting devices, absorbent products, external collection devices, etc., be checked (and changed as needed) on a schedule based upon the resident's voiding pattern, accepted standards of practice, and the manufacturer's recommendations.

Skin-Related Complications

Skin problems associated with incontinence and moisture can range from irritation to increased risk of skin breakdown. Moisture may make the skin more susceptible to damage from friction and shear during repositioning.

One form of early skin breakdown is maceration or the softening of tissue by soaking. Macerated skin has a white appearance and a very soft, sometimes "soggy" texture.

The persistent exposure of perineal skin to urine and/or feces can irritate the epidermis and can cause severe dermatitis or skin erosion. Skin erosion is the loss of some or all of the epidermis (comparable to a deep chemical peel) leaving a slightly depressed area of skin.

One key to preventing skin breakdown is to keep the perineal skin clean and dry. Research has shown that a soap and water regimen alone may be less effective in preventing skin breakdown compared with moisture barriers and no-rinse incontinence cleansers.[7] Because frequent washing with soap and water can dry the skin, the use of a perineal rinse may be indicated. Moisturizers help preserve the moisture in the skin by either sealing in existing moisture or adding moisture to the skin. Moisturizers include creams, lotions, or pastes. However, moisturizers should be used sparingly—if at all—on already macerated or excessively moist skin.

CATHETERIZATION

42 CFR 483.25 (d) (1) Urinary Incontinence requires that a resident who enters the facility without an indwelling catheter is not catheterized unless the resident's clinical condition demonstrates that catheterization was necessary. Some residents are admitted to the facility with indwelling catheters that were placed elsewhere (e.g., during a recent acute hospitalization). The facility is responsible for the assessment of the resident at risk for urinary catheterization and/or the ongoing assessment for the resident who currently has a catheter. This is followed by implementation of appropriate individualized interventions and monitoring for the effectiveness of the interventions.

Assessment

A resident may be admitted to the facility with or without an indwelling urinary catheter (urethral or suprapubic) and may be continent or incontinent of urine. Regardless of the admission status, a comprehensive assessment should address those factors that predispose the resident to the development of urinary incontinence and the use of an indwelling urinary catheter.

An admission evaluation of the resident's medical history and a physical examination helps identify the resident at risk for requiring the use of an indwelling urinary catheter. This evaluation is to include detection of reversible causes of incontinence and identification of individuals with incontinence caused by conditions that may not be reversible, such as bladder tumors and spinal cord diseases. (See the assessment factors discussed under incontinence.) The assessment of continence/incontinence is based upon an interdisciplinary review. The comprehensive assessment should include underlying factors supporting the medical justification for the initiation and continuing need for catheter use, determination of which factors can be modified or reversed (or rationale for why those factors should not be modified), and the development of a plan for removal. The clinician's decision to use an indwelling catheter in the elderly should be based on valid clinical indicators.

For the resident with an indwelling catheter, the facility's documented assessment and staff knowledge of the resident should include information to support the use of an indwelling catheter. Because of the risk of substantial complications with the use of indwelling urinary catheters, they should be reserved primarily for short-term decompression of acute urinary retention. The assessment should include consideration of the risks and benefits of an indwelling (suprapubic or urethral) catheter; the potential for removal of the catheter; and consideration of complications resulting from the use of an indwelling catheter, such as symptoms of blockage of the catheter with associated bypassing of urine, expulsion of the catheter, pain, discomfort, and bleeding.

Intermittent Catheterization

Intermittent catheterization can often manage overflow incontinence effectively. Residents who have new onset incontinence from a transient, hypotonic/atonic bladder (usually seen following indwelling catheterization in the hospital) may benefit from intermittent bladder catheterization until the bladder tone returns (e.g., up to approximately 7 days). A voiding trial and post void residual can help identify when bladder tone has returned.

Indwelling Catheter Use

The facility's documented assessment and staff approach to the resident should be based on evidence to support the use of an indwelling catheter. Appropriate indications for continuing use of an indwelling catheter beyond 14 days may include:[8]

- Urinary retention that cannot be treated or corrected medically or surgically, for which alternative therapy is not feasible, and which is characterized by:

  ✧ Documented PVR volumes in a range over 200 ml;
  ✧ Inability to manage the retention/incontinence with intermittent catheterization; and
  ✧ Persistent overflow incontinence, symptomatic infections, and/or renal dysfunction.

- Contamination of Stage III or IV pressure ulcers with urine which has impeded healing, despite appropriate personal care for the incontinence; and
- Terminal illness or severe impairment, which makes positioning or clothing changes uncomfortable, or which is associated with intractable pain.

Catheter-Related Complications

An indwelling catheter may be associated with significant complications, including bacteremia, febrile episodes, bladder stones, fistula formation, erosion of the urethra, epididymitis, chronic renal inflammation, and pyelonephritis. In addition, indwelling catheters are prone to blockage. Risk factors for catheter blockage include alkaline urine, poor urine flow, proteinuria, and pre-existing bladder stones. In the absence of evidence indicating blockage, catheters need not be changed routinely as long as monitoring is adequate. Based on the resident's individualized assessment, the catheter may need to be changed more or less often than every 30 days.

Some residents with indwelling catheters experience persistent leakage around the catheter. Examples of factors that may contribute to leakage include irritation by a large balloon or by catheter materials, excessive catheter diameter, fecal impaction, and improper catheter positioning. Because leakage around the catheter is frequently caused by bladder spasm, leakage should generally not be treated by using increasingly larger catheter sizes, unless medically justified. Current standards indicate that catheterization should be accomplished with the narrowest, softest tube that will serve the purpose of draining the bladder. Additional care practices related to catheterization include:

- Educating the resident or responsible party on the risks and benefits of catheter use;
- Recognizing and assessing for complications and their causes, and maintaining a record of any catheter-related problems;
- Attempts to remove the catheter as soon as possible when no indications exist for its continuing use;
- Monitoring for excessive PVR, after removing a catheter that was inserted for obstruction or overflow incontinence;
- Keeping the catheter anchored to prevent excessive tension on the catheter, which can lead to urethral tears or dislodging the catheter; and
- Securing the catheter to facilitate flow of urine.

Research has shown that catheterization is an important, potentially modifiable, risk factor for UTI. By the 30th day of catheterization, bacteriuria is nearly universal.[9] The potential for complications can be reduced by:

- Identifying specific clinical indications for the use of an indwelling catheter;
- Assessing whether other treatments and services would appropriately address those conditions; and
- Assessing whether residents are at risk for other possible complications resulting from the continuing use of the catheter, such as obstruction resulting from catheter encrustation, urethral erosion, bladder spasms, hematuria, and leakage around the catheter.

URINARY TRACT INFECTIONS

Catheter-Related Bacteriuria and UTIs/Urosepsis

Most individuals with indwelling catheters for more than 7 days have bacteriuria. Bacteriuria alone in a catheterized individual should not be treated with antibiotics.

A long-term indwelling catheter (>2 to 4 weeks) increases the chances of having a symptomatic UTI and urosepsis. The incidence of bacteremia is 40 times greater in individuals with a long-term indwelling catheter than in those without one. For suspected UTIs in a catheterized individual, the literature recommends removing the current catheter and inserting a new one and obtaining a urine sample via the newly inserted catheter.[10]

Clinical Evidence That May Suggest UTI

Clinically, an acute deterioration in stable chronic symptoms may indicate an acute infection. Multiple co-existing findings such as fever with hematuria are more likely to be from a urinary source.

No one lab test alone proves that a UTI is present. For example, a positive urine culture will show bacteriuria but that alone is not enough to diagnose a symptomatic UTI. However, several test results in combination with clinical findings can help to identify UTIs such as the presence of pyuria (more than minimal white cells in the urine) on microscopic urinalysis, or a positive urine dipstick test for leukocyte esterase (indicating significant pyuria) or for nitrites (indicating the presence of Enterobacteriaceae). A negative leukocyte esterase or the absence of pyuria strongly suggests that a UTI is not present. A positive leukocyte esterase test alone does not prove that the individual has a UTI.[11]

In someone with nonspecific symptoms such as a change in function or mental status, bacteriuria alone does not necessarily warrant antibiotic treatment. Additional evidence that could confirm a UTI may include hematuria, fever (which could include a variation from the individual's normal or usual temperature range), or evidence of pyuria (either by microscopic examination or by dipstick test). In the absence of fever, hematuria, pyuria, or local urinary tract symptoms, other potential causes of nonspecific general symptoms, such as fluid and electrolyte imbalance or adverse drug reactions, should be considered instead of, or in addition to, a UTI. Although sepsis, including urosepsis, can cause dizziness or falling, there is not clear evidence linking bacteriuria or a localized UTI to an increased fall risk.[12]

Indications to Treat a UTI

Because many residents have chronic bacteriuria, the research-based literature suggests treating only symptomatic UTIs. Symptomatic UTIs are based on the following criteria:[13]

- Residents without a catheter should have at least three of the following signs and symptoms:

  ⬥ Fever (increase in temperature of >2 degrees F (1.1 degrees C) or rectal temperature >99.5 degrees F (37.5 degrees C) or single measurement of temperature >100 degrees F (37.8 degrees C));[14]
  ⬥ New or increased burning pain on urination, frequency, or urgency;
  ⬥ New flank or suprapubic pain or tenderness;
  ⬥ Change in character of urine (e.g., new bloody urine, foul smell, or amount of sediment) or as reported by the laboratory (new pyuria or microscopic hematuria); and/or

♦ Worsening of mental or functional status (e.g., confusion, decreased appetite, unexplained falls, incontinence of recent onset, lethargy, decreased activity).[15]

• Residents with a catheter should have at least two of the following signs and symptoms:

♦ Fever or chills;
♦ New flank pain or suprapubic pain or tenderness;
♦ Change in character of urine (e.g., new bloody urine, foul smell, or amount of sediment) or as reported by the laboratory (new pyuria or microscopic hematuria); and/or
♦ Worsening of mental or functional status. Local findings such as obstruction, leakage, or mucosal trauma (hematuria) may also be present.[16]

Follow-Up of UTIs

The goal of treating a UTI is to alleviate systemic or local symptoms, not to eradicate all bacteria. Therefore, a post-treatment urine culture is not routinely necessary but may be useful in select situations. Continued bacteriuria without residual symptoms does not warrant repeat or continued antibiotic therapy. Recurrent UTIs (2 or more in 6 months) in a noncatheterized individual may warrant additional evaluation (such as a determination of an abnormal PVR urine volume or a referral to a urologist) to rule out structural abnormalities such as enlarged prostate, prolapsed bladder, periurethral abscess, strictures, bladder calculi, polyps, and tumors.

Recurrent symptomatic UTIs in a catheterized or noncatheterized individual should lead the facility to check whether perineal hygiene is performed consistently to remove fecal soiling in accordance with accepted practices. Recurrent UTIs in a catheterized individual should lead the facility to look for possible impairment of free urine flow through the catheter, to re-evaluate the techniques being used for perineal hygiene and catheter care, and to reconsider the relative risks and benefits of continuing the use of an indwelling catheter.

Because the major factors (other than an indwelling catheter) that predispose individuals to bacteriuria, including physiological aging changes and chronic co-morbid illnesses, cannot be modified readily, the facility should demonstrate that they:

• Employ standard infection control practices in managing catheters and associated drainage system;
• Strive to keep the resident and catheter clean of feces to minimize bacterial migration into the urethra and bladder (e.g., cleaning fecal material away from, rather than towards, the urinary meatus);
• Take measures to maintain free urine flow through any indwelling catheter; and
• Assess for fluid needs and implement a fluid management program (using alternative approaches as needed) based on those assessed needs.

ENDNOTES

1. Geurrero, P. & Sinert, R. (November 18, 2004). Urinary Incontinence. Retrieved November 29, 2004 from E-Medicine. Website: www.emedicine.com/emerg/topic791.htm.

2. Delafuente, J.C. & Stewart, R.B. (Eds.). (1995). Therapeutics in the Elderly (2nd ed., pp. 471). Cincinnati, OH: Harvey Whitney Books.

3. Newman, D.K. (2002). Managing and Treating Urinary Incontinence (pp.106–107). Baltimore, MD: Health Professions Press.

4. Newman, D.K. (2002). Managing and Treating Urinary Incontinence.

5. Ouslander, J.G., Schnelle, J.F., Uman, G., Fingold, S., Nigam, J.G., Tuico, E., et al. (1995). Predictors of Successful Prompted Voiding Among Incontinent Nursing Home Residents. Journal of the American Medical Association, 273(17), 1366–1370.

6. Armstrong, E.P. & Ferguson, T.A. (1998). Urinary Incontinence: Healthcare Resource Consumption in Veteran Affair Medical Centers. Veteran's Health System Journal, October, 37–42.

7. Byers, P.H., Ryan, P.A., Regan, M.B., Shields, A., & Carta, S.G. (1995). Effects of Incontinence Care Cleansing Regimens on Skin Integrity. Continence Care, 22(4), 187–192.

8. Niël-Weise, B.S., van den Broek, P.J. Urinary catheter policies for long-term bladder drainage. The Cochrane Database of Systematic Reviews 2005, Issue 1. Art. No.: CD004201. DOI: 10.1002/14651858.CD004201.pub2.

9. Maki, D.G. & Tambyah, P.A. (2001). Engineering Out the Risk of Infection with Urinary Catheters. Emerging Infectious Diseases, 7(2), 342–347.

10. Grahn, D., Norman, D.C., White, M.L., Cantrell, M. & Thomas, T.T. (1985). Validity of Urinary Catheter Specimen for Diagnosis of Urinary Tract Infection in the Elderly. Archives of Internal Medicine, 145,1858.

11. Nicolle, L.E. (1999). Urinary Tract Infections in the Elderly. In W.R. Hazzard, J.P. Blass., W.H. Ettinger, J.B. Halter & J.G. Ouslander (Eds.), Principles of Geriatric Medicine and Gerontology (4th ed., pp. 823–833). New York: McGraw-Hill.

12. Nicolle, L.E. & SHEA Long-term Care Committee. (2001). Urinary Tract Infections in Long-Term Care Facilities. Infection Control Hospital Epidemiology, 22, 167–175.

13. McGreer, A., Campbell, B., Emori, T.G., Hierholzer, W.J., Jackson, M.M., Nicolle, L.E., et al. (1991). Definitions of Infections for Surveillance in Long Term Care Facilities. American Journal of Infection Control, 19(1), 1–7.

14. AMDA: Common Infections in the Long-term Care Setting. Clinical practice guideline. Adapted from Bentley D.W., Bradley S., High K., et al. Practice guideline for evaluation of fever and infection in long-term care facilities. Guidelines from the Infectious Diseases Society of America. J Am Med Dir Assoc 2001; 2(5): 246–258.

15. Ouslander, J.G., Osterweil, D., Morley, J. (1997). Medical Care in the Nursing Home. (2nd ed., pp. 303–307). New York: McGraw-Hill.

16. Nicolle, L.E. (1997). Asymptomatic Bacteriuria in the Elderly. Infectious Disease Clinics of North America, 11, 647–662.

INVESTIGATIVE PROTOCOL

URINARY CONTINENCE AND CATHETERS

Objectives

- To determine whether the initial insertion or continued use of an indwelling catheter is based upon clinical indication for use of a urinary catheter;
- To determine the adequacy of interventions to prevent, improve, and/or manage urinary incontinence; and
- To determine whether appropriate treatment and services have been provided to prevent and/or treat UTIs.

Use

Use this protocol for a sampled resident with an indwelling urinary catheter or for a resident with urinary incontinence.

Procedures

Briefly review the assessment, care plan, and orders to identify facility interventions and to guide observations to be made. Staff are expected to assess and provide appropriate care from the day of admission, for residents with urinary incontinence or a condition that may contribute to incontinence or the presence of an indwelling urinary catheter (including newly admitted residents). Corroborate observations by interview and record review.

NOTE: Criteria established in this protocol provide general guidelines and best practices which should be considered when making a determination of compliance, and is not an exhaustive list of mandatory elements.

1. Observation

Observe whether staff consistently implemented care plan interventions across various shifts. During observations of the interventions, note and/or follow up on deviations from the care plan or from current standards of practice, as well as potential negative outcomes.

Observe whether staff make appropriate resident accommodations consistent with the assessment, such as placing the call bell within reach and responding to the call bell, in relation to meeting toileting needs; maintaining a clear pathway and ready access to toilet facilities; providing (where indicated) elevated toilet seats, grab bars, adequate lighting, and assistance needed to use devices such as urinals, bedpans and commodes.

Observe whether assistance has been provided to try to prevent incontinence episodes, such as whether prompting, transfer, and/or stand-by assist to ambulate were provided as required for toileting.

For a resident who is on a program to restore continence or is on a prompted void or scheduled toileting program, note:

- The frequency of breakthrough or transient incontinence;
- How staff respond to the incontinence episodes; and
- Whether care is provided in accord with standards of practice (including infection control practices) and with respect for the resident's dignity.

For a resident who has been determined by clinical assessment to be unable to participate in a program to restore continence or in a scheduled toileting program and who requires care due to incontinence of urine, observe:

- Whether the resident is on a scheduled check and change program; and
- Whether staff check and change in a timely fashion.

For a resident who has experienced an incontinent episode, observe:

- The condition of the pads/sheets/clothing (a delay in providing continence care may be indicated by brown rings/circles, saturated linens/clothing, odors, etc.);
- The resident's physical condition (such as skin integrity, maceration, erythema, erosion);
- The resident's psychosocial outcomes (such as embarrassment or expressions of humiliation, resignation, about being incontinent);
- Whether staff implemented appropriate hygiene measures (e.g., cleansing, rinsing, drying and applying protective moisture barriers or barrier films as indicated) to try to prevent skin breakdown from prolonged exposure of the skin to urine; and
- Whether the staff response to incontinence episodes and the provision of care are consistent with standards of practice (including infection control practices) and with respect for the resident's dignity.

For a resident with an indwelling catheter, observe the delivery of care to evaluate:

- Whether staff use appropriate infection control practices regarding hand washing, catheter care, tubing, and the collection bag;
- Whether staff recognize and assess potential evidence of symptomatic UTI or other related changes in urine condition (such as onset of bloody urine, cloudiness, or oliguria, if present);
- How staff manage and assess urinary leakage from the point of catheter insertion to the bag, if present;
- If the resident has catheter-related pain, how staff assess and manage the pain; and
- What interventions (such as anchoring the catheter, avoiding excessive tugging on the catheter during transfer and care delivery) are being used to prevent inadvertent catheter removal or tissue injury from dislodging the catheter.

For a resident experiencing incontinence and who has an indwelling or intermittent catheter, observe whether the resident is provided and encouraged to take enough fluids to meet the resident's hydration needs, as reflected in various measures of hydration status (approximately

30ml/kg/day or as indicated based on the resident's clinical condition). For issues regarding hydration, see Guidance at 42 CFR 483.25(j), F327.

2. Interviews

Interview the resident, family, or responsible party to the degree possible to identify:

- Their involvement in care plan development including defining the approaches and goals, and whether interventions reflect preferences and choices;
- Their awareness of the existing continence program and how to use devices or equipment;
- If timely assistance is provided as needed for toileting needs, hydration, and personal hygiene and if continence care and/or catheter care is provided according to the care plan;
- If the resident comprehends and applies information and instructions to help improve or maintain continence (where cognition permits);
- Presence of urinary tract-related pain, including causes and management;
- If interventions were refused, whether consequences and/or other alternative approaches were presented and discussed; and
- Awareness of any current UTI, history of UTIs, or perineal skin problems.

If the resident has a skin problem that may be related to incontinence, or staff are not following the resident's care plan and continence/catheter care program, interview the nursing assistants to determine if they:

- Are aware of, and understand, the interventions specific to this resident (such as the bladder or bowel restorative/management programs);
- Have been trained and know how to handle catheters, tubing, and drainage bags and other devices used during the provision of care; and
- Know what, when, and to whom to report changes in status regarding bowel and bladder function, hydration status, urine characteristics, and complaints of urinary-related symptoms.

3. Record Review

Assessment and Evaluation. Review the RAI, the history and physical, and other information such as physician orders, progress notes, nurses' notes, pharmacist reports, lab reports, and any flow sheets or forms the facility uses to document the resident's voiding history, including the assessment of the resident's overall condition, risk factors, and information about the resident's continence status, rationale for using a catheter, environmental factors related to continence programs, and the resident's responses to catheter/continence services. Request staff assistance, if the information is not readily available.

Determine if the facility assessment is consistent with or corroborated by documentation within the record and comprehensively reflects the status of the resident for:

- Patterns of incontinent episodes, daily voiding patterns, or prior routines;
- Fluid intake and hydration status;
- Risks or conditions that may affect urinary continence;

- Use of medications that may affect continence and impaired continence that could reflect adverse drug reactions;
- Type of incontinence (stress, urge, overflow, mixed, functional, or transient incontinence) and contributing factors;
- Environmental factors that might facilitate or impede the ability to maintain bladder continence, such as access to the toilet, call bell, type of clothing and/or continence products, ambulation devices (walkers, canes), use of restraints, side rails;
- Type and frequency of physical assistance necessary to facilitate toileting;
- Clinical rationale for use of an indwelling catheter;
- Alternatives to extended use of an indwelling catheter (if possible); and
- Evaluation of factors possibly contributing to chronically recurring or persistent UTIs.

Care Plan. If the care plan refers to a specific facility treatment protocol that contains details of the treatment regimen, the protocol must be available to the direct care staff, so that they may be familiar with it and use it. The care plan should clarify any significant deviations from such a protocol for a specific resident. If care plan interventions that address aspects of continence and skin care related to incontinence are integrated within the overall care plan, the interventions do not need to be repeated in a separate continence care plan.

Review the care plan to determine if the plan is based upon the goals, needs, and strengths specific to the resident and reflects the comprehensive assessment. Determine if the plan:

- Identifies quantifiable, measurable objectives with time frames to be able to assess whether the objectives have been met;
- Identifies interventions specific enough to guide the provision of services and treatment (e.g., toilet within an hour prior to each meal and within 30 minutes after meals, or check for episodes of incontinence within 30 minutes after each meal or specific times based upon the assessment of voiding patterns);
- Is based upon resident choices and preferences;
- Promotes maintenance of resident dignity;
- Addresses potential psychosocial complications of incontinence or catheterization such as social withdrawal, embarrassment, humiliation, isolation, resignation;
- Includes a component to inform the resident and representative about the risks and benefits of catheter use, on continence management approaches, medications selected, etc.;
- Addresses measures to promote sufficient fluid intake, including alternatives such as food substitutes that have a high liquid content, if there is reduced fluid intake;
- Defines interventions to prevent skin breakdown from prolonged exposure to urine and stool;
- Identifies and addresses the potential impact on continence of medication and urinary tract stimulants or irritants (e.g., caffeine) in foods and beverages;
- Identifies approaches to minimize risk of infection (personal hygiene measures and catheter/tubing/bag care); and
- Defines environmental approaches and devices needed to promote independence in toileting, to maintain continence, and to maximize independent functioning.

For the resident who is not on a scheduled toileting program or a program to restore normal bladder function to the extent possible, determine if the care plan provides specific approaches for a check and change program.

For the resident who is on a scheduled toileting or restorative program (e.g., retraining, habit training, scheduled voiding, prompted voiding, toileting devices), determine whether the care plan:

- Identifies the type of urinary incontinence and bases the program on the resident's voiding/elimination patterns; and
- Has been developed by considering the resident's medical/health condition, cognitive and functional ability to participate in a relevant continence program, and needed assistance.

For the resident with a catheter, determine whether the care plan:

- Defines the catheter, tubing, and bag care, including indications, according to facility protocol, for changing the catheter, tubing, or bag;
- Provides for assessment and removal of the indwelling catheter when no longer needed; and
- Establishes interventions to minimize catheter-related injury, pain, encrustation, excessive urethral tension, accidental removal, or obstruction of urine outflow.

Care Plan Revision. Determine if the resident's condition and effectiveness of the care plan interventions have been monitored and care plan revisions were made (or justifications for continuing the existing plan) based upon the following:

- The outcome and/or effects of goals and interventions;
- A decline or lack of improvement in continence status;
- Complications associated with catheter usage;
- Resident failure to comply with a continence program and alternative approaches that were offered to try to maintain or improve continence, including counseling regarding the potential consequences of not following the program;
- Change in condition, ability to make decisions, cognition, medications, behavioral symptoms, or visual problems;
- Input by the resident and/or the responsible person; and
- An evaluation of the resident's level of participation in, and response to, the continence program.

4. Interviews with Health Care Practitioners and Professionals

If inconsistencies in care or potential negative outcomes have been identified, or care is not in accord with standards of practice, interview the nurse responsible for coordinating or overseeing the resident's care. Determine:

- How the staff monitor implementation of the care plan, changes in continence, skin condition, and the status of UTIs;

- If the resident resists toileting, how staff have been taught to respond;
- Types of interventions that have been attempted to promote continence (i.e., special clothing, devices, types and frequency of assistance, change in toileting schedule, environmental modifications);
- If the resident is not on a restorative program, how it was determined that the resident could not benefit from interventions such as a scheduled toileting program;
- For the resident on a program of toileting, whether the nursing staff can identify the programming applicable to the resident, and:

  ✧ The type of incontinence;
  ✧ The interventions to address that specific type;
  ✧ How it is determined that the schedule and program is effective (i.e., how continence is maintained or if there has been a decline or improvement in continence, how the program is revised to address the changes); and
  ✧ Whether the resident has any physical or cognitive limitations that influence potential improvement of his/her continence;

- For residents with urinary catheters, whether the nursing staff:

  ✧ Can provide appropriate justification for the use of the catheter;
  ✧ Can identify previous attempts made (and the results of the attempts) to remove a catheter; and
  ✧ Can identify a history of UTIs (if present), and interventions to try to prevent recurrence.

If the interventions defined or care provided do not appear to be consistent with recognized standards of practice, interview one or more health care practitioners and professionals as necessary (e.g., physician, charge nurse, director of nursing) who, by virtue of training and knowledge of the resident, should be able to provide information about the causes, treatment, and evaluation of the resident's condition or problem. Depending on the issue, ask about:

- How it was determined that the chosen interventions were appropriate;
- Risks identified for which there were no interventions;
- Changes in condition that may justify additional or different interventions; or how they validated the effectiveness of current interventions; and
- How they monitor the approaches to continence programs (e.g., policies/procedures, staffing requirements, how staff identify problems, assess the toileting pattern of the resident, develop and implement continence-related action plans, how staff monitor and evaluate resident's responses, etc.).

If the attending physician is unavailable, interview the medical director, as appropriate.

DETERMINATION OF COMPLIANCE (Task 6, Appendix P)

Synopsis of regulation (F315)

The urinary incontinence requirement has three aspects. The first aspect requires that a resident who does not have an indwelling urinary catheter does not have one inserted unless the resident's clinical condition demonstrates that it was necessary. The second aspect requires the facility to provide appropriate treatment and services to prevent urinary tract infections; and the third is that the facility attempt to assist the resident to restore as much normal bladder function as possible.

Criteria for Compliance

- Compliance with 42 CFR 483.25(d)(1) and (2), F315, Urinary Incontinence

  ✧ For a resident who was admitted with an indwelling urinary catheter or who had one placed after admission, the facility is in compliance with this requirement, if staff have:

    - Recognized and assessed factors affecting the resident's urinary function and identified the medical justification for the use of an indwelling urinary catheter;

    - Defined and implemented pertinent interventions to try to minimize complications from an indwelling urinary catheter, and to remove it if clinically indicated, consistent with resident conditions, goals, and recognized standards of practice;

    - Monitored and evaluated the resident's response to interventions; and

    - Revised the approaches as appropriate.

If not, the use of an indwelling urinary catheter is not medically justified, and/or the ongoing treatment and services for catheter care were not provided consistent with the resident's needs. Cite F315.

  ✧ For a resident who is incontinent of urine, the facility is in compliance with this requirement if they:

    - Recognized and assessed factors affecting the risk of symptomatic urinary tract infections and impaired urinary function;

    - Defined and implemented interventions to address correctable underlying causes of urinary incontinence and to try to minimize the occurrence of symptomatic urinary tract infections in accordance with resident needs, goals, and recognized standards of practice;

    - Monitored and evaluated the resident's response to preventive efforts and treatment interventions; and

    - Revised the approaches as appropriate.

If not, the facility is not in compliance with the requirement to assist the resident to maintain or improve the continence status, and/or prevent the decline of the condition of urinary incontinence for the resident. Cite F315.

✧ For a resident who has or has had a symptomatic urinary tract infection, the facility is in compliance with this requirement if they have:

- Recognized and assessed factors affecting the risk of symptomatic urinary tract infections and impaired urinary function;

- Defined and implemented interventions to try to minimize the occurrence of symptomatic urinary tract infections and to address correctable underlying causes, in accordance with resident needs, goals, and recognized standards of practice;

- Monitored and evaluated the resident's responses to preventive efforts and treatment interventions; and

- Revised the approaches as appropriate.

If not, the development of a symptomatic urinary tract infection, and/or decline of the resident with one, was not consistent with the identified needs of the resident. Cite F315.

Non-compliance for F315

After completing the Investigative Protocol, analyze the data in order to determine whether or not non-compliance with the regulation exists. Non-compliance for F315 may include (but is not limited to) one or more of the following, including failure to:

- Provide care and treatment to prevent incontinence and/or improve urinary continence and restore as much normal bladder function as possible;
- Provide medical justification for the use of a catheter or provide services for a resident with a urinary catheter;
- Assess, prevent (to the extent possible) and treat a symptomatic urinary tract infection (as indicated by the resident's choices, clinical condition, and physician treatment plan);
- Accurately or consistently assess a resident's continence status on admission and as indicated thereafter;
- Identify and address risk factors for developing urinary incontinence;
- Implement interventions (such as bladder rehabilitative programs) to try to improve bladder function or prevent urinary incontinence, consistent with the resident's assessed need and current standards of practice;
- Provide clinical justification for developing urinary incontinence or for the failure of existing urinary incontinence to improve;
- Identify and manage symptomatic urinary tract infections, or explain adequately why they could or should not do so;
- Implement approaches to manage an indwelling urinary catheter based upon standards of practice, including infection control procedures;
- Identify and apply relevant policies and procedures to manage urinary incontinence, urinary catheters, and/or urinary tract infections;
- Notify the physician of the resident's condition or changes in the resident's continence status or development of symptoms that may represent a symptomatic UTI (in contrast to asymptomatic bacteriuria).

Potential Tags for Additional Investigation

During the investigation of 42 CFR 483.25(d)(1) and (2), the surveyor may have identified concerns related to outcome, process, and/or structure requirements. The surveyor should investigate these requirements before determining whether non-compliance may be present. The following are examples of related outcome, process and/or structure requirements that should be considered:

- 42 CFR 483.10(b)(11), F157, Notification of Changes

  ◇ Determine if staff notified the physician of significant changes in the resident's continence, catheter usage, or the development, treatment and/or change in symptomatic UTIs; or notified the resident or resident's representative (where one exists) of significant changes as noted above.

- 42 CFR 483.15(a), F241, Dignity

  ◇ Determine if staff provide continence care and/or catheter care to the resident in a manner that respects his/her dignity, strives to meet needs in a timely manner, monitors and helps the resident who cannot request assistance, and strives to minimize feelings of embarrassment, humiliation, and/or isolation related to impaired continence.

- 42 CFR 483.20(b)(1), F272, Comprehensive Assessments

  ◇ Determine if the facility comprehensively assessed the resident's continence status and resident-specific risk factors (including potential causes), and assessed for the use of continence-related devices, including an indwelling catheter.

- 42 CFR 483.20(k), F279, Comprehensive Care Plans

  ◇ Determine if the facility developed a care plan (1) that was consistent with the resident's specific conditions, risks, needs, behaviors, and preferences and with current standards of practice and (2) that includes measurable objectives, approximate timetables, specific interventions and/or services needed to prevent or address incontinence, provide catheter care; and to prevent UTIs to the extent possible.

- 42 CFR 483.20(k)(2)(iii), F280, Comprehensive Care Plan Revision

  ◇ Determine if the care plan was reviewed and revised periodically, as necessary, related to preventing, managing, or improving incontinence, managing an indwelling urinary catheter, possible discontinuation of an indwelling catheter, and attempted prevention and management of UTIs.

- 42 CFR 483.20(k)(3)(i), F281, Services Provided Meet Professional Standards

  ◇ Determine if services and care were provided for urinary incontinence, catheter care and/or symptomatic UTIs in accordance with accepted professional standards.

- 42 CFR 483.25, F309, Quality of Care

  ✧ Determine if staff identified and implemented appropriate measures to address any pain related to the use of an indwelling urinary catheter or skin complications such as maceration, and to provide the necessary care and services in accordance with the comprehensive assessment plan of care.

- 42 CFR 483.25 (a)(3), F312, Quality of Care

  ✧ Determine if staff identified and implemented appropriate measures to provide good personal hygiene for the resident who cannot perform relevant activities of daily living, and who has been assessed as unable to achieve and/or restore normal bladder function.

- 42 CFR 483.40(a), F385, Physician Supervision

  ✧ Determine if the physician has evaluated and addressed, as indicated, medical issues related to preventing or managing urinary incontinence, catheter usage, and symptomatic UTIs.

- 42 CFR 483.65(b)(3), F444, Infection Control: Hand Washing

  ✧ Determine if staff wash their hands after providing incontinence care, and before and after providing catheter care.

- 42 CFR 483.75(f), F498, Proficiency of Nurse Aides

  ✧ Determine if nurse aides correctly deliver continence and catheter care, including practices to try to minimize skin breakdown, UTIs, catheter-related injuries, and dislodgement.

- 42 CFR 483.30(a), F353, Sufficient Staff

  ✧ Determine if the facility had qualified staff in sufficient numbers to provide necessary care and services on a 24-hour basis, based upon the comprehensive assessment and care plan, to prevent, manage, and/or improve urinary incontinence where possible.

- 42 CFR 483.75(i)(2), F501, Medical Director

  ✧ Determine whether the medical director, in collaboration with the facility and based on current standards of practice, has developed policies and procedures for the prevention and management of urinary incontinence, for catheter care, and for the identification and management of symptomatic urinary tract infections; and whether the medical director interacts, if requested by the facility, with the physician supervising the care of the resident related to the management of urinary incontinence, catheter, or infection issues.

V. DEFICIENCY CATEGORIZATION (Part V, Appendix P)

Once the team has completed its investigation, analyzed the data, reviewed the regulatory requirements, and determined that non-compliance exists, the team must determine the severity of each deficiency, based on the resultant effect or potential for harm to the resident.

The key elements for severity determination for F315 are as follows:

1. Presence of harm/negative outcome(s) or potential for negative outcomes because of lack of appropriate treatment and care. Actual or potential harm/negative outcome for F315 may include, but is not limited to:

- Development, recurrence, persistence, or increasing frequency of urinary incontinence, which is not the result of underlying clinical conditions;
- Complications such as urosepsis or urethral injury related to the presence of an indwelling urinary catheter that is not clinically justified;
- Significant changes in psychosocial functioning, such as isolation, withdrawal, or embarrassment, related to the presence of un-assessed or unmanaged urinary incontinence and/or a decline in continence, and/or the use of a urinary catheter without a clinically valid medical justification; and
- Complications such as skin breakdown that are related to the failure to manage urinary incontinence;

2. Degree of harm (actual or potential) related to the non-compliance. Identify how the facility practices caused, resulted in, allowed, or contributed to the actual or potential for harm:

- If harm has occurred, determine if the harm is at the level of serious injury, impairment, death, compromise, or discomfort; and
- If harm has not yet occurred, determine the potential for serious injury, impairment, death, or compromise or discomfort to occur to the resident; and

3. The immediacy of correction required. Determine whether the non-compliance requires immediate correction in order to prevent serious injury, harm, impairment, or death to one or more residents.

The survey team must evaluate the harm or potential for harm based upon the following levels of severity for tag F315. First, the team must rule out whether Severity Level 4, Immediate Jeopardy to a resident's health or safety exists by evaluating the deficient practice in relation to immediacy, culpability, and severity. (Follow the guidance in Appendix Q, Immediate Jeopardy.)

Severity Level 4 Considerations: Immediate Jeopardy to Resident Health or Safety

Immediate Jeopardy is a situation in which the facility's non-compliance with one or more requirements of participation:

- Has allowed/caused/resulted in, or is likely to allow/cause/result in serious injury, harm, impairment, or death to a resident; and
- Requires immediate correction, as the facility either created the situation or allowed the situation to continue by failing to implement preventative or corrective measures.

Examples of possible negative outcomes as a result of the facility's deficient practices may include:

- Complications resulting from utilization of urinary appliance(s) without medical justification: As a result of incorrect or unwarranted (i.e., not medically indicated) utilization of a urinary catheter, pessary, etc., the resident experiences injury or trauma (e.g., urethral tear) that requires surgical intervention or repair.
- Extensive failure in multiple areas of incontinence care and/or catheter management: As a result of the facility's non-compliance in multiple areas of continence care or catheter management, the resident developed urosepsis with complications leading to prolonged decline or death.

NOTE: If immediate jeopardy has been ruled out based upon the evidence, then evaluate whether actual harm that is not immediate jeopardy exists at Severity Level 3.

Severity Level 3 Considerations: Actual Harm That Is Not Immediate Jeopardy

Level 3 indicates non-compliance that results in actual harm, and can include but may not be limited to clinical compromise, decline, or the resident's ability to maintain and/or reach his/her highest practicable well-being.

Examples of avoidable negative outcomes may include, but are not limited to:

- The development of a symptomatic UTI: As a result of the facility's non-compliance, the resident developed a symptomatic UTI, without long-term complications, associated with the use of an indwelling catheter for which there was no medical justification.
- The failure to identify, assess, and mange urinary retention: As a result of the facility's non-compliance, the resident had persistent overflow incontinence and/or developed recurrent symptomatic UTIs.
- The failure to provide appropriate catheter care: As a result of the facility's non-compliance, the catheter was improperly managed, resulting in catheter-related pain, bleeding, urethral tears, or urethral erosion.
- Medically unjustified use of an indwelling catheter with complications: As a result of the facility's non-compliance, a resident who was admitted with a urinary catheter had the catheter remain for an extended period of time without a valid medical justification for its continued use, or a urinary catheter was inserted after the resident was in the facility and used for an extended time without medical justification, during which the resident experienced significant complications such as recurrent symptomatic UTIs.

Decline or failure to improve continence status: As a result of the facility's failure to assess and/or re-assess the resident's continence status, utilize sufficient staffing to implement continence programs and provide other related services based on the resident's assessed needs, and/ or to evaluate the possible adverse effects of medications on continence status, the resident failed to maintain or improve continence status.

- Complications due to urinary incontinence: As a result of the facility's failure to provide care and services to a resident who is incontinent of urine, in accordance with resident need and accepted standards of practice, the resident developed skin maceration and/or erosion or declined to attend or participate in social situations (withdrawal) due to embarrassment or humiliation related to unmanaged urinary incontinence.

NOTE: If Severity Level 3 (actual harm that is not immediate jeopardy) has been ruled out based upon the evidence, then evaluate as to whether Level 2 (no actual harm with the potential for more than minimal harm) exists.

Severity Level 2 Considerations: No Actual Harm with Potential for More Than Minimal Harm That Is Not Immediate Jeopardy

Level 2 indicates non-compliance that results in a resident outcome of no more than minimal discomfort and/or has the potential to compromise the resident's ability to maintain or reach his or her highest practicable level of well-being. The potential exists for greater harm to occur if interventions are not provided.

Examples of potentially avoidable negative outcomes may include, but are not limited to:

- Medically unjustified use of an indwelling catheter: As a result of the facility's non-compliance, the resident has the potential for experiencing complications, such as symptomatic UTIs, bladder stones, pain, etc.
- Complications associated with inadequate care and services for an indwelling catheter: As a result of the facility's non-compliance, the resident has developed potentially preventable non-life-threatening problems related to the catheter, such as leaking of urine due to blockage of urine outflow, with or without skin maceration and/or dermatitis.
- Potential for decline or complications: As a result of the facility's failure to consistently implement a scheduled voiding program defined in accordance with the assessed needs, the resident experiences repeated episodes of incontinence but has not demonstrated a decline or developed complications.

Severity Level 1: No Actual Harm with Potential for Minimal Harm

The failures of the facility to provide appropriate care and services to improve continence, manage indwelling catheters, and minimize negative outcome places residents at risk for more than minimal harm. Therefore, Severity Level 1 does not apply for this regulatory requirement.

F317 Range of motion

§483.25(e) Range of Motion

Based on the comprehensive assessment of a resident, the facility must ensure that (see Tag F318 for intent, guidelines, procedures, and probes for §483.25(e))

§483.25(e)(1) A resident who enters the facility without a limited range of motion does not experience reduction in range of motion unless the resident's clinical condition demonstrates that a reduction in range of motion is unavoidable; and

SEE INTERPRETIVE GUIDELINES AT TAG F318

F318 Treatment of residents with limited range of motion

§483.25(e)(2) A resident with a limited range of motion receives appropriate treatment and services to increase range of motion and/or to prevent further decrease in range of motion

Intent §483.25(e)

The intent of this regulation is to ensure that the resident reaches and maintains his or her highest level of range of motion and to prevent avoidable decline of range of motion.

Interpretive Guidelines §483.25(e)

This corresponds to MDS 2.0 sections G and P when specified for use by the State.

"Range of motion (ROM)" is defined as the extent of movement of a joint.

The clinical condition that may demonstrate that a reduction in ROM is unavoidable is: limbs or digits immobilized because of injury or surgical procedures (e.g., surgical adhesions).

Adequate preventive care may include active ROM performed by the resident's passive ROM performed by staff; active-assistive ROM exercise performed by the resident and staff; and application of splints and braces, if necessary.

Examples of clinical conditions that are the primary risk factors for a decreased range of motion are:

- Immobilization (e.g., bedfast);
- Deformities arising out of neurological deficits (e.g., strokes, multiple sclerosis, cerebral palsy, and polio); and
- Pain, spasms, and immobility associated with arthritis or late state Alzheimer's disease.

This clinical condition may demonstrate that a reduction in ROM is unavoidable only if adequate assessment, appropriate care planning, and preventive care was provided, and resulted in limitation in ROM or muscle atrophy.

Procedures §483.25(e)

For each resident selected for a comprehensive review, or focused review, as appropriate, who needs routine preventive care:

- Observe staff providing routine ROM exercises. Are they done according to the care plan?

Probes §483.25(e)

Is there evidence that there has been a decline in sampled residents' ROM or muscle atrophy that was avoidable?

- Was the resident at risk for decline in ROM? If so, why?
- What care did the facility provide, including routine preventive measures that addressed the resident's unique risk factors (e.g., use muscle strengthening exercises in residents with muscle atrophy)?
- Was this care provided consistently?

For all sampled residents who have limited ROM, what is the facility doing to prevent further declines in ROM?

- Are passive ROM exercises provided and active ROM exercises supervised per the plan of care?
- Have care plan objectives identified resident's needs and has resident progress been evaluated?

"Mental and psychosocial adjustment difficulties" refer to problems residents have in adapting to changes in life's circumstances. The former focuses on internal thought processes; the latter, on the external manifestations of these thought patterns.

Mental and psychosocial adjustment difficulties are characterized primarily by an overwhelming sense of loss of one's capabilities; of family and friends; of the ability to continue to pursue activities and hobbies; and of one's possessions. This sense of loss is perceived as global and uncontrollable and is supported by thinking patterns that focus on helplessness and hopelessness; that all learning and essentially all meaningful living ceases once one enters a nursing home. A resident with a mental adjustment disorder will have a sad or anxious mood, or a behavioral symptom such as aggression.

The "Diagnostic and Statistical Manual of Mental Disorders, Fourth Edition (DSM/IV)," specifies that adjustment disorders develop within 3 months of a stressor (e.g., moving to another room) and are evidenced by significant functional impairment. Bereavement with the death of a loved one is not associated with adjustment disorders developed within 3 months of a stressor.

- Is there evidence that care planning is changed as the resident's condition changes?
- Identify if resident triggers RAPs for ADL functional/rehabilitation potential, visual function, and communication. Consider whether the RAPs used to assess causal factors for decline, potential for decline, or lack of improvement.

F319 Mental and psychosocial functioning

§483.25(f) Mental and Psychosocial Functioning

Based on the comprehensive assessment of a resident, the facility must ensure that—

(See Tag F319 for intent, guidelines, and probes for §483.25(f))

§483.25(f)(1) A resident who displays mental or psychosocial adjustment difficulty, receives appropriate treatment, and services to correct the assessed problem; and

Intent §483.25(f)

The intent of this regulation is that the resident receives care and services to assist him or her to reach and maintain the highest level of mental and psychosocial functioning.

Interpretive Guidelines §483.25(f)

This corresponds to MDS 2.0 sections B, F, E, and I when specified for use by the State.

Other manifestations of mental and psychosocial adjustment difficulties may, over a period of time, include:

- Impaired verbal communication;
- Social isolation (e.g., loss or failure to have relationships);
- Sleep pattern disturbance (e.g., disruptive change in sleep/rest pattern as related to one's biological and emotional needs);
- Spiritual distress (disturbances in one's belief system);
- Inability to control behavior and potential for violence (aggressive behavior directed at self or others); and
- Stereotyped response to any stressor (i.e., the same characteristic response, regardless of the stimulus).

Appropriate treatment and services for psychosocial adjustment difficulties may include providing residents with opportunities for self-governance; systematic orientation programs; arrangements to keep residents in touch with their communities, cultural heritage, former lifestyle, and religious practices; and maintaining contact with friends and family. Appropriate treatment for mental adjustment difficulties may include crisis intervention services; individual, group or family psychotherapy; drug therapy and training in monitoring of drug therapy; and other rehabilitative services. (See §483.45(a).)

Clinical conditions that may produce apathy, malaise, and decreased energy levels that can be mistaken for depression associated with mental or psychosocial adjustment difficulty are: (This list is not all inclusive.)

- Metabolic diseases (e.g., abnormalities of serum glucose, potassium, calcium, and blood urea nitrogen, hepatic dysfunction);
- Endocrine diseases (e.g., hypothyroidism, hyperthyroidism, diabetes, hypoparathyroidism, hyperparathyroidism, Cushing's disease, Addison's disease);
- Central nervous system diseases (e.g., tumors and other mass lesions, Parkinson's disease, multiple sclerosis, Alzheimer's disease, vascular disease);
- Miscellaneous diseases (e.g., pernicious anemia, pancreatic disease, malignancy, infections, congestive heart failure);
- Over-medication with anti-hypertensive drugs; and
- Presence of restraints.

Probes §483.25(f)(1)

For sampled residents selected for a comprehensive or focused review, determine, as appropriate, for those residents exhibiting difficulties in mental and psychosocial adjustment:

- Is there a complete accurate assessment of resident's usual and customary routines?
- What evidence is there that the facility makes accommodations for the resident's usual and customary routines?
- What programs/activities has the resident received to improve and maintain maximum mental and psychosocial functioning?
- Has the resident's mental and psychosocial functioning been maintained or improved (e.g., fewer symptoms of distress)? Have treatment plans and objectives been re-evaluated?
- Has the resident received a psychological or psychiatric evaluation to evaluate, diagnose, or treat her/his condition, if necessary?
- Identify if resident triggers RAPs for activities, mood state, psychosocial well-being, and psychotropic drug use. Consider whether the RAPs were used to assess the causal factors for decline, potential for decline, or lack of improvement.
- How are mental and psychosocial adjustment difficulties addressed in the care plan?

See §483.45(a), F406 for health rehabilitative services for mental illness and mental retardation.

 Psychosocial adjustment difficulty does not display a pattern of decreased social interaction and/or increased withdrawn, angry, or depressive behaviors, unless the resident's clinical condition demonstrates that such a pattern was unavoidable.

F320 Avoidance of pattern of decreased social interaction

§483.25(f)(2)

(2) A resident whose assessment did not reveal a mental or psychosocial adjustment difficulty does not display a pattern of decreased social interaction and/or increased withdrawn, angry, or

depressive behaviors, unless the resident's clinical condition demonstrates that such a pattern is unavoidable.

Procedures §483.25(f)(2)

For sampled residents whose assessment did not reveal a mental or psychosocial adjustment difficulty, but who display decreased social interaction or increased withdrawn, angry, or depressed behaviors, determine, as appropriate, was this behavior unavoidable?

Probes §483.25(f)(2)

- Did the facility attempt to evaluate whether this behavior was attributable to organic causes or other risk factors not associated with adjusting to living in the nursing facility?
- What care did the resident receive to maintain his/her mental or psychosocial functioning?
- Were individual objectives of the plan of care periodically evaluated, and if progress was not made in reducing, maintaining, or increasing behaviors that assist the resident to have his/her needs met, were alternative treatment approaches developed to maintain mental or psychosocial functioning?
- Identify if resident triggers RAPs for behavior problem, cognitive loss/dementia, and psychosocial well-being. Consider whether the RAPs were used to assess causal factors for decline, potential for decline, or lack of improvement.
- Did the facility use the RAPs for behavior problems, cognitive loss/dementia, and psychosocial well-being to assess why the behaviors or change in mental or psychosocial functioning was occurring?

§483.25(g) Naso-Gastric Tubes

Based on the comprehensive assessment of a resident, the facility must ensure that—

(See Tag F322 for intent, guidelines, and probes for §483.25(g))

F321 Conditions for using naso-gastric tubes

§483.25(g)(1) A resident who has been able to eat enough alone or with assistance is not fed by naso-gastric tube unless the resident's clinical condition demonstrates that use of a naso-gastric tube was unavoidable; and

F322 Naso-gastric tube requirement for preventing aspiration, restoration of normal eating

§483.25(g)(2) A resident who is fed by a naso-gastric or gastrostomy tube receives the appropriate treatment and services to prevent aspiration pneumonia, diarrhea, vomiting, dehydration, metabolic abnormalities, and nasal-pharyngeal ulcers and to restore, if possible, normal eating skills.

Intent §483.25(g)

The intent of this regulation is that a naso-gastric tube feeding is utilized only after adequate assessment, and the resident's clinical condition makes this treatment necessary.

Interpretive Guidelines §483.25(g)

This corresponds to MDS 2.0 sections G, K, P when specified for use by the State.

This requirement is also intended to prevent the use of tube feeding when ordered over the objection of the resident. Decisions about the appropriateness of tube feeding for a resident are developed with the resident or his/her family, surrogate, or representative as part of determining the care plan.

Complications in tube feeding are not necessarily the result of improper care, but assessment for the potential for complications and care and treatment are provided to prevent complications in tube feeding by the facility.

Clinical conditions demonstrating that nourishment via a naso-gastric tube is unavoidable include:

- The inability to swallow without choking or aspiration, i.e., in cases of Parkinson's disease, pseudobulbar palsy, or esophageal diverticulum;
- Lack of sufficient alertness for oral nutrition (e.g., resident comatose); and
- Malnutrition not attributable to a single cause or causes that can be isolated and reversed. There is documented evidence that the facility has not been able to maintain or improve the resident's nutritional status through oral intake.

Probes §483.25(g)

For sampled residents who, upon admission to the facility, were not tube fed and now have a feeding tube, was tube feeding unavoidable? To determine if the tube feeding was unavoidable, assess the following:

- Did the facility identify the resident at risk for malnutrition?
- What did the facility do to maintain oral feeding, prior to inserting a feeding tube? Did staff provide enough assistance in eating? Did staff cue resident as needed, assist with the use of assistive devices, or feed the resident, if necessary?

- Is the resident receiving therapy to improve or enhance swallowing skills, as need is identified in the comprehensive assessment?
- Was an assessment done to determine the cause of decreased oral intake/weight loss or malnutrition?
- If there was a dietitian consultation, were recommendations followed?

For all sampled residents who are tube fed:

- Is the naso-gastric tube properly placed?
- Are staff responsibilities for providing enteral feedings clearly assigned (i.e., who administers the feeding, formula, amount, feeding intervals, flow rate)?
- Do staff monitor feeding complications (e.g., diarrhea, gastric distension, aspiration) and administer corrective actions to allay complications (e.g., changing rate of formula administration)?
- Are there negative consequences of tube use (e.g. agitation, depression, self-extubation, infections, aspiration, and restraint use without a medical reason for the restraint)?
- When long-term use is anticipated, is gastric tube placement considered?

Is the potential for complications from feedings minimized by:

- Use of a small bore, flexible naso-gastric tube, unless contraindicated;
- Securely attached tube to the nose/face;
- Checking for correct tube placement prior to beginning a feeding or administering medications and after episodes of vomiting or suctioning;
- Checking a resident with a newly inserted gastric tube for gastric residual volume every 2–4 hours until the resident has demonstrated an ability to empty his/her stomach;
- Properly elevating the resident's head;
- Providing the type, rate, and volume of the feeding as ordered;
- Using universal precautions and clean technique and as per facility/manufacturer's directions when stopping, starting, flushing, and giving medications through the tube;
- Using hang time recommendations by the manufacturer to prevent excessive microbial growth;
- Implement the procedures to ensure cleanliness of supplies, e.g. irrigating syringes changed on a regular bases as per facility policy. It is not necessary to change the irrigating syringe each time it is used;
- Using a pump equipped with a functional alarm (if pump used);
- The facility's criteria for determining that a resident may be able to return to eating by mouth (e.g., a resident whose Parkinson's symptoms have been controlled);
- There are sampled residents meet these criteria;
- If so, the facility has assisted them in returning to normal eating; and
- Identify if resident triggers RAPs for feeding tubes, nutritional status, and dehydration/fluid maintenance. Consider whether the RAPs were used to assess causal factors for decline, potential for decline, and lack of improvement.

F323 Resident environment free of accident hazards

§483.25(h) Accidents

The facility must ensure that—

§483.25(h)(1) The resident environment remains as free of accident hazards as is possible; and

Intent §483.25(h)(1)

The intent of this provision is that the facility prevents accidents by providing an environment that is free from hazards over which the facility has control.

Interpretive Guidelines §483.25(h)(1)

This corresponds to MDS version 2.0 section J, when specified for use by the State.

"Accident hazards" are defined as physical features in the NF environment that can endanger a resident's safety, including but not limited to:

- Physical restraints (see physical restraints §483.13);
- Equipment or devices that are defective, poorly maintained, or not used in accordance with manufacturer's specifications (e.g., wheelchairs or geri-chairs with nonworking brakes, and loose nuts and bolts on walkers);
- Bathing facilities that do not have nonslip surfaces;
- Hazards (e.g., electrical appliances with frayed wires, cleaning supplies easily accessible to cognitively impaired residents, wet floors that are not obviously labeled and to which access is not blocked);
- Defective or improperly latched side rails or spaces within side rails, between upper and lower rails, between rails and the mattress, between side rails and the bed frame, or spaces between side rails and the head or foot board of the bed that can entrap limbs, neck, or thorax, and can cause injury or death;
- Handrails not securely fixed to the wall, difficult to grasp, and/or with sharp edges/splinters; and
- Water temperatures in hand sinks or bathtubs which can scald or harm residents.

Probes §483.25(h)(1)

(See F221 for guidance concerning the use of bedrails.) See also §483.70(h), Safe Environment.

F324 Adequate resident supervision and assistive devices to prevent accidents

§483.25(h)(2) Each resident receives adequate supervision and assistance devices to prevent accidents.

Intent §483.25(h)(2)

The intent of this provision is that the facility identifies each resident at risk for accidents and/or falls, and adequately plans care and implements procedures to prevent accidents.

An "accident" is an unexpected, unintended event that can cause a resident bodily injury. It does not include adverse outcomes associated as a direct consequence of treatment or care (e.g., drug side effects or reactions).

Procedures §483.25(h)(2)

- If a resident(s) selected for a comprehensive or focused review has had an accident, review the facility's investigation of that accident and their response to prevent the accident from recurring.
- Identify if the resident triggers RAPs for falls, cognitive loss/dementia, physical restraints, and psychotropic drug use and whether the RAPs were used to assess causal factors for decline or lack of improvement.
- If the survey team identifies a number of or pattern of accidents, in Phase II sampling, review the quality assurance activities of the facility to determine the facility's response to accidents.

Probes §483.25(h)(2)

1. Are there a number of accidents or injuries of a specific type or on any specific shift (e.g., falls, skin injuries)?

2. Are residents who smoke properly supervised and monitored?

3. If the survey team identifies residents repeatedly involved in accidents or sampled residents who have had an accident:

   a. Is the resident assessed for being at risk for falls?

   b. What care-planning and implementation is the facility doing to prevent accidents and falls for those residents identified at risk?

   c. How did the facility fit, and monitor, the use of that resident's assistive devices?

   d. How were drugs that may cause postural hypotension, dizziness, or visual changes monitored?

§483.25(i) Nutrition

Based on a resident's comprehensive assessment, the facility must ensure that a resident—

(See F326 for intent, guidelines, procedures, and probes for §483.25(i))

F325 Maintain acceptable parameters of nutritional status for each resident

(1) Maintains acceptable parameters of nutritional status, such as body weight and protein levels, unless the resident's clinical condition demonstrates that this is not possible; and

F326 Provide therapeutic diets for each nutritional problem

§483.25(i)(2) Receives a therapeutic diet when there is a nutritional problem

Intent §483.25(i)

The intent of this regulation is to assure that the resident maintains acceptable parameters of nutritional status, taking into account the resident's clinical condition or other appropriate intervention, when there is a nutritional problem.

Interpretive Guidelines §483.25(i)

This corresponds to MDS 2.0 sections G, I, J, K, and L when specified for use by the State.

Parameters of nutritional status which are unacceptable include unplanned weight loss as well as other indices such as peripheral edema, cachexia, and laboratory tests indicating malnourishment (e.g., serum albumin levels).

Weight

Since ideal body weight charts have not yet been validated for the institutionalized elderly, weight loss (or gain) is a guide in determining nutritional status. An analysis of weight loss or gain should be examined in light of the individual's former lifestyle as well as the current diagnosis.

Suggested parameter for evaluating significance of unplanned and undesired weight loss are:

Interval	Significant Loss	Severe Loss
1 month	5%	Greater than 5%
3 months	7.5%	Greater than 7.5%
6 months	10%	Greater than 10%

The following formula determines percentage of loss:

$$\% \text{ of body weight loss} = \frac{\text{usual weight} - \text{actual weight}}{\text{usual weight}} \times 100$$

In evaluating weight loss, consider the resident's usual weight through adult life; the assessment of potential for weight loss; and care plan for weight management. Also, was the resident on a calorie restricted diet, or if newly admitted and obese, and on a normal diet, are fewer calories provided than prior to admission? Was the resident edematous when initially weighed, and with treatment, no longer has edema? Has the resident refused food?

Suggested laboratory values are:

Albumin >60 yr.: 3.4–4.8 g/dl (good for examining marginal protein depletion).
Plasma Transferrin >60 yr.: 180–380 g/dl. (Rises with iron deficiency anemia. More persistent indicator of protein status.)

Hemoglobin Males: 14–17 g/dl; Females: 12–15 g/dl

Hematocrit Males: 41–53 Females: 36–46

Potassium: 3.5–5.0 mEq/L

Magnesium 1.3–2.0 mEg/L

Some laboratories may have different "normals." Determine range for the specific laboratory.

Because some healthy elderly people have abnormal laboratory values, and because abnormal values can be expected in some disease processes, do not expect laboratory values to be within normal ranges for all residents. Consider abnormal values in conjunction with the resident's clinical condition and baseline normal values.

NOTE: There is no requirement that facilities order the tests referenced above.

Clinical Observations

Potential indicators of malnutrition are pale skin, dull eyes, swollen lips, swollen gums, swollen and/or dry tongue with scarlet or magenta hue, poor skin turgor, cachexia, bilateral edema, and muscle wasting.

Risk factors for malnutrition are:

1. Drug therapy that may contribute to nutritional deficiencies such as:

    a. Cardiac glycosides;
    b. Diuretics;
    c. Anti-inflammatory drugs;
    d. Antacids (antacid overuse);
    e. Laxatives (laxative overuse);
    f. Psychotropic drug overuse;
    g. Anticonvulsants;
    h. Antineoplastic drugs;
    i. Phenothiazines;
    j. Oral hypoglycemics;

2. Poor oral health status or hygiene, eyesight, motor coordination, or taste alterations;

3. Depression or dementia;

4. Therapeutic or mechanically altered diet;

5. Lack of access to culturally acceptable foods;

6. Slow eating pace resulting in food becoming unpalatable, or in staff removing the tray before resident has finished eating; and

7. Cancer.

Clinical conditions demonstrating that the maintenance of acceptable nutritional status may not be possible include, but are not limited to:

- Refusal to eat and refusal of other methods of nourishment;
- Advanced disease (i.e., cancer, malabsorption syndrome);
- Increased nutritional/caloric needs associated with pressure sores and wound healing (e.g., fractures, burns);
- Radiation or chemotherapy;
- Kidney disease, alcohol/drug abuse, chronic blood loss, hyperthyroidism;
- Gastrointestinal surgery; and
- Prolonged nausea, vomiting, diarrhea not relieved by treatment given according to accepted standards of practice.

"Therapeutic diet" means a diet ordered by a physician as part of treatment for a disease or clinical condition, to eliminate or decrease certain substances in the diet, (e.g., sodium) or to increase certain substances in the diet (e.g., potassium), or to provide food the resident is able to eat (e.g., a mechanically altered diet).

Procedures §483.25(i)

Determine if residents selected for a comprehensive review or focused review as appropriate, have maintained acceptable parameters of nutritional status. Where indicated by the resident's medical status, have clinically appropriate therapeutic diets been prescribed?

Probes §483.25(i)

For sampled residents whose nutritional status is inadequate, do clinical conditions demonstrate that maintenance of inadequate nutritional status was unavoidable:

- Did the facility identify factors that put the resident at risk for malnutrition?
- Identify if resident triggered RAPs for nutritional status, ADL functional/rehabilitation potential, feeding tubes, psychotropic drug use, and dehydration/fluid balance. Consider whether the RAPs were used to assess the causal factors for decline, potential for decline, or lack of improvement.
- What routine preventive measures and care did the resident receive to address unique risk factors for malnutrition (e.g., provision of an adequate diet with supplements or modifications as indicated by nutrient needs)?
- Were staff responsibilities for maintaining nutritional status clear, including monitoring the amount of food the resident is eating at each meal and offering substitutes?
- Was this care provided consistently?
- Were individual goals of the plan of care periodically evaluated and if not met, were alternative approaches considered or attempted?

F327 Resident hydration

§483.25(j) Hydration

§483.25(j) Hydration. The facility must provide each resident with sufficient fluid intake to maintain proper hydration and health.

Intent §483.25(j)

The intent of this regulation is to assure that the resident receives sufficient amount of fluids based on individual needs to prevent dehydration.

Interpretive Guidelines §483.25(j)

This corresponds to MDS 2.0 sections G, K, I, J, and L when specified for use by the State.

"Sufficient fluid" means the amount of fluid needed to prevent dehydration (output of fluids far exceeds fluid intake) and maintain health. The amount needed is specific for each resident, and fluctuates as the resident's condition fluctuates (e.g., increase fluids if resident has fever or diarrhea).

Risk factors for the resident becoming dehydrated are:

- Coma/decreased sensorium;
- Fluid loss and increased fluid needs (e.g., diarrhea, fever, uncontrolled diabetes);
- Fluid restriction secondary to renal dialysis;
- Functional impairments that make it difficult to drink, reach fluids, or communicate fluid needs (e.g., aphasia);
- Dementia in which resident forgets to drink or forgets how to drink;
- Refusal of fluids; and
- Did the MDS trigger RAPs on hydration? What action was taken based on the RAP?

Consider whether assessment triggers RAPs and are RAPs used to assess the causal factors for decline, potential for decline, or lack of improvement.

A general guideline for determining baseline daily fluid needs is to multiply the resident's body weight in kg times 30cc (2.2 lbs = 1kg), except for residents with renal or cardiac distress. An excess of fluids can be detrimental for these residents.

Procedures §483.25(j)

Identify if resident triggers RAPs for dehydration/fluid maintenance, and cognitive loss.

Probes §483.25(j)

Do sampled residents show clinical signs of possible insufficient fluid intake (e.g., dry skin and mucous membranes, cracked lips, poor skin turgor, thirst, fever), abnormal laboratory values (e.g., elevated hemoglobin and hematocrit, potassium, chloride, sodium, albumin, transferrin, blood urea nitrogen (BUN), or urine specific gravity)?

Has the facility provided residents with adequate fluid intake to maintain proper hydration and health? If not:

- Did the facility identify any factors that put the resident at risk of dehydration?
- What care did the facility provide to reduce those risk factors and ensure adequate fluid intake (e.g., keep fluids next to the resident at all times and assisting or cuing the resident to drink)? Is staff aware of need for maintaining adequate fluid intake?
- If adequate fluid intake is difficult to maintain, have alternative treatment approaches been developed, attempt to increase fluid intake by the use of popsicles, gelatin, and other similar non-liquid foods?

F328 Special needs: injections, parenteral and enteral fluids, colostomy, ureterostomy or ileostomy care, tracheostomy care, tracheal suctioning, respiratory care, foot care, and prostheses

§483.25(k) Special Needs

The facility must ensure that residents receive proper treatment and care for the following special services

Intent 483.25(k)

The intent of this provision is that the resident receives the necessary care and treatment including medical and nursing care and services when they need the specialized services as listed below.

Interpretive Guidelines §483.25(k)

This corresponds to MDS 2.0 section P when specified by for use by the State.

The non-availability of program funding does not relieve a facility of its obligation to ensure that its residents receive all needed services listed in §1819(b)(4)(A) of the Act for Medicare and §1919(b)(4)(A) of the Act for Medicaid. For services not covered, a facility is required to assist the resident in securing any available resources to obtain the needed services.

§483.25(k)(1) Injections

Probes §483.25(k)(1)

For sampled residents receiving one or more of these services within 7 days of the survey:

- Is proper administration technique used (i.e., maintenance of sterility; correct needle size, route)?
- Are there signs of redness, swelling, lesions from previous injections?
- If appropriate, is resident observed for adverse reaction after the injection?
- Are syringes and needles disposed of according to facility policy and accepted Practice (e.g., Centers for Disease Control and Prevention and Occupational Safety and Health Administration guidelines)?
- Do nursing notes indicate, as appropriate, the resident's response to treatment (e.g., side effects/adverse actions; problems at the injection site(s); relief of pain)?

§483.25(k)(2) Parenteral and Enteral Fluids

Probes §483.25(k)(2)

This corresponds to MDS 2.0 sections K5 and 6 and P1 when specified for use by the State.

For residents selected for a comprehensive review, or focused review as appropriate, receiving one or more of these services within 7 days of the survey:

- Are there signs of inflammation or infiltration at the insertion site?
- If the IV site, tubing, or bottle/bag is changed, is sterile technique maintained?
- Is the rate of administration that which is ordered by the physician?
- Has the resident received the amount of fluid during the past 24 hours that he/she should have received according to the physician's orders (allow flexibility up to 150cc unless an exact fluid intake is critical for the resident)?

Procedures §483.25(k)(2)

See §483.25(g) for enteral feedings (includes gastrostomy).

§483.25(k)(3) Colostomy, Ureterostomy, or Ileostomy care

Procedures §483.25(k)(3)

This corresponds to MDS 2.0 sections G, H, and P when specified for use by the State.

Identify if resident triggers RAPs for urinary incontinence, nutritional status, pressure ulcers (skin care).

Probes §483.25(k)(3)

- If appropriate, is the resident provided with self-care instructions?

Does the staff member observe and respond to any signs of resident's discomfort about the ostomy or its care?

- Is skin surrounding the ostomy free of excoriation (abrasion, breakdown)?
- If excoriation is present, does the clinical record indicate an onset and a plan of care to treat the excoriation?

§483.25(k)(4) Tracheostomy Care

Procedures §483.25(k)(4) (Includes care of the tracheostomy site)

This corresponds to MDS 2.0 sections M and P when specified for use by the State.

Observations for tracheostomy care are most appropriate for residents with new or relatively new tracheostomies, and may not be appropriate for those with tracheostomies of long standing.

Probes §483.25(k)(4) (Includes care of the tracheostomy site)

- Is the skin around the tracheostomy clean and dry? Are the dressing and the ties clean and dry, with the cannula secure?

- Does the resident have signs of an obstructed airway or need for suctioning (e.g., secretions draining from mouth or tracheotomy; unable to cough to clear chest; audible crackles or wheezes; dyspneic; restless or agitated)?
- If appropriate for a specific resident, is there a suction machine and catheter immediately available?
- Is there an extra cannula of the correct size at the bedside or other place easily accessible if needed in an emergency?

For sampled residents receiving one or more of these services within 7 days of the survey:

- Is suction machine available for immediate use, clean, working, and available to a source of emergency power?
- Is there an adequate supply of easily accessible suction catheters?

§483.25(k)(5) Standard: Tracheal Suctioning

Probes §483.25(k)(5)

This corresponds to MDS 2.0 section P when specified for use by the State

§483.25(k)(6) Standard: Respiratory Care

Procedures §483.25(k)(6)

This corresponds to MDS 2.0 section P when specified for use by the State.

Includes use of respirators/ventilators, oxygen, intermittent positive pressure breathing (IPPB) or other inhalation therapy, pulmonary care, humidifiers, and other methods to treat conditions of the respiratory tract.

Identify if resident triggers RAPs for delirium and dehydration/fluid maintenance.

Probes §483.25(k)(6)

For sampled residents receiving one or more of these services within 7 days of the survey:

- If oxygen is in use, are precautions observed (e.g., proper storage and handling of oxygen cylinders secured)? Secondary "No Smoking" signs are not required in facilities that prohibit smoking and have signs at all major entrances that the facility does not allow smoking.
- If the survey team observes a treatment being administered, is the resident encouraged and instructed on how to assist in the treatment?
- Is the staff following the facility's protocol and/or written procedures for ventilators (e.g., functioning alarms); frequency of staff monitoring; monitoring of resident response (e.g., use of accessory muscles to breathe, cleanliness of mouth, skin irritation); and availability of manual resuscitators?

- If the resident is ventilator dependent, is routine machine maintenance and care done (e.g., water changes/tubing changes, safety checks on alarms, and machine functioning checks)?

§483.25(k)(7) Foot Care

Procedures §483.25(k)(7)

This corresponds with MDS 2.0 sections G and M when specified for use by the State.

Includes treatment of foot disorders—by qualified persons, e.g., podiatrist, Doctor of Medicine, Doctor of Osteopathy—including, but not limited to, corns, neuroma, calluses, bunions, heel spurs, nail disorders, and preventive care to avoid foot problems in diabetic residents and residents with circulatory disorders.

Probes §483.25(k)(7)

For residents selected for a comprehensive review, or focused review, as appropriate:

- Do nails, corns, calluses, and other foot problems appear unattended; do these foot problems interfere with resident mobility?
- Are residents able to see a qualified person when they want?
- What preventive foot care do staff provide diabetic residents?

§483.25(k)(8) Prostheses

Probes §483.25(k)(8)

MDS 2.0 sections D, G, L, M, and P when specified for use by the State.

Includes artificial limbs, eyes, teeth.

For residents selected for a comprehensive review, or focused review, as appropriate:

- Is resident able to put on the prosthesis by himself/herself or with some assistance?
- Are residents wearing their prostheses?
- Does the prosthesis fit correctly?
- Is skin/mucous membrane in contact with the prosthesis free of abrasions, wounds, irritation?

F329 Unnecessary drugs

(Rev. 12, Issued: 10-14-05, Effective: 10-14-05, Implementation: 10-14-05)

§483.25(l) Unnecessary Drugs

1. General. Each resident's drug regimen must be free from unnecessary drugs. An unnecessary drug is any drug when used:

(i) In excessive dose (including duplicate therapy); or

(ii) For excessive duration; or

(iii) Without adequate monitoring; or

(iv) Without adequate indications for its use; or

(v) In the presence of adverse consequences which indicate the dose should be reduced or discontinued; or

(vi) Any combinations of the reasons above.

Interpretive Guidelines §483.25(l)(1)

It is important to note that these regulations and interpretive guidelines are not meant to cast a negative light on the use of psychopharmacological drugs in long-term care facilities. The use of psychopharmacological drugs can be therapeutic and enabling for residents suffering from mental illnesses such as schizophrenia or depression. The goal of these regulations and guidelines is to stimulate appropriate differential diagnosis of "behavioral symptoms" so the underlying cause of the symptoms is recognized and treated appropriately. This treatment may include the use of environmental and/or behavioral therapy, as well as, psychopharmacological drugs. The goal of these regulations is also to prevent the use of psychopharmacological drugs when the "behavioral symptom" is caused by conditions such as: (1) environmental stressors (e.g., excessive heat, noise, overcrowding); (2) psychosocial stressors (e.g., abuse, taunting, not following a resident's customary daily routine); or (3) treatable medical conditions (e.g., heart disease, diabetes, Chronic Obstructive Pulmonary Disease). Behavioral symptoms resulting from these causes should not be "covered up" with sedating drugs.

An excellent differential diagnostic process for behavioral symptoms is described in the RAP on Behavior Problems (soon to be known as behavioral symptoms). Also, a number of very practical manuals are now available that teach nursing personnel how to assess and provide individualized care for behavioral symptoms, which leads to the avoidance of physical restraints, and unnecessary drugs. These manuals include, but are not limited to, the following list:

1. "Managing Behavior Problems in Nursing Home Residents"
   Department of Preventive Medicine
   Vanderbilt University School of Medicine

2. "Retrain, Don't Restrain"
   American Association of Homes and Services for the Aging, or
   The American Health Care Association

3. "Innovations in Restraint Reduction"
   American Health Care Association

4. "Avoiding Physical Restraint Use: New Standards in Care"
   National Citizens' Coalition for Nursing Home Reform

5. "Avoiding Drugs Used as Chemical Restraints: New Standards in Care"
   National Citizens' Coalition for Nursing Home Reform

Interpretive Guidelines §483.25(l)(1)

A. Long-Acting Benzodiazepine Drugs

The following long-acting benzodiazepine drugs should not be used in residents unless an attempt with a shorter-acting drug (i.e., those listed under B. Benzodiazepine or Other Anxiolytic/Sedative Drugs, and under C. Drugs Used for Sleep Induction) has failed.

After an attempt with a shorter-acting benzodiazepine drug has failed, a long-acting benzodiazepine drug should not be used unless:

- Evidence exists that other possible reasons for the resident's distress have been considered and ruled out. (See §483.25(l)(1)(iv).);
- Its use results in maintenance or improvement in the resident's functional status (to evaluate functional status, see §483.25(a) through (k) and MDS 2.0 sections B through P). (See §483.25(l)(1)(iv).);
- Daily use is less than four continuous months unless an attempt at a gradual dose reduction is unsuccessful. (See §483.25(l)(1)(ii).); and
- Its use is less than, or equal to, the following listed total daily doses unless higher doses (as evidenced by the resident's response and/or the resident's clinical record) are necessary for the maintenance, or improvement in the resident's functional status. (See §483.25(l)(1)(i).)

Long-Acting Benzodiazepines — Not Maximum Doses

LONG-ACTING BENZODIAZEPINES		NOT MAXIMUM DOSES
Generic	Brand	Daily Oral Dosage
Flurazepam	(Dalmane®)	15mg
Chlordiazepoxide	(Librium®)	20mg
Clorazepate	(Tranxene®)	15mg
Diazepam	(Valium®)	5mg
Clonazepam	(Klonopin®)	1.5mg
Quazepam	(Doral®)	7.5mg
Halazepam	(Paxipam®)	40mg

NOTES: When diazepam is used for neuromuscular syndromes (e.g., cerebral palsy, tardive dyskinesia, or seizure disorders), this guideline does not apply.

When long-acting benzodiazepine drugs are being used to withdraw residents from short-acting benzodiazepine drugs, this guideline does not apply.

When clonazepam is used in bi-polar disorders, management of tardive dyskinesia, nocturnal myoclonus, or seizure disorders, this guideline does not apply.

The daily doses listed under long-acting Benzodiazepines are doses (usually administered in divided doses) for "geriatric" or "elderly" residents. The facility is encouraged to initiate therapy with lower doses and when necessary only gradually increase doses. The facility may exceed these doses if it provides evidence (see Survey Procedures and Probes) to show why it was necessary for the maintenance or improvement in the resident's functional status.

"Duplicate drug therapy" is any drug therapy that duplicates a particular drug effect on the resident. For example, any two or more drugs, whether from the same drug category or not, which have a sedative effect. Duplicate drug therapy should prompt the facility to evaluate the resident for accumulation of the adverse effects.

For drugs in this category, a gradual dose reduction should be attempted at least twice within one year before one can conclude that the gradual dose reduction is clinically contraindicated.

B. Benzodiazepine or Other Anxiolytic/Sedative Drugs

Use of listed Anxiolytic/Sedative drugs for purposes other than sleep induction should only occur when:

1. Evidence exists that other possible reasons for the resident's distress have been considered and ruled out. (See §483.25(l)(1)(iv));

2. Use results in a maintenance or improvement in the resident's functional status (to evaluate functional status, see §483.25(a) through (k) and MDS 2.0 sections B through P). (See §483.25(l)(1)(iv));

3. Daily use (at any dose) is less than four continuous months unless an attempt at a gradual dose reduction is unsuccessful. (See §483.25(l)(1)(ii));

4. Use is for one of the following indications as defined by the Diagnostic and Statistical Manual of Mental Disorders, Fourth Edition (DSM-IV) or subsequent editions. (See §483.25(l)(1)(iv)):

   a. Generalized anxiety disorder;

   b. Organic mental syndromes (now called "delirium, dementia, and amnestic and other cognitive disorders" by DSM-IV) with associated agitated behaviors, which are quantitatively and objectively documented (see note number one) which are persistent and not due to preventable reasons and which constitute sources of distress or dysfunction to the resident or represent a danger to the resident or others;

    c. Panic disorder;

    d. Symptomatic anxiety that occurs in residents with another diagnosed psychiatric disorder (e.g., depression, adjustment disorder); and

5. Use is equal to or less than the following listed total daily doses, unless higher doses (as evidenced by the resident response and/or the resident's clinical record) are necessary for the improvement or maintenance in the resident's functional status. (See §483.25(l)(1)(i), F342.)

Short-Acting Benzodiazepines — Not Maximum Doses

SHORT-ACTING BENZODIAZEPINES / NOT MAXIMUM DOSES

Generic	Brand	Daily Oral Dosage
Lorazepam	(Ativan®)	2 mg
Oxazepam	(Serax®)	30 mg
Alprazolam	(Xanex®)	0.75 mg
Estazolam	(ProSom®)	0.5 mg

OTHER ANXIOLYTIC AND SEDATIVE DRUGS

Generic	Brand	Daily Oral Dosage
Diphenhydramine	(Benadryl®)	50 mg
Hydroxyzine	(Atarax®, Vistaril®)	50 mg
Chloral Hydrate	(many brands)	750 mg

NOTES

1. This documentation is often referred to as "behavioral monitoring charts" and is necessary to assist in: (a) assessing whether the resident's behavioral symptom is in need of some form of intervention, (b) determining whether the behavioral symptom is transitory or permanent, (c) relating the behavioral symptom to other events in the resident's life in order to learn about potential causes (e.g., death in the family, not adhering to the resident's customary daily routine), (d) ruling out environmental causes such as excessive heat, noise, overcrowding, etc., (e) ruling out medical causes such as pain, constipation, fever, infection. For a more complete description of behavioral monitoring charts and how they can assist in the differential diagnosis of behavioral symptoms see the RAP on behavior problems (soon to be know as behavioral symptoms).

2. The daily doses listed under Short-Acting Benzodiazepines are doses (usually administered in divided doses) for "geriatric" or "elderly" residents. The facility is encouraged to initiate therapy with lower doses and, when necessary, only **gradually** increase doses. The facility may exceed these doses if it provides evidence (see survey procedures and probes) to show why it was necessary for the maintenance or improvement in the resident's functional status.

3. For drugs in this category, a gradual dose reduction should be attempted at least twice within one year before one can conclude that a gradual dose reduction is clinically contraindicated.

4. Diphenhydramine, hydroxyzine and chloral hydrate are not necessarily drugs of choice for treatment of anxiety disorders. They are only listed here in the event of their potential use.

C. Drugs for Sleep Induction

Drugs used for sleep induction should only be used if:

- Evidence exists that other possible reasons for insomnia (e.g., depression, pain, noise, light, caffeine) have been ruled out. (See §483.25(1)(1)(iv));
- The use of a drug to induce sleep results in the maintenance or improvement of the resident's functional status (to evaluate functional status, see §483.25(a) through (k) and MDS 2.0 sections B through P). (See §483.25(1)(1)(iv);)
- Daily use of the drug is less than ten continuous days unless an attempt at a gradual dose reduction is unsuccessful. (See §483.25(1)(1)(ii);) and
- The dose of the drug is equal or less than the following listed doses unless higher doses (as evidenced by the resident response and/or the resident's clinical record) are necessary for maintenance or improvement in the resident's functional status. (See §483.25(1)(1)(i).)

HYPNOTIC DRUGS		NOT MAXIMUM DOSES
Generic	**Brand**	**Dose by Mouth**
Temazepam	(Restoril®)	7.5 mg
Triazolam	(Halcion®)	0.125 mg
Lorazepam	(Ativan®)	1 mg
Oxazepam	(Serax®)	15 mg
Alpraxolam	(Xanax®)	0.25 mg
Estazolam	(ProSom®)	0.5 mg
Diphenhydramine	(Benadryl®)	25 mg
Hydroxyzine	(Atarax®, Vistaril®)	50 mg
Chloral Hydrate	(many brands)	500 mg
Zolpidem	(Ambien®)	5 mg

NOTES

1. Diminished sleep in the elderly is not necessarily pathological.

2. The doses listed are doses for "geriatric" or "elderly" residents. The facility is encouraged to initiate therapy with lower doses and when necessary only **gradually** increase doses. The facility may exceed these doses if it provides evidence (see survey procedures and probes) to show why it was necessary for the maintenance or improvement in the resident's functional status.

3. Diphenhydramine, hydroxyzine, and chloral hydrate are not necessarily drugs of choice for sleep disorders. They are listed here only in the event of their potential use.

4. For drugs in this category, a gradual dose reduction should be attempted at least three times within six months before one can conclude that a gradual dose reduction is clinically contraindicated.

D. Miscellaneous Hypnotic/Sedative/Anxiolytic Drugs

The **initiation** of the following hypnotic/sedative/anxiolytic drugs should not occur in any dose for any resident. (See Notes for exceptions.) Residents currently using these drugs or residents admitted to the facility while using these drugs should receive **gradual** dose reductions as part of a plan to eliminate or modify the symptoms for which they are prescribed. A gradual dose reduction should be attempted at least twice within one year before one can conclude that the gradual dose reduction is clinically contraindicated. Newly admitted residents using these drugs may have a period of adjustment before a **gradual** dose reduction is attempted.

(CAUTION: DO NOT ENCOURAGE RAPID WITHDRAWAL OF THESE DRUGS. THIS MIGHT RESULT IN SEVERE PHYSIOLOGICAL WITHDRAWAL SYMPTOMS.)

BARBITURATES (EXAMPLES)

Generic	Brand
Amobarbital	(Amytal®)
Butabarbital	(Butisol®, others)
Pentobarbital	(Nembutal®)
Secobarbital	(Seconal®)
Phenobarbital	(many brands)
Amobarbital-Secobarbital	(Tuinal®)
Barbiturates with other drugs	(e.g., Fiorinal®)

MISCELLANEOUS HYPNOTIC/SEDATIVE/ANXIOLYTICS

Generic	Brand
Glutethimide	(Doriden®)
Methprylon	(Noludar®)
Ethchlorvynol	(Placidyl®)
Meprobamate	(Equinal®, Miltown®)
Paraldehyde	(many brands)

1. Any sedative drug is excepted from this Guideline when used as a single dose sedative for dental or medical procedures.

2. Phenobarbital is excepted from this Guideline when used in the treatment of seizure disorders.

3. When Miscellaneous Hypnotic/Sedative/Anxiolytic Drugs are used outside these Guidelines they may be unnecessary drugs as a result of inadequate indications for use. (See Survey Procedures and Probes.)

E. Antipsychotic Drug Dosage Levels

Screen for Higher Doses of Antipsychotic Drugs

These dose levels are NOT MAXIMUM DOSES. These daily dose levels are given to establish a point at which higher doses should be explained. If a resident is prescribed a higher dose than shown, the facility should explain the specific clinical circumstance requiring the higher dose.

ANTIPSYCHOTIC DRUGS		DAILY ANTIPSYCHOTIC ORAL DOSAGE FOR RESIDENTS WITH ORGANIC MENTAL SYNDROMES MG/DAY
Generic	**Brand**	
Chlorpromazine	(Thorazine®)	75
Promazine	(Sparine®)	150
Triflupromazine	(Vesprin®)	20
Thioridazine	(Mellaril®)	75
Mesoridazine	(Serentil®)	25
Acetophenazine	(Tindal®)	20
Perphenazine	(Trilafon®)	8
Fluphenazine	(Prolixin®, Permitil®)	4
Trifluoperazine	(Stelazine®)	8
Chlorprothixene	(Taractan®)	75
Thiothixene	(Navane®)	7
Halperidol	(Haldol®)	4
Molindone	(Moban®)	10
Loxapine	(Loxitane®)	10
Clozapine	(Clozaril®)	50
Prochlorperazine	(Compazine®)	10
Risperidone	(Risperidal®)	2
Olanzapine	(Zyprexa®)	10
Quetiapine	(Seroquel®)	200

1. The doses listed are daily doses (usually administered in divided doses) for residents with organic mental syndromes (now called "Delirium, Dementia, and Amnestic" and other cognitive disorders by DSM-IV). The facility is encouraged to initiate therapy with lower doses and when necessary only gradually increase doses. The facility may exceed these doses if it provides evidence (see Survey Procedures and Probes) to show why it is necessary for the maintenance or improvement in the resident's functional status.

2. The "specific conditions" for use of antipsychotic drugs are listed under the Guideline for §§483.25(l)(1) and (2).

3. The dose of prochlorperazine may be exceeded for short-term (seven days) treatment of nausea and vomiting. Residents with nausea and vomiting secondary to cancer or cancer chemotherapy can also be treated with higher doses for longer periods of time.

4. When antipsychotic drugs are used outside these Guidelines without valid reasons for the higher dose, they may be deemed unnecessary drugs as a result of excessive dose.

F. Monitoring for Antipsychotic Drug Side Effects

The facility assures that residents who are undergoing antipsychotic drug therapy receive adequate monitoring for significant side effects of such therapy with emphasis on the following:

- Tardive dyskinesia;
- Postural (orthostatic) hypotension;
- Cognitive/behavior impairment;
- Akathisia; and
- Parkinsonism.

NOTES: For a more detailed description of these side effects, see the RAP: Psychotropic Drug Use, pg. C-91, "Revised Long Term Care Resident Assessment Instrument User's Manual," Version 2.0, December 2002.

When antipsychotic drugs are used without monitoring for these side effects, they may be unnecessary drugs because of inadequate monitoring.

G. Antidepressant Drugs

The under diagnosis and under treatment of depression in nursing homes has been documented in a Journal of the American Medical Association paper entitled "Depression and Mortality in the Nursing Home" (JAMA, February 27, 1991-vol. 265, No. 8). CMS continues to support the accurate identification and treatment of depression in nursing homes.

The following is a list of commonly used antidepressant drugs:

ANTIDEPRESSANT DRUGS

Generic	Brand
Amitriptyline*	(Elavil®)
Amoxapine	(Asendin®)
Desipramine	(Norpramin®, Pertofrane®)
Doxepin*	(Sinequan®)
Imipramine*	(Tofranil®)
Maprotiline	(Ludiomil®)
Nortriptyline	(Aventyl®, Pamelor®)
Protriptyline	(Vivactil®)
Trimipramine*	(Surmontil®)
Fluoxetine	(Prozac®)
Sertraline	(Zoloft®)
Trazodone	(Desyrel®)
Clomipramine*	(Anafranil®)
Paroxetine	(Paxil®)
Bupropion	(Wellbutrin®)
Isocarboxazid*	(Marplan®)

Phenelzine*	(Nardil®)
Tranylcypromine*	(Parnate®)
Venlafaxine	(Effexor®)
Nefazodone	(Serzone®)
Fluvoxamine	(Luvox®)

* These are not necessarily drugs of choice for depression in the elderly. They are listed here only in the event of their potential use.

Procedures 483.25(l)(1)

Consider drug therapy "unnecessary" only after determining that the facility's use of the drug is:

- In excessive dose (including duplicate drug therapy);
- For excessive duration;
- Without adequate monitoring;
- Without adequate indications of use;
- Any combination of the reasons above.

Allow the facility the opportunity to provide a rationale for the use of drugs prescribed outside the preceding Guidelines. The facility may not justify the use of a drug prescribed outside the proceeding Guidelines solely on the basis of "the doctor ordered it." This justification would render the regulation meaningless. The rationale must be based on sound risk-benefit analysis of the resident's symptoms and potential adverse effects of the drug.

Examples of evidence that would support a justification of why a drug is being used outside these Guidelines but in the best interests of the resident may include, but are not limited to:

- A physician's note indicating for example, that the dosage, duration, indication, and monitoring are clinically appropriate, **and the reasons why they are clinically appropriate;** this note should demonstrate that the physician has carefully considered the risk/benefit to the resident in using drugs outside the Guidelines.
- A medical or psychiatric consultation or evaluation (e.g., Geriatric Depression Scale) that confirms the physician's judgment that use of a drug outside the Guidelines is in the best interest of the resident.
- Physician, nursing, or other health professional documentation indicating that the resident is being monitored for adverse consequences or complications of the drug therapy;
- Documentation confirming that previous attempts at dosage reduction have been unsuccessful;
- Documentation (including MDS documentation) showing resident's subjective or objective improvement, or maintenance of function while taking the medication;
- Documentation showing that a resident's decline or deterioration is evaluated by the interdisciplinary team to determine whether a particular drug, or a particular dose, or duration of therapy, may be the cause;
- Documentation showing why the resident's age, weight, or other factors would require a unique drug dose or drug duration, indication, monitoring; and
- Other evidence the survey team may deem appropriate.

If the survey team determines that there is a deficiency in the use of antipsychotics, cite the facility under either the "unnecessary drug" regulation or the "antipsychotic drug" regulation, but not both.

NOTE: The unnecessary drug criterion of "adequate indications for use" does not simply mean that the **physician's order** must include a reason for using the drug (although such order writing is encouraged). It means that the **resident** lacks a valid clinical reason for use of the drug as evidenced by the survey team's evaluation of some, but not necessarily all, of the following: resident assessment, plan of care, reports of significant change, progress notes, laboratory reports, professional consults, drug orders, observation and interview of the resident, and other information.

H. Miscellaneous Drugs That are Potentially Inappropriate in the Elderly:

The following list of drugs and diagnoses/drug combinations have been partially adapted from a paper entitled "Explicit Criteria for Determining Inappropriate Medication Use by the Elderly" by Mark H. Beers, M.D. This paper was published in the *Archives of Internal Medicine*, Vol. 157, July 28, 1997. The paper lists numerous drugs and diagnosis/drug combinations that are judged to place a person over the age of 65 at greater risk of adverse drug outcomes (ADR). The judgments in this paper were arrived at through an extensive review of the literature by a panel of experts. There are two important quotations from the paper that the surveyor should keep in mind at all times:

1. "These criteria were developed to predict when the potential for adverse outcomes is greater than the potential for benefit"; and

2. "Without measuring outcomes, criteria cannot determine whether adverse outcomes have occurred; they can only determine that they are more likely to occur."

These criteria are divided into two broad categories. Drug therapy that is classified as having "high severity" and therapy that is considered as not having "high severity." Severity is defined as: "a combination of both the likelihood that an adverse outcome would occur and the clinical significance of that outcome should it occur." The survey guidelines are located in two parts, F329 and F429. The surveyor has the option to cite at either or both tags depending on the situation.

1. Drug Therapy With High Potential for Severe Adverse Outcomes in Persons Over 65 that are to be used to determine compliance with 483.25(1)(1), Unnecessary Drug (F329); and

2. Drug Therapy With High Potential for Less Severe Adverse Outcomes In Persons Over 65 that are to be used to determine compliance with 483.60(c)(1), Drug Regimen Review Report, (F429) which are located under guidance to surveyors for drug regimen review.

It should be noted that medication alterations may not be appropriate for some short-term residents. Many residents arrive in the long-term care setting already on medications that they have managed to tolerate for years or that have been prescribed in the hospital. For some short-stay residents, it is difficult to change these medications without a period of observation and information gathering. Therefore, review by the surveyor is not necessary for drug therapy given the first seven consecutive days upon admission/readmission, unless there is an immediate threat to health and safety. These guidelines do not supercede the unnecessary drug guidelines and drug regimen review guidelines.

List of Drugs With High Potential for Severe Adverse Outcomes

1. Pentazocine (Talwin)

Risk: "Pentazocine is a narcotic analgesic that causes more central nervous system side effects, including confusion and hallucinations, more commonly than other narcotic drugs." Dizziness, lightheadedness, euphoria, and sedation are also common side effects of pentazocine.

2. Long-Acting Benzodiazepines

NOTE: Surveyor guidance for unnecessary drugs (§483.25(1)(1), F329) already has guidelines for Long Acting Benzodiazepine Drugs. The Surveyor should use that guideline. This guideline is repeated here to give emphasis to potential side effects of these drugs.

Risk: "These benzodiazepine drugs have an extremely long half-life in the elderly (often days), producing prolonged sedation and increased incidence of falls and fractures." Other common side effects of benzodiazepine drugs include drowsiness, ataxia, fatigue, confusion, weakness, dizziness, vertigo, syncope, and psychological changes.

3. Amitriptyline (Elavil) Also include combination products such as: Amitriptyline and chlordiazepoxide (Limbitrol) Amitriptyline and Perphenazine (Triavil).

Risk: "Because of its strong anticholinergic and sedating properties, amitriptyline is rarely the antidepressant of choice in the elderly." Anticholinergic side effects are indicated by symptoms such as dry mouth, blurred vision, urinary retention, constipation, confusion, and sometimes, delirium or hallucinations. Amitriptyline can also cause cardiac arrhythmias and orthostatic hypotension.

Exception: Surveyor review is not required if:

- The resident is being treated for neurogenic pain (that is trigeminal neuralgia, peripheral neuropathy);
- There is evidence in the record that the resident has experienced this type of pain; and
- That a risk/benefit has been considered, including alternative pain therapies that may have fewer side effects in the individual.

4. Doxepin (Sinequan)

Risk: "Because of its strong anticholinergic and sedating properties, doxepin is rarely the antidepressant of choice in the elderly." Anticholinergic side effects are indicated by symptoms such as dry mouth, blurred vision, urinary retention, constipation, confusion, and sometimes delirium or hallucinations. Doxepin may also cause cardiac arrhythmias.

5. Meprobamate (Miltown), (Equanil)

NOTE: Surveyor guidance for unnecessary drugs (483.25(1)(1), F329) already has guidelines for this drug under "D. Miscellaneous Hypnotic/Sedative/Anxiolytic Drugs." This guideline is provided here to further emphasize the risk of using this drug.

Risk: "Meprobamate is a highly addictive and sedating anxiolytic (i.e., antianxiety drug). Avoid in elderly patients. Those using meprobamate for prolonged periods may be addicted and may need to be withdrawn slowly." The most frequent side effects of meprobamate are drowsiness and ataxia.

6. Disopyramide (Norpace), (Norpace CR)

Risk: "Disopyramide, of all antiarrhythmic drugs, is the most potent negative inotrope (decreased force of heart contraction) and therefore may induce heart failure in the elderly. It is also strongly anticholinergic." Anticholinergic side effects are indicated by symptoms such as dry mouth, blurred vision, urinary retention, constipation, confusion, and sometimes delirium or hallucinations. In addition to the anticholinergic side effects, disopyramide has the following cardiovascular side effects: edema, weight gain, chest pain, dyspnea, syncope and hypotension.

7. Digoxin (Lanoxin)

Risk: Because of decreased renal clearance of digoxin, doses in the elderly should rarely exceed 0.125 mg daily, except when treating atrial arrhythmias. (NOTE: the panelists' review of the literature has revealed countless studies showing that low dose digoxin is effective, but higher dose digoxin adds risks without improving outcomes.) Side effects may include anorexia, nausea and vomiting are the common early signs of digoxin toxicity. Nervous system symptoms include headache, fatigue, malaise, drowsiness, depression, and generalized muscle weakness. Visual disturbances also occur, including blurred vision, yellow or green vision, diplopia, photophobia, and flashing lights.

High Severity: Yes, if recently started. The panelists for the Beers' study believed that the severity of adverse reaction would be substantially greater when these drugs were recently started. **In general,** the greatest risk would be within **about** a 1-month period. If the surveyor encounters the use of this drug within the first month, they should treat it as a High Potential for Severe Outcomes drug under F329. After 1 month, it should be treated as a High Potential for Less Severe Outcomes under F429. It should be noted that validating when the drug was started is often a complex issue, and may be too much of a burden for the facility to accurately determine.

If there is a diagnosis of an atrial arrhythmia (e.g., atrial flutter, atrial fibrillation, supraventricular tachycardia), the survey must view the higher dose as acceptable.

Exception: Higher doses may be used for up to seven days before the facility would have to justify the risk versus benefit in writing. The surveyor need not review the higher dose during the seven day period unless an immediate threat to health and safety, for example, digoxin toxicity, is suspected.

8. Methyldopa (Aldomet)

Also combination products such as: Methyldopa and hydrochlorothiazide (Aldoril).

Risk: "Methyldopa may cause bradycardia and exacerbate depression in the elderly. Alternate treatments for hypertension are generally preferred."

High Severity: Yes if recently started. The panelists for the Beers' study believed that the severity of adverse reaction would be substantially greater when these drugs were recently started. **In general,** the greatest risk would be within **about** a 1-month period. If the surveyor encounters the use of this drug within the first month, they should treat it as a High Potential for Severe Outcomes drug under F329. After 1 month it should be treated as a High Potential for Less Severe Outcomes under F429. It should be noted that validating when the drug was started is often a complex issue, and may be too much of a burden for the facility to accurately determine.

9. Chlorpropamide (Diabinese)

Risk: "Chlorpropamide has a prolonged half-life in the elderly and can cause prolonged and serious hypoglycemia. Hypoglycemic symptoms are as follows:

Hypoglycemic Symptoms: Weakness, sweating, tachycardia, palpitations, tremor, nervousness, irritability, tingling in the mouth and tongue, hunger, nausea (unusual) and vomiting (unusual), headache, hypothermia, visual disturbances, mental dullness, confusion, amnesia, seizures, coma.

Additionally, chlorpropamide is the only hypoglycemic agent that causes SIADH (syndrome of inappropriate antidiuretic hormone release). SIADH causes hyponatremia. Chlorpropamide should be avoided in the elderly.

10. Gastrointestinal antispasmodic drugs such as: Dicyclomine (Bentyl), Hyoscyamine (Levsin, Levsinex), Propantheline (Probanthine), Belladonna Alkaloids (Donnatal & others), Clidinium and chlordiazepoxide (Librax)

Risk: "Gastrointestinal antispasmodic drugs are highly anticholinergic and generally produce substantial toxic effects in the elderly. Additionally, their effectiveness at doses tolerated by the elderly is questionable. All these drugs are best avoided in the elderly, especially for long term use." Anticholinergic side effects can include symptoms such as dry mouth, blurred vision, urinary retention, constipation, confusion, and sometimes delirium or hallucinations.

Exception: Review by the surveyor is not necessary if these drugs are used periodically (once every three months) for a short period (not over seven days) for symptoms of an acute, self-limiting illness.

11. Barbiturates

NOTE: Surveyor guidance for unnecessary drugs (483.25(1)(1), F329) already has guidelines for these drugs under: D. Miscellaneous Hypnotic/Sedative/Anxiolytic Drugs. This guideline is provided here to further emphasize the risk of using these drugs.

Risk: "Barbiturates cause more side effects than most other sedative or hypnotic drugs in the elderly and are highly addictive. They should not be started as new therapy in the elderly except when used to control seizures." Common side effects from barbiturates include: drowsiness, lethargy, vertigo, headache, severe CNS depression, mental depression, nausea, vomiting, diarrhea, and constipation. When discontinued, these drugs must be tapered very slowly to avoid potentially life-threatening withdrawal effects.

12. Meperidine (Demerol)

Risk: "Meperidine is not an effective analgesic when administered orally, and has many disadvantages to other narcotic drugs. Avoid oral use in the elderly." Respiratory, the greatest risk would be within **about** a 1-month period. If the surveyor encounters the use of this drug within the first month, they should treat it as a High Potential for Severe Outcomes drug under F329. After 1 month it should be treated as a High Potential for Less Severe Outcomes under F429.

13. Ticlopidine (Ticlid)

Risk: "Ticlopidine has been shown to be no better than aspirin in preventing clotting and is considerably more toxic. Avoid in the elderly." The most serious side effects of eyor is not necessary in individuals who receive ticlopidine because they have had a previous stroke or have evidence of stroke precursors, that is, transient ischemic attacks (TIAs), and cannot tolerate aspirin.

List of Diagnosis/Drug Combinations With High Potential for Severe Adverse Outcomes

1. Chronic Obstructive Pulmonary Disease (COPD)

Drugs(s): Hypnotic/sedatives such as:

- Long-Acting Benzodiazepines such as Flurazepam (Dalmane), Chlordiazepoxide (Librium), Clorazepate (Tranxene), Diazepam (Valium), Clonazepame (Klonopin), Quazepam (Doral), and Halazepam (Paxipam).
- Barbiturates such as Amobarbital (Amytal), Butabarbital (Butisol), Pentobarbital (Nembutal), and Secobarbital (Seconal).
- Miscellaneous Hypnotic/sedatives such as Glutethimide (Doriden), Methprylon (Noludar), Ethchlorvynol (Placidyl), Meprobamate (Equinal, Miltown), Paraldehyde (many brands), and Chloral Hydrate (Noctec).

Risk: "May slow respirations and increase carbon dioxide retention in persons with chronic obstructive pulmonary disease (COPD)."

NOTE: After review of the literature, the Panelists, in consultation with pulmonologists, determined, despite common usage of hypnotic/sedative drug use in persons with COPD, there is no data to support this practice, and pulmonologists virtually all agree that such drugs should be avoided in COPD patients for the reasons mentioned above.

Potential Side Effects: Exacerbation of COPD symptoms. The most common symptoms of COPD are cough, increased sputum production, shortness of breath, tightness in the chest, burning sensation, and wheezing.

Exception: The use of Short Acting Benzodiazepines such as Lorazapam (Ativan), Oxazepam (Serax) Alprazolam (Xanax) to relieve anxiety, preferably on an as needed basis, after thorough assessment and optimal treatment of the symptoms of COPD.

2. Active or recurrent gastritis, peptic ulcer disease or gastroesophageal reflux disease (GERD).

Drugs: Non-Steroidal Anti-inflammatory Drugs (NSAIDs) such as Diclofenac (Cataflam & Voltaren), Diflunisal (Dolobid), Etodolac (Lodine), Fenoprofen (Nalfon), Ibuprofen (Motrin & Advil), Indomethacin (Indocin), Ketoprofen (Orudis), Nabumetone (Relafen), Naproxen (Anaprox), Oxaprozin (Daypro), Phenylbutazone (many brands), Piroxicam (Feldene), Sulindac (Clinoril), Tolmetin (Tolectin).

Risk: "May exacerbate ulcer disease, gastritis, and gastroesophageal reflux disease (GERD)."

Potential Side Effects: Nausea, Dyspepsia, vomiting, abdominal pain, heartburn, epigastric pain, diarrhea, and flatulence.

3. Seizures or epilepsy.

Drug: Metoclopramide (Reglan).

Risk: May Lower seizure threshold.

4. Blood Clotting Disorders.

Drugs: Aspirin, NSAIDs (see #2 above for list), Dipyridamole (Persantine) and Ticlopidine (Ticlid).

Risk: "May cause bleeding in those using anticoagulants."

Potential Side Effects: Bleeding (e.g., from gums while brushing teeth or from small abrasions or contusions), and GI bleeding, indicated by black tarry stools, occult blood in the stool, or coffee ground like vomitus. A low hematocrit could be a sign of internal bleeding.

5. Benign Prostatic Hypertrophy (BPH)

Drugs: Anticholinergic antihistamines such as Chlorpheniramine (Chlor-Trimeton), Diphenhydramine (Benadryl), Hydroxyzine (Vistaril and Atarax), Cyproheptadine (Periactin), Promethazine (Phenergan), Tripelanamine (PBZ), Dexchlorpheniramine (Polaramine);

Exception: Review by the surveyor is not necessary if these drugs are used periodically (once every three months) for a short duration (not over seven days) for symptoms of an acute, self-limiting illness.

Anti-Parkinson medications such as Benztropine (Cogentin), Trihexyphenidyl (Artane), Procyclidine (Kemardren), Biperiden (Akineton);

GI antispasmodics such as dicyclomine (Bentyl) Hyoscyamine (Levsin & Levsinex), Propantheline (Probanthine), belladonna alkaloids (Donnatal), Clidinium containing products such as Librax;

Exception: Review by the surveyor is not necessary if these drugs are used periodically (once every three months) for a short duration (not over seven days) for symptoms of an acute, self-limiting illness.

Anticholinergic antidepressant drugs such as Amitriptyline (Elavil), Amoxapine (Asendin), Clomipramine (Anafranil), Desipramine (Pertofrane), Doxepin (Adapin, Sinequan), Imipramine (Tofranil), Maprotiline (Ludiomil), Nortriptyline (Aventyl, Pamelor), Protriptyline (Vivactil).

Risk: "Anticholinergic drugs may impair micturition and cause obstruction in persons with Benign Prostatics Hypertrophy (BPH)."

Potential Side Effects: Urinary retention, urinary incontinence, reflux, pyelonephritis, nephritis, low grade temperature, and low back pain.

6. Arrhythmias

Drugs: Tricyclic antidepressant drugs such as Amitriptyline (Elavil), Amoxapine (Asendin), Clomipramine (Anafranil), Desipramine (Pertofrane), Doxepin (Adapin, Sinequan), Imipramine (Tofranil), Maprotiline (Ludiomil), Nortriptyline (Aventyl, Pamelor), Protriptyline (Vivactil).

Risk: "May induce arrhythmias."

Potential Side Effects: Cardiac arrhythmias.

High Severity: YES, if recently started. The panelists for the Beers' study believed that the severity of adverse reaction would be substantially greater when these drugs were recently started. **In general,** the greatest risk would be within **about** a 1-month period. If the surveyor encounters the use of this drug within the first month, they should treat it as a High Potential for Severe Outcomes drug under F329. After 1 month, it should be treated as a high potential for less severe outcomes drug under F429.

---

§483.25(l)(2) Antipsychotic drugs

Based on a comprehensive assessment of a resident, the facility must assure that-

Guidelines § 483.25(l)(2)(i)

For a list of examples of commonly used antipsychotic drugs, see E. Under Interpretive Guidelines for § 483.25(l)(1), Unnecessary Drug.

F330 Minimization of antipsychotic drugs

§483.25(l)(2)(i)

Residents who have not used antipsychotic drugs are not given these drugs unless antipsychotic drug therapy is necessary to treat a specific condition as diagnosed and documented in the clinical record; and

Antipsychotic drugs should not be used unless the clinical record documents that the resident has one or more of the following "specific conditions":

1. Schizophrenia;
2. Schizo-affective disorder;
3. Delusional disorder;
4. Psychotic mood disorders (including mania and depression with psychotic features);
5. Acute psychotic episodes;
6. Brief reactive psychosis;
7. Schizophreniform disorder;
8. Atypical psychosis;
9. Tourette's disorder;
10. Huntington's disease;
11. Organic mental syndromes (now called delirium, dementia, and amnestic and other cognitive disorders by DSM-IV) **with associated psychotic and/or agitated behaviors:**

a. Which have been quantitatively and objectively documented. This documentation is necessary to assist in:

(1) Assess whether the resident's behavioral symptom is in need of some form of intervention,
(2) Determining whether the behavioral symptom is transitory or permanent,
(3) Relating the behavioral symptom to other events in the resident's life in order to learn about potential causes (e.g., death in the family, not adhering to the resident's customary daily routine),
(4) Ruling out environmental causes such as excessive heat, noise, overcrowding,
(5) Ruling out medical causes such as pain, constipation, fever, infection. For a more complete description of behavioral monitoring charts and how they can assist in the differential diagnosis of behavioral symptoms see the RAP on behavior problems (soon to be known as behavioral symptoms); and

b. Which are persistent, and
c. Which are not caused by preventable reasons; and
d. Which are causing the resident to:

(1) Present a danger to himself/herself or to others, or
(2) **Continuously** scream, yell, or pace if these specific behaviors cause an impairment in functional capacity (to evaluate functional capacity, see §483.25 (a) through (k) and MDS 2.0 sections B through P), or
(3) Experience psychotic symptoms (hallucinations, paranoia, delusions) not exhibited as dangerous behaviors or as screaming, yelling, or pacing but which cause the resident distress or impairment in functional capacity; or

12. Short-term (7 days) symptomatic treatment of hiccups, nausea, vomiting or pruritus. Residents with nausea and vomiting secondary to cancer or cancer chemotherapy can be treated for longer periods of time.

Antipsychotics should not be used if one or more of the following is/are the **only** indication:

- Wandering;
- Poor self care;
- Restlessness;
- Impaired memory;
- Anxiety;
- Depression (without psychotic features);
- Insomnia;
- Unsociability;
- Indifference to surroundings;
- Fidgeting;
- Nervousness;
- Uncooperativeness; or
- Agitated behaviors which **do not** represent danger to the resident or others.

F331 Antipsychotic drugs: discontinuance efforts

§483.25(l)(2)(ii)

Residents who use antipsychotic drugs receive gradual dose reductions, and behavioral interventions, unless clinically contraindicated, in an effort to discontinue these drugs.

Interpretive Guidelines §483.25(l)(2)(ii)

Residents must, unless clinically contraindicated, have gradual dose reductions of the antipsychotic drug. The gradual dose reduction should be under close supervision. If the gradual dose reduction is causing an adverse effect on the resident and the gradual dose reduction is discontinued, documentation of this decision and the reasons for it should be included in the clinical record. Gradual dose reductions consist of tapering the resident's daily dose to determine if the resident's symptoms can be controlled by a lower dose or to determine if the dose can be eliminated altogether.

"**Behavioral interventions**" means modification of the resident's behavior or the resident's environment, including staff approaches to care, to the largest degree possible to accommodate the resident's behavioral symptoms.

"**Clinically contraindicated**" means that a resident NEED NOT UNDERGO a "gradual dose reduction" or "behavioral interventions" IF:

1. The resident has a "specific condition" (as listed under 1 through 10 on page P-185) and has a history of recurrence of psychotic symptoms (e.g., delusions, hallucinations), which

have been stabilized with a maintenance dose of an antipsychotic drug without incurring significant side effects;

2. The resident has organic mental syndrome (now called "Delirium, Dementia, and Amnestic and other Cognitive Disorders" by DSM IV) and has had a gradual dose reduction attempted TWICE in one year and that attempt resulted in the return of symptoms for which the drug was prescribed to a degree that a cessation in the gradual dose reduction, or a return to previous dose reduction was necessary; or

3. The resident's physician provides a justification why the continued use of the drug and the dose of the drug is clinically appropriate. This justification should include:

   (a) a diagnosis, but not simply a diagnostic label or code, but the description of symptoms;

   (b) a discussion of the differential psychiatric and medical diagnosis (e.g., why the resident's behavioral symptom is thought to be a result of a dementia with associated psychosis and/or agitated behaviors, and not the result of an unrecognized painful medical condition of a psychosocial or environmental stressor);

   (c) a description of the justification for the choice of a particular treatment, or treatments; and

   (d) a discussion of why the present dose is necessary to manage the symptoms of the resident. This information need not necessarily be in the physician's progress notes, but must be a part of the resident's clinical record.

Procedures §483.25(l)(2)(i) and (ii)

In determining whether an antipsychotic drug is without a specific condition or that gradual dose reduction and behavioral interventions have not been performed, allow the facility an opportunity to justify why using the drug outside the Guidelines is in the best interest of the resident.

Examples of evidence that would support a justification of why a drug is being used outside the Guidelines, but in the best interest of the resident, may include, but are not limited to:

- A physician's note indicating that the use of the drug, or continued use of the drug is clinically appropriate, and the reasons why this use is clinically appropriate. This note must demonstrate that the physician has carefully considered the risk/benefit to the resident in using drugs outside these Guidelines.
- A medical or psychiatric consultation or evaluation (e.g., Geriatric Depression Scale) that confirms the physician's judgment that use of a drug outside the Guidelines is in the best interest of the resident.
- Physician, nursing, or other health professional documentation indicating that the resident is being monitored for adverse consequences or complications of the drug therapy.
- Documentation confirming that previous attempts at dosage reduction have been unsuccessful.
- Documentation (including MDS documentation) showing resident's subjective or objective improvement or maintenance of function while taking the medication.

- Documentation showing that a resident's decline or deterioration is evaluated by the inter-disciplinary team to determine whether a particular drug, a particular dose, or duration of therapy, may be the cause.
- Documentation showing why the resident's age, weight, or other factors would require a unique drug dose or drug duration.
- Other evidence the surveyor may deem appropriate.

The facility can refer to a prescriber's (or appropriately trained health professional's) justification as a valid justification for the use of a drug. It may not justify the use of a drug, its dose, or its duration, solely on the basis that "it was ordered" without supportive information. If the survey team determines that there is a deficiency in the use of antipsychotics, cite the facility under either the unnecessary drug regulation or the antipsychotic drug regulation, but not both quality of care tags.

F332 Medication error rate under five percent
and
F333 Residents free of significant medication errors

(Rev. 5, Issued: 11-19-04, Effective: 11-19-04, Implementation: 11-19-04)

§483.25(m) Medication Errors

The facility must ensure that—

[F332] §483.25(m)(1) It is free of medication error rates of 5 percent or greater; and

[F333] §483.25(m)(2) Residents are free of any significant medication errors.

Interpretive Guidelines §483.25(m)

Medication Error — The observed preparation or administration of drugs or biologicals which is not in accordance with:

1. Physician's orders;

2. Manufacturer's specifications (not recommendations) regarding the preparation and administration of the drug or biological;

3. Accepted professional standards and principles which apply to professionals providing services. Accepted professional standards and principles include the various practice regulations in each State, and current commonly accepted health standards established by national organizations, boards, and councils.

"Significant medication error" means one which causes the resident discomfort or jeopardizes his or her health and safety. Criteria for judging significant medication errors as well as examples are provided under significant and non-significant medication errors. Discomfort may be a subjective or relative term used in different ways depending on the individual situation. (Constipation that is unrelieved by an ordered laxative that results in a drug error that is omitted for one day may be slightly uncomfortable or perhaps not uncomfortable at all. When the constipation persists for greater than three days, the constipation may be more significant. Constipation causing obstruction or fecal impaction can jeopardize the resident's health and safety.)

"Medication error rate" is determined by calculating the percentage of errors. The numerator in the ratio is the total number of errors that the survey team observes, both significant and non-significant. The denominator is called "opportunities for errors" and includes all the doses the survey team observed being administered plus the doses ordered but not administered. The equation for calculating a medication error rate is as follows:

Medication Error Rate = Number of Errors Observed divided by the Opportunities for Errors (doses given plus doses ordered but not given) X 100.

"Medication error rate" — A medication error rate of 5% or greater includes both significant and non-significant medication errors. It indicates that the facility may have systemic problems with its drug distribution system and a deficiency should be written.

The error rate must be 5% or greater. Rounding of a lower rate (e.g., 4.6%) to a 5% rate is not permitted.

Significant and Non-Significant Medication Errors

"Determining Significance" — The relative significance of medication errors is a matter of professional judgment. Follow three general guidelines in determining whether a medication error is significant or not:

"Resident Condition" — The resident's condition is an important factor to take into consideration. For example, a fluid pill erroneously administered to a dehydrated resident may have serious consequences, but if administered to a resident with a normal fluid balance may not. If the resident's condition requires rigid control, a single missed or wrong dose can be highly significant.

"Drug Category" — If the drug is from a category that usually requires the resident to be titrated to a specific blood level, a single medication error could alter that level and precipitate a reoccurrence of symptoms or toxicity. This is especially important with a drug that has a Narrow Therapeutic Index (NTI) (i.e., a drug in which the therapeutic dose is very close to the toxic dose). Examples of drugs with NTI are as follows: Anticonvulsant: phenytoin (Dilantin), carbamazepine (Tegretol); Anticoagulants: warfarin (Coumadin); Antiarrhythmic: digoxin (Lanoxin); Antiasthmatics: theophylline (TheoDur); Antimanic Drugs: lithium salts (Eskalith, Lithobid).

"Frequency of Error" — If an error is occurring with any frequency, there is more reason to classify the error as significant. For example, if a resident's drug was omitted several times, as verified by reconciling the number of tablets delivered with the number administered, classifying that error as significant would be more in order. This conclusion should be considered in concert with the resident's condition and the drug category.

"Examples of Significant and Non-Significant Medication Errors" — Some of these errors are identified as significant. This designation is based on expert opinion without regard to the status of the resident. Most experts concluded that the significance of these errors, in and of themselves, have a high potential for creating problems for the typical long-term care facility resident. Those errors identified as non-significant have also been designated primarily on the basis of the nature of the drug. Resident status and frequency of error could classify these errors as significant.

Examples of Medication Errors Detected

Omissions Examples (Drug ordered but not administered at least once):

DRUG ORDER	SIGNIFICANCE
Haldol 1 mg BID	NS*
Motrin 400 mg TID	NS
Quinidine 200 mg TID	S**
Tearisol Drops 2 both eyes TID	NS
Metamucil one packet BID	NS
Multivitamin one daily	NS
Mylanta Susp. one oz., TID AC	NS
Nitrol Oint. one inch	S

*Not significant
**Significant

Unauthorized Drug Examples (Drugs administered without a physician's order):

DRUG ORDER	SIGNIFICANCE
Feosol	NS
Coumadin 4 mg	S
Zyloprim 100 mg	NS
Tylenol 5 gr.	NS
Motrin 400 mg	NS

Wrong Dose Examples:

DRUG ORDER	ADMINISTERED	SIGNIFICANCE
Timoptic 0.25% one drop in the left eye TID	Three drops in each eye	NS
Digoxin 0.125 mg every day	0.25 mg	S
Amphojel 30 ml QID	15 ml	NS
Dilantin 125 SUSP 12 ml	2 ml	S

Wrong Route of Administration Examples:

DRUG ORDER	ADMINISTERED	SIGNIFICANCE
Hydergine 0.5 SL.L BID	Resident swallowed	NS
Cortisporin Otic drops 4 to 5 leaf ear QID	Left eye	S

Wrong Dosage Form Examples:

DRUG ORDER	ADMINISTERED	SIGNIFICANCE
Colace Liquid 100 mg BID	Capsule	NS
Mellaril 10 mg	Concentrate	NS[†]
Dilantin Kapseals 100 mg three Kapseals po HS	Prompt Phenytoin 100 mg three capsules po	S[‡]

[†] If correct dose was given.
[‡] Parke Davis Kapseals have an extended rate of absorption. Prompt Phenytoin capsules do not.

Wrong Drug Examples:

DRUG ORDER	ADMINISTERED	SIGNIFICANCE
Tums	Oscal	NS[†]
Vibramycin	Vancomycin	S

Wrong Time Examples:

DRUG ORDER	ADMINISTERED	SIGNIFICANCE
Digoxin 0.25 daily at 8 a.m.	at 9:30 a.m.	NS
Percoset 2 Tabs 20 min before painful treatment	2 Tabs given 3 hrs after treatment	S

[§] PC After meals
[§§] AC Before meals

Medication Errors Due to Failure to Follow Manufacturer's Specifications or Accepted Professional Standards

The following situations in drug administration may be considered medication errors:

- Failure to "Shake Well": The failure to "shake" a drug product that is labeled "shake well." This may lead to an under dose or overdose depending on the drug product and the elapsed time since the last "shake." The surveyor should use common sense in determining the adequacy of the shaking of the medication. Some drugs, for example dilantin, are more critical to achieve correct dosage delivery than others.
- Insulin Suspensions: Also included under this category is the failure to "mix" the suspension without creating air bubbles. Some individuals "roll" the insulin suspension to mix it without creating air bubbles. Any motion used is acceptable so long as the suspension is mixed and does not have air bubbles in it prior to the administration.
- Crushing Medications That Should Not Be Crushed: Crushing tablets or capsules that the manufacturer states "do not crush."

Exceptions to the "Do Not Crush" rule:

If the prescriber orders a drug to be crushed which the manufacturer states should not be crushed, the prescriber or the pharmacist must explain, in the clinical record, why crushing the medication will not adversely affect the resident. Additionally, the pharmacist should inform the facility staff to observe for pertinent adverse effects.

If the facility can provide literature from the drug manufacturer or from a reviewed health journal to justify why modification of the dosage form will not compromise resident care.

- Adequate Fluids with Medications: The administration of medications without adequate fluid when the manufacturer specifies that adequate fluids be taken with the medication. For example:

  ◇ Bulk laxatives (e.g. Metamucil®, Fibril®, Serration®, Counsel®, Citrucel®;
  ◇ Nonsteroidal Anti-inflammatory Drugs (NSAIDs) should be administered with adequate fluid. Adequate fluid is not defined by the manufacturer but is usually 4–8 ounces. The surveyor should count fluids consumed during meals or snacks (such as coffee, juice, milk, soft drinks, etc.) as fluids taken with the medication, as long as they [are] consumed within a reasonable time of taking the medication (e.g., within approximately 30 minutes). If the resident refuses to take adequate fluid, the facility should not be at fault so long as they made a good faith effort to offer fluid and provided any assistance that may be necessary to drink the fluid. It is important that the surveyor not apply this rule to residents who are fluid restricted; and
  ◇ Potassium supplements (solid or liquid dosage forms) such as: Kaochlor, Klorvess, Kaon, K-Lor, K-Tab, K-Dur, K-Lyte, Slow K, Klotrix, Micro K, or Ten-K should be administered with or after meals with a full glass (e.g. approximately 4–8 ounces of water or fruit juice). This will minimize the possibility of gastrointestinal irritation and saline cathartic effect. If the resident refuses to take adequate fluid, the facility should

not be at fault so long as they made a good faith effort to offer fluid, and provided any assistance that may be necessary to drink the fluid. It is important that the surveyor not apply this rule to residents who are fluid restricted.

- Medications That Must Be Taken with Food or Antacids: The administration of medications without food or antacids when the manufacturer specifies that food or antacids be taken with or before the medication is considered a medication error. The most commonly used drugs that should be taken with food or antacids are the Nonsteroidal Anti-Inflammatory Drugs (NSAIDs). There is evidence that elderly, debilitated persons are at greater risk of gastritis and GI bleeds, including silent GI bleeds. Determine if the time of administration was selected to take into account the need to give the medication with food.

  ✧ Examples of commonly used NSAID's are as follows:

GENERIC NAME	BRAND NAME
Diclofenac	Voltaren, Cataflam
Diflunisal	Dolobid
Etodolac	Lodine
Fenoprofen	Nalfon
Ibuprofen	Motrin, Advil
Indomethacin	Indocin
Ketoprofen	Orudis, Oruvail
Mefenamic Acid	Ponstel
Nabumetone	Relafen
Naproxen	Naprosyn, Aleve
Piroxicam	Feldene
Sulindac	Clinoril
Tolmetin	Tolectin

- Medications Administered with Enteral Nutritional Formulas: Administering medications immediately before, immediately after, or during the administration of enteral nutritional formulas (ENFs) without achieving the following minimum objectives:

  ✧ Check the placement of the naso-gastric or gastrostomy tube in accordance with the facility's policy on this subject. NOTE: If the placement of the tube is not checked, this is not a medication error; it is a failure to follow accepted professional practice and should be evaluated under F Tag 281 requiring the facility to meet professional standards of quality.
  ✧ Flush the enteral feeding tube with at least 30 ml of preferably warm water before and after medications are administered. While it is noted that some facility policies ideally adopt flushing the tube after each individual medication is given, as opposed to after the group of multiple medications is given, unless there are known compatibility problems between medicines being mixed together, a minimum of one flushing before and after giving the medications is all the surveyor need review. There may be cases where flushing with 30 ml after each single medication is given may overload an indi-

vidual with fluid, raising the risk of discomfort or stress on body functions. Failure to flush, before and after, would be counted as one medication error and would be included in the calculation for medication errors exceeding 5 percent.

◇ The administration of enteral nutrition formula and administration of dilantin should be separated to minimize interaction. The surveyor should look for appropriate documentation and monitoring if the two are administered simultaneously. If the facility is not aware that there is a potential for an interaction between the two when given together, and is not monitoring for outcome of seizures or unwanted side effects of dilantin, then the surveyor should consider simultaneous administration a medication error.

- Medications Instilled into the Eye: The administration of eye drops without achieving the following critical objectives:

  ◇ Eye Contact: The eye drop, but not the dropper, must make full contact with the conjunctival sac and then be washed over the eye when the resident closes the eyelid; and
  ◇ Sufficient Contact Time: The eye drop must contact the eye for a sufficient period of time before the next eye drop is instilled. The time for optimal eye drop absorption is approximately 3 to 5 minutes. (It should be encouraged that when the procedures are possible, systemic effects of eye medications can be reduced by pressing the tear duct for one minute after eye drop administration or by gentle eye closing for approximately three minutes after the administration.)

- Allowing Resident to Swallow Sublingual Tablets: If the resident persists in swallowing a sublingual tablet (e.g., nitroglycerin) despite efforts to train otherwise, the facility should endeavor to seek an alternative dosage form for this drug.
- Medication Administered Via Metered Dose Inhalers (MDI): The use of MDI in other than the following ways (this includes use of MDI by the resident). This is an error if the person administering the drug did not do all the following:

  ◇ Shake the container well;
  ◇ Position the inhaler in front of or in the resident's mouth. Alternatively a spacer may be used;
  ◇ For cognitively impaired residents, many clinicians believe that the closed mouth technique is easier for the resident and more likely to be successful. However, the open mouth technique often results in better and deeper penetration of the medication into the lungs, when this method can be used; and
  ◇ If more than one puff is required (whether the same medication or a different medication), wait approximately a minute between puffs.

NOTE: If the person administering the drug follows all the procedures outlined above, and there is a failure to administer the medication because the resident can't cooperate (for example, a resident with dementia may not understand the procedure), this should not be called a medication error. The surveyor should evaluate the facility's responsibility to assess the resident's circumstance, and possibly attempt other dosage forms such as oral dosage forms or nebulizers.

Determining Medication Errors

Timing Errors — If a drug is ordered before meals (AC) and administered after meals (PC), always count this as a medication error. Likewise, if a drug is ordered PC and is given AC, count as a medication error. Count a wrong time error if the drug is administered 60 minutes earlier or later than its scheduled time of administration, BUT ONLY IF THAT WRONG TIME ERROR CAN CAUSE THE RESIDENT DISCOMFORT OR JEOPARDIZE THE RESIDENT'S HEALTH AND SAFETY. Counting a drug with a long half-life (e.g., digoxin) as a wrong time error when it is 15 minutes late is improper because this drug has a long half-life (beyond 24 hours) and 15 minutes has no significant impact on the resident. The same is true for many other wrong time errors (except AC AND PC errors).

To determine the scheduled time, examine the facility's policy relative to dosing schedules. The facility's policy should dictate when it administers a.m. doses, or when it administers the first dose in a 4-times-a-day dosing schedule.

Prescriber's Orders — the latest recapitulation of drug orders is sufficient for determining whether a valid order exists provided the prescriber has signed the "recap." The signed "recap," if the facility uses the "recap" system and subsequent orders constitute a legal authorization to administer the drug.

Procedures §483.25(m)

Medication Error Detection Methodology — Use an observation technique to determine medication errors. The survey team should observe the administration of drugs, on several different drug "passes," when necessary. Record what is observed; and reconcile the record of observation with the prescriber's drug orders to determine whether or not medication errors have occurred.

Do not rely solely on a paper review to determine medication errors. Detection of blank spaces on a medication administration record does not constitute the detection of actual medication errors. Paper review only identifies possible errors in most cases. In some cases paper review can help identify actual errors but research has shown that the procedure is time consuming for the number of actual errors detected.

Observation Technique — The survey team must know without doubt, what drugs, in what strength, and dosage forms, are being administered. This is accomplished prior to drug administration and may be done in a number of ways depending on the drug distribution system used (e.g. unit dose, vial system, punch card).

1. Identify the drug product. There are two principal ways to do this. In most cases, they are used in combination: Identify the product by its size, shape, and color. Many drug products are identifiable by their distinctive size, shape, or color. This technique is problematic because not all drugs have distinctive sizes, shapes, or color. Identify the product by observing the label. When the punch card or the unit dose system is

used, the survey team can usually observe the label and adequately identify the drug product. When the vial system is used, observing the label is sometimes more difficult. Ask the nurse to identify the medication being administered.

2. Observe and record the administration of drugs ("pass"). Follow the person administering drugs and observe residents receiving drugs (e.g., actually swallowing oral dosage forms). Be neutral and as unobtrusive as possible during this process.

    • Make every effort to observe residents during several different drug "passes," if possible, so the survey team will have an assessment of the entire facility rather than one staff member on one drug pass.
    • Identifying residents can present a problem. The surveyor should ask appropriate staff to explain the facility policy or system for the identification of residents.

3. Reconcile the surveyor's record of observation with physician's orders. Compare the record of observation with the most current orders for drugs. This comparison involves two distinct activities:

    • For each drug on the surveyor's list: Was it administered according to the prescriber's orders? For example, in the correct strength, by the correct route? Was there a valid order for the drug? Was the drug the correct one?
    • For drugs not on the surveyor's list: Are there orders for drugs that should have been administered, but were not? Examine the record for drug orders that were not administered and should have been. Such circumstances may represent omitted doses, one of the most frequent types of errors.
    • Ask the person administering drugs, if possible, to describe the system for administering the drugs given. Occasionally, a respiratory therapist may administer inhalers, a designated treatment person may only administer topical treatments, a hospice nurse may administer hospice medications, another person may administer eye drops or as needed drugs, etc. Sometimes people may share medication carts. Under these circumstances, these individuals should be interviewed about the omitted dose, if they were involved, if possible. When persons that were actually responsible for administering the drugs are not available, ask their supervisor for clarification.

The surveyor should now have a complete record of what was observed and what should have occurred according to the prescribers' orders. Determine the number of errors by adding the errors on each resident. Before concluding for certain that an error has occurred, discuss the apparent error with the person who administered the drugs if possible. There may be a logical explanation for an apparent error. For example, the surveyor observed that a resident had received Lasix 20 mg, but the order was for 40 mg. This was an apparent error in dosage. But the nurse showed the surveyor another more recent order which discontinued the 40 mg order and replaced it with a 20 mg order.

4. Reporting Errors — Describe to the facility each error that the survey team detects (e.g., Mary Jones received digoxin in 0.125 instead of 0.25 mg). The survey team is not

required to analyze the errors and come to any conclusions on how the facility can correct them. Do not attempt to categorize errors into various classifications (e.g., wrong dose, wrong resident). Stress that an error occurred and that future errors must be avoided.

5.   Observe Many Individuals Administering Medications. Strive to observe as many individuals administering medications as possible. This provides a better picture of accuracy of the facility's entire drug distribution system.

Dose Reconciliation Technique Supplement to the Observation Technique — When an omission error has been detected through the observation technique, the dose reconciliation technique can sometimes enable the survey team to learn how frequently an error has occurred in the past. Learning about the frequency of an error can assist in judging the significance of the error. (See Significant and Non Significant Medication Errors above.) The dose reconciliation technique requires a comparison of the number of doses remaining in a supply of drugs with the number of days the drug has been in use and the directions for use. For example, if a drug were in use for 5 days with direction to administer the drug 4 times a day, then 20 doses should have been used. If a count of the supply of that drug shows that only 18 doses were used (i.e., two extra doses exist) and no explanation for the discrepancy exists (e.g., resident refused the dose, or resident was hospitalized), then two omission errors may have occurred.

Use the dose reconciliation technique in facilities that indicate the number of drugs received, and the date and the specific "pass" when that particular drug was started. Unless this information is available, do not use this technique. If this information is not available, there is no Federal authority under which the survey team may require it, except for controlled drugs.

(Rev. 19, Issued: 06-01-06, Effective/Implementation: 06-01-06) §483.25(n)

Influenza and pneumococcal immunizations—

(1)   Influenza. The facility must develop policies and procedures that ensure that—
   (i)   Before offering the influenza immunization, each resident or the resident's legal representative receives education regarding the benefits and potential side effects of the immunization;
   (ii)   Each resident is offered an influenza immunization October 1 through March 31 annually, unless the immunization is medically contraindicated or the resident has already been immunized during this time period;
   (iii) The resident or the resident's legal representative has the opportunity to refuse immunization; and
   (iv)   The resident's medical record includes documentation that indicates, at a minimum, the following:
      (A)   That the resident or resident's legal representative was provided education regarding the benefits and potential side effects of influenza immunization; and
      (B)   That the resident either received the influenza immunization or did not receive the influenza immunization due to medical contraindications or refusal.

(2) Pneumococcal disease. The facility must develop policies and procedures that ensure that—

   (i)   Before offering the pneumococcal immunization, each resident or the resident's legal representative receives education regarding the benefits and potential side effects of the immunization;

   (ii) Each resident is offered an pneumococcal immunization, unless the immunization is medically contraindicate or the resident has already been immunized;

   (iii) The resident or the resident's legal representative has the opportunity to refuse immunization; and

   (iv) The resident's medical record includes documentation that indicates, at a minimum, the following:

         (A) That the resident or resident's legal representative was provided education regarding the benefits and potential side effects of pneumococcal immunization; and

         (B) That the resident either received the pneumococcal immunization or did not receive the pneumococcal immunization due to medical contraindication or refusal.

   (v)   Exception. As an alternative, based on an assessment and practitioner recommendation, a second pneumococcal immunization may be given after 5 years following the first pneumococcal immunization, unless medically contraindicated or the resident or the resident's legal representative refuses the second immunization.

F353 Nursing Services

§483.30 Nursing Services

The facility must have sufficient nursing staff to provide nursing and related services to attain or maintain the highest practicable physical, mental, and psychosocial well-being of each resident, as determined by resident assessments and individual plans of care.

Intent §483.30

To assure that sufficient qualified nursing staff are available on a daily basis to meet residents' needs for nursing care in a manner and in an environment which promote each resident's physical, mental, and psychosocial well-being, thus enhancing their quality of life.

Procedures §483.30

§483.30(a) and (b) are to be reviewed during the standard survey whenever quality of care problems have been discovered (see Appendix P, Survey Protocol, Task 4, for further information and Task 5C for the investigative protocol to complete this review). In addition, fully review requirements of nursing services during an extended survey or when a waiver of RN and/or licensed nurse (RN/LPN) staffing has been requested or granted. Except as licensed nursing personnel are specifically required by the regulation (e.g., an RN for 8 consecutive hours a day, 7 days a week), the determination of sufficient staff will be made based on the staff's ability to provide needed care to residents that enable them to reach their highest practicable physical, mental and psychosocial well being.

The ability to meet the requirements of §§483.13, 483.15(a), 483.20, 483.25 and 483.65 determines sufficiency of nurse staffing.

§483.30(a) Sufficient Staff

§483.30(a)(1) The facility must provide services by sufficient numbers of each of the following types of personnel on a 24-hour basis to provide nursing care to all residents in accordance with resident care plans:

(i) Except when waived under paragraph (c) of this section, licensed nurses; and
(ii) other nursing personnel.

§483.30(a)(2) Except when waived under paragraph (c) of this section, the facility **must** designate a licensed nurse to serve as a charge nurse on each tour of duty. For Interpretive Guidelines and Probes on §483.30(a) see tag F354.

F354 Registered nurse

§483.30(b) Registered Nurse

§483.30(b)(1) Except when waived under paragraph (c) or (d) of this section, the facility must use the services of a registered nurse for at least 8 consecutive hours a day, 7 days a week.

§483.30(b)(2) Except when waived under paragraph (c) or (d) of this section, the facility must designate a registered nurse to serve as the director of nursing (DON) on a full time basis.

§483.30(b)(3) The director of nursing may serve as a charge nurse only when the facility has an average daily occupancy of 60 or fewer residents.

Interpretive Guidelines §483.30(a) and (b)

At a minimum, "**staff**" is defined as licensed nurses (RNs and/or LPNs/LVNs), and nurse aides. Nurse aides must meet the training and competency requirements described in §483.75(e).

"Full time" is defined as working 35 or more hours a week.

Except for licensed staff noted above, the determining factor in sufficiency of staff (including both numbers of staff and their qualifications) will be the ability of the facility to provide needed care for residents. A deficiency concerning staffing should ordinarily provide examples of care deficits caused by insufficient quantity and quality of staff. If, however, inadequate staff (either the number or category) presents a clear threat to residents reaching their highest practicable level of well-being, cite this as a deficiency. Provide specific documentation of the threat.

The facility is required to designate an RN to serve as DON on a full time basis. This requirement can be met when RNs share the position. If RNs share the DON position, the total hours per week must equal 40. Facility staff must understand the shared responsibilities. The facility can only be waived from this requirement if it has a waiver under subsection (c) or (d).

Probes §483.30(a) and (b)

Determine nurse staffing sufficiency for each unit:

- Is there adequate staff to meet direct care needs, assessments, planning, evaluation, supervision?
- Do work loads for direct care staff appear reasonable?
- Do residents, family, and ombudsmen report insufficient staff to meet resident needs?
- Are staff responsive to residents' needs for assistance, and call bells answered promptly?
- Do residents call out repeatedly for assistance?
- Are residents, who are unable to call for help, checked frequently (e.g., each half hour) for safety, comfort, positioning, and to offer fluids and provision of care?
- Are identified care problems associated with a specific unit or tour of duty?
- Is there a licensed nurse that serves as a charge nurse (e.g., supervises the provision of resident care) on each tour of duty (if facility does not have a waiver of this requirement)?
- What does the charge nurse do to correct problems in nurse staff performance?
- Does the facility have the services of an RN available 8 consecutive hours a day, 7 days a week (if this requirement has not been waived)?
- How does the facility assure that each resident receives nursing care in accordance with his/her plan of care on weekends, nights, and holidays?
- How does the sufficiency (numbers and categories) of nursing staff contribute to identified quality of care, resident rights, quality of life, or facility practices problems?

F355 – Nursing Waivers

§483.30(c) Nursing facilities

Waiver of requirement to provide licensed nurses on a 24-hour basis. To the extent that a facility is unable to meet the requirements of paragraphs (a)(2) and (b)(1) of this section, a State may waive such requirements with respect to the facility if—

(1) The facility demonstrates to the satisfaction of the State that the facility has been unable, despite diligent efforts (including offering wages at the community prevailing rate for nursing facilities), to recruit appropriate personnel;

(2) The State determines that a waiver of the requirement will not endanger the health or safety of individuals staying in the facility;

(3) The State finds that, for any periods in which licensed nursing services are not available, a registered nurse or a physician is obligated to respond immediately to telephone calls from the facility;

(4) A waiver granted under the conditions listed in paragraph (c) of this section is subject to annual State review;

(5) In granting or renewing a waiver, a facility may be required by the State to use other qualified, licensed personnel;

(6) The State agency granting a waiver of such requirements provides notice of the waiver to the State long-term care ombudsman (established under section 307 (a)(12) of the Older Americans Act of 1965) and the protection and advocacy system in the State for the mentally ill and mentally retarded; and

(7) The nursing facility that is granted such a waiver by a State notifies residents of the facility (or, where appropriate, the guardians or legal representatives of such residents) and members of their immediate families of the waiver.

Intent §483.30(c)

To give the facility flexibility, in limited circumstances, when the facility cannot meet nurse staffing requirements.

Interpretive Guidelines §483.30(c)

The facility may request a waiver of the RN requirement, and/or the 24-hour licensed nurse requirement. If the facility is Medicaid-certified only, the State has the authority to grant the waiver. If the facility is dually-participating, CMS has the delegated authority to grant the waiver. (See guidelines for §483.30(d).)

A survey of Nursing Services must be conducted if a waiver has been granted or requested.

Probes §483.30(c)

Before granting a continuation of this waiver, or during the annual review, at a minimum, determine:

- Is a continuing effort being made to obtain licensed nurses?
- How does the facility ensure that residents' needs are being met?
- Are all nursing policies and procedures followed on each shift during times when licensed services are waived?
- Is there a qualified person to assess, evaluate, plan, and implement resident care?
- Is care being carried out according to professional practice standards on each shift?

- Can the survey team ensure the State that the absence of licensed nurses will NOT endanger the health or safety of residents?
- Are there trends in the facility, which might be indicators of decreased quality of care as a result of insufficient staffing to meet resident needs (e.g., increases in incident reports, the infection rate, hospitalizations)?
- Are there increases in loss of function, pressure sores, tube feedings, catheters, weight loss, mental status?
- Is there evidence that preventive measures (e.g., turning, ambulating) are taken to avoid poor quality of care outcomes and avoidable sudden changes in health status?
- Is there evidence that sudden changes in resident health status and emergency needs are being properly identified and managed by appropriate facility staff and in a timely manner?
- If the facility has a waiver of the requirement to provide licensed nurses on a 24-hour basis, have they notified the ombudsman, residents, surrogates or legal representatives, and members of their immediate families of the waiver, and are there services residents need that are not provided because licensed nurses are not available?
- Is there an increase in hospitalizations because licensed personnel are not available to provide appropriate services?
- Does the facility meet all applicable requirements to continue to receive a waiver?
- Does the staff indicate that an RN or physician is available to respond immediately to telephone calls when licensed nurses are not available?

§483.30(d)

SNFs Waiver of the requirement to provide services of a registered nurse for more than 40 hours a week.

§483.30(d)(1) The Secretary may waive the requirement that a SNF provide the services of a registered nurse for more than 40 hours a week, including a director of nursing specified in paragraph (b) of this section, if the Secretary finds that —

(i) The facility is located in a rural area and the supply of skilled nursing facility services in the area is not sufficient to meet the needs of individuals residing in the area;
(ii) The facility has one full-time registered nurse who is regularly on duty at the facility 40 hours a week; and
(iii) The facility either —

(A) Has only patients whose physicians have indicated (through physicians' orders or admission notes) that they do not require the services of a registered nurse or a physician for a 48-hour period or;
(B) Has made arrangements for a registered nurse or a physician to spend time at the facility, as determined necessary by the physician, to provide necessary skilled nursing services on days when the regular full-time registered nurse is not on duty;

(iv) The Secretary provides notice of the waiver to the State long-term care ombudsman (established under section 307(a)(12) of the Older Americans Act of 1965) and the protection and advocacy system in the State for the mentally ill and mentally retarded; and

(v) The facility that is granted such a waiver notifies residents of the facility (or, where appropriate, the guardians or legal representatives of such residents) and members of their immediate families of the waiver.

(2) A waiver of the registered nurse requirement under paragraph (d)(1) of this section is subject to annual renewal by the Secretary.

Interpretive Guidelines §483.30(d)

CMS is delegated the waiver authority for SNFs, including dually-participating facilities (SNF/NFs). The Medicare waiver authority is far more limited than is the State's authority under Medicaid since a State may waive any element of the nurse staffing requirement, whereas the Secretary may waive only the RN requirement. The requirements that a registered nurse provide services for 8 hours a day, 7 days a week (more than 40 hours a week), and that there be an RN designated as director of nursing on a full-time basis, may be waived by the Secretary in the following circumstances:

- The facility is located in a rural area with an inadequate supply of SNF services to meet area needs. Rural is defined as "all areas not delineated as 'urban' by the Bureau of Census, based on the most recent census;
- The facility has one full-time registered nurse regularly working 40 hours a week. This may be the same individual or part-time individuals. This nurse may or may not be the DON, and may perform some DON and some clinical duties if the facility so desires; **and either**;
- The facility has only residents whose physicians have noted, in writing, do not need RN or physician care for a 48-hour period. This does not relieve the facility from responsibility for providing for emergency availability of a physician, when necessary, nor does it relieve the facility from being responsible for meeting all needs of the residents during those 48 hours; OR
- A physician or RN will spend the necessary time at the facility to provide care residents need during the days that an RN is not on duty. This requirement refers to clinical care of the residents that need skilled nursing services.
- If a waiver of this requirement has been granted, conduct a survey of nursing services during each certification survey. Dually-participating facilities must meet the waiver provisions of the SNF.

Probes §483.30(d)

If the SNF has a waiver of the more than 40 hours a week RN requirement:

- Does each clinical record have documentation by the physician that the resident does not need services of a physician or an RN for a 48-hour period each week?
- Are there any emergency or routine services that should be, but are not, provided to residents during the days that a registered nurse is not on duty?
- If specific skilled care is necessary for a resident during the time that an RN is not on duty, does an RN or physician provide that service on an "as needed" basis? See also probes at §483.30(c).

- Is there an RN on duty 40 hours a week?
- If more than one RN provides the 40 hour per week coverage, how is information exchanged that maintains continuity of resident care?
- Did the facility notify residents (or their legal guardians), their immediate families, and the ombudsman about the waiver?

If the SNF requests continuation of the waiver to provide the services of a registered nurse for more than 40 hours a week, the survey team is to provide the Secretary with information needed to grant this continuation.

- Does the SNF meet all requirements necessary for continuation of the waiver?

Procedures §483.30(a)-(d)

If the facility has an approved nurse staffing waiver, it is **not** considered a deficiency. The facility does not need to submit a POC. The following procedure should be used to document that a facility has a waiver of nurse staffing requirements. When a facility does not meet the nurse staffing requirements, cite the appropriate tag. If the facility does have a waiver, reference the tag number based on the type of facility. The type of facility (SNF, NF, or SNF/NF) determines what type of waiver is granted:

- For SNFs and SNF/NFs which may be waived from the requirement to provide more than 40 hours of registered nurse services a week, and for NFs which have been granted a waiver from the 56-hour registered nurse requirement, cite F354;
- For NFs that have a waiver of the 24-hour licensed nursing requirement, cite F353; or
- Both facility types could be waived for the requirement to designate a registered nurse as the director of nursing on a full-time basis. Cite F355. When the Form CMS-2567 is entered into OSCAR, code the waived tag as a "W." Enter the tag number, leave the correction date blank, and enter a "W" in the CP field. This will indicate that this is not a deficiency—that the requirement has been waived.

F356

(Rev. 19, Issued: 06-01-06, Effective/Implementation: 06-01-06)

§483.30(e)

Nurse Staffing Information—

(1) Data requirements.

The facility must post the following information on a daily basis:

(i) Facility name

(ii) The current date

(iii) The total number and the actual hours worked by the following categories of licensed and unlicensed nursing staff directly responsible for resident care per shift:

(A) Registered nurses.

(B) Licensed practical nurses or licensed vocational nurses (as defined under State law).

(C) Certified nurse aides.

(iv) Resident census.

(2) Posting requirements.

(i) The facility must post the nurse staffing data specified in paragraph (e)(1) of this section on a daily basis at the beginning of each shift.

(ii) Data must be posted as follows:

(A) Clear and readable format.

(B) In a prominent place readily accessible to residents and visitors.

(3) Public access to posted nurse staffing data. The facility must, upon oral or written request, make nurse staffing data available to the public for review at a cost not to exceed the community standard.

(4) Facility data retention requirements. The facility must maintain the posted daily nurse staffing data for a minimum of 18 months, or as required by State law, whichever is greater.

§483.35 Dietary Services Tags 360 – 372

§483.35(a) Staffing
§483.35 (b) Standard Sufficient Staff
§483.35(c) Standard Menus and Nutritional Adequacy
§483.35(d) Food
§483.35(e) Therapeutic Diets
§483.35(f) Frequency of Meals
§483.35(g) Assistive Devices
§483.35(h) Sanitary Conditions

F360 Dietary services: nourishing, nutritionally sound diets

§483.35 Dietary Services

The facility must provide each resident with a nourishing, palatable, well-balanced diet that meets the daily nutritional and special dietary needs of each resident.

F361 Dietary: adequate staffing §483.35(a)

(a) Staffing

The facility must employ a qualified dietitian either full-time, part-time, or on a consultant basis.

(1) If a qualified dietitian is not employed full-time, the facility must designate a person to serve as the director of food service who receives frequently scheduled consultation from a qualified dietitian.

(2) A qualified dietitian is one who is qualified based upon either registration by the Commission on Dietetic Registration of the American Dietetic Association, or on the basis of education, training, or experience in identification of dietary needs, planning, and implementation of dietary programs.

§483.35(a)
Intent:

The intent of this regulation is to ensure that a qualified dietitian is utilized in planning, managing, and implementing dietary service activities in order to assure that the residents receive adequate nutrition.

A director of food services has no required minimum qualifications, but must be able to function collaboratively with a qualified dietitian in meeting the nutritional needs of the residents.

§483.35(a)
Guidelines to Surveyors:

A dietitian qualified on the basis of education, training, or experience in identification of dietary needs, planning, and implementation of dietary programs has experience or training which includes:

- Assessing special nutritional needs of geriatric and physically impaired persons;
- Developing therapeutic diets;
- Developing "regular diets" to meet the specialized needs of geriatric and physically impaired persons;
- Developing and implementing continuing education programs for dietary services and nursing personnel;
- Participating in interdisciplinary care planning;
- Budgeting and purchasing food and supplies; and
- Supervising institutional food preparation, service, and storage.

§483.35(a)
Procedures:

If resident reviews determine that residents have nutritional problems, determine if these nutritional problems relate to inadequate or inappropriate diet nutrition/assessment and monitoring. Determine if these are related to dietitian qualifications.

§483.35(a)
Probes:

If the survey team finds problems in resident nutritional status:

- Do practices of the dietitian or food services director contribute to the identified problems in residents' nutritional status? If yes, what are they?
- What are the educational, training, and experience qualifications of the facility's dietitian?

F362 Dietary: sufficient staff

§483.35(b)

(b) Sufficient staff

The facility must employ sufficient support personnel competent to carry out the functions of the dietary service.

§483.35(b)
Guidelines to Surveyors:

"Sufficient support personnel" is defined as enough staff to prepare and serve palatable, attractive, nutritionally adequate meals at proper temperatures and appropriate times and support proper sanitary techniques being utilized.

§483.35(b)
Procedures:

For residents who have been triggered for a dining review, do they report that meals are palatable, attractive, served at the proper temperatures, and at appropriate times?

§483.35(b)
Probes:

Sufficient staff preparation:
- Is food prepared in scheduled time frames in accordance with established professional practices?

Observe food service:
- Does food leave kitchen in scheduled time frames? Is food served to residents in scheduled time frames?

F363 Menus: meet nutritional needs, be prepared in advance, be followed

§483.35(c)

(c) Menus and nutritional adequacy

Menus must—

(1) Meet the nutritional needs of residents in accordance with the recommended dietary allowances of the Food and Nutrition Board of the National Research Council, National Academy of Sciences;

§483.35(c)(1)(2)(3)
Intent:

The intent of this regulation is to assure that the meals served meet the nutritional needs of the resident in accordance with the recommended dietary allowances (RDAs) of the Food and Nutrition Board of the National Research Council, of the National Academy of Sciences. This regulation also assures that there is a prepared menu by which nutritionally adequate meals have been planned for the resident and followed.

§483.35(c)(1)
Procedures:

- For sampled residents who have a comprehensive review or a focused review, as appropriate, observe if meals served are consistent with the planned menu and care plan in the amounts, types, and consistency of foods served.

If the survey team observes deviation from the planned menu, review appropriate documentation from diet card, record review, and interviews with food service manager or dietitian to support reasons for deviation from the written menu.

§483.35(c)(1)
Probes:

- Are residents receiving food in the amount, type, consistency, and frequency to maintain normal body weight and acceptable nutritional values?
- If food intake appears inadequate based on meal observations, or resident's nutritional status is poor based on resident review, determine if menus have been adjusted to meet the caloric and nutrient intake needs of each resident.
- If a food group is missing from the resident's daily diet, does the facility have an alternative means of satisfying the resident's nutrient needs? If so, does the facility perform a follow-up?

(Menu adequately provides the daily basic food groups)
Does the menu meet basic nutritional needs by providing daily food in the groups of the food pyramid system and based on individual nutritional assessment taking into account current nutritional recommendations?

Note: A standard meal planning guide (e.g., food pyramid) is used primarily for menu planning and food purchasing. It is not intended to meet the nutritional needs of all residents. This guide must be adjusted to consider individual differences. Some residents will need more due to age, size, gender, physical activity, and state of health. There are many meal planning guides from reputable sources, e.g., American Diabetes Association, American Dietetic Association, American Medical Association, or U.S. Department of Agriculture, that are available and appropriate for use when adjusted to meet each resident's needs.

(2) Be prepared in advance; and

§483.35(c)(2)
Probes:

(Menu prepared in advance)
Are there preplanned menus for both regular and therapeutic diets?

(3) Be followed.

§483.35(c)(3)
Probes:

(Menu followed)
Is food served as planned? If not, why? There may be legitimate and extenuating circumstances why food may not be available on the day of the survey and must be considered before a concern is noted.

F364 Food: conservation of nutritive value, flavor, appearance, attractive, proper temperature

§483.35(d)(1)(2)

(d) Food

Each resident receives and the facility provides—

(1) Food prepared by methods that conserve nutritive value, flavor, and appearance;

§483.35(d)(1)(2)
Intent:

The intent of this regulation is to assure that the nutritive value of food is not compromised and destroyed because of prolonged food storage, light, and air exposure; prolonged cooking of foods in a large volume of water and prolonged holding on steam table, and the addition of baking soda. Food should be palatable, attractive, and at the proper temperature as determined by the type of food to ensure resident's satisfaction. Refer to §483.15(e) and/or §483.15(a)

§483.35(d)(1)
Guidelines to Surveyors:

"Food-palatability" refers to the taste and/or flavor of the food.

"Food attractiveness" refers to the appearance of the food when served to residents.

§483.35(d)(1)
Procedures:

Evidence for palatability and attractiveness of food, from day to day and meal to meal, may be strengthened through sources such as additional observation, resident and staff interviews, and review of resident council minutes. Review nutritional adequacy in §483.25(i)(1).

(2) Food that is palatable, attractive, and at the proper temperature;

§483.35(d)(1)(2)
Probes:

Does food have a distinctively appetizing aroma and appearance, which is varied in color and texture?

Is food generally well seasoned (use of spices, herbs, etc.) and acceptable to residents?

(Conserves nutritive value)
Is food prepared in a way to preserve vitamins? Method of storage and preparation should cause minimum loss of nutrients.

(Food temperature)
Is food served at preferable temperature (hot foods are served hot and cold foods are served cold) as discerned by the resident and customary practice? Not to be confused with the proper holding temperature.

F365 Food prepared to meet individual needs

§483.35(d)(3)

(3) Food prepared in a form designed to meet individual needs; and

---

F366 Substitutes offered of similar nutritive value

§483.35(d)(4)

(4) Substitutes offered of similar nutritive value to residents who refuse food served.

§483.35(d)(3)(4)
Intent:

The intent of this regulation is to assure that food is served in a form that meets the resident's needs and satisfaction; and that the resident receives appropriate nutrition when a substitute is offered.

§483.35(d)(3)(4)
Procedures:

Observe trays to assure that food is appropriate for resident according to assessment and care plan. Ask the resident how well the food meets their taste needs. Ask if the resident is offered or is given the opportunity to receive substitutes when refusing food on the original menu.

§483.35(d)(3)(4)
Probes:

Is food cut, chopped, or ground for individual resident's needs?

Are residents who refuse food offered substitutes of similar nutritive value?

§483.35(d) (4)
Guidelines to Surveyors:

A food substitute should be consistent with the usual and ordinary food items provided by the facility. For example if a facility never serves smoked salmon, they would not be required to serve this as a food substitute; or the facility may, instead of grapefruit juice, substitute another citrus juice or vitamin C-rich juice that the resident likes.

F367 Therapeutic Diets

§483.35(e)

Therapeutic Diets

§483.35(e)
Intent:

The intent of this regulation is to assure that the resident receives and consumes foods in the appropriate form and/or the appropriate nutritive content as prescribed by a physician and/or assessed by the interdisciplinary team to support the treatment and plan of care.

§483.35(e)
Interpretive Guidelines:

"Therapeutic Diet" is defined as a diet ordered by a physician as part of treatment for a disease or clinical condition, or to eliminate or decrease specific nutrients in the diet, (e.g., sodium) or to increase specific nutrients in the diet (e.g., potassium), or to provide food the resident is able to eat (e.g., a mechanically altered diet).

"Mechanically altered diet" is one in which the texture of a diet is altered. When the texture is modified, the type of texture modification must be specific and part of the physicians' order.

§483.35(e)
Procedures:

If the resident has inadequate nutrition or nutritional deficits that manifests into and/or are a product of weight loss or other medical problems, determine if there is a therapeutic diet that is medically prescribed.

Probes: §483.35(e)

Is the therapeutic diet that the resident receives prescribed by the physician?

Also, see §483.25(i). Nutritional Status.

(Rev. 19, Issued: 06-01-06, Effective/Implementation: 06-01-06) Therapeutic diets must be prescribed by the attending physician.

F368 Frequency of meals

§483.35(f)

(f) Frequency of meals.

(1) Each resident receives and the facility provides at least three meals daily, at regular times comparable to normal mealtimes in the community.

(2) There must be no more than 14 hours between a substantial evening meal and breakfast the following day, except as provided in (4) below.

(3) The facility must offer snacks at bedtime daily.

(4) When a nourishing snack is provided at bedtime, up to 16 hours may elapse between a substantial evening meal and breakfast the following day if a resident group agrees to this meal span, and a nourishing snack is served.

§483.35(f)(1)(2)(3)(4)
Intent:

The intent of this regulation is to assure that the resident receives his/her meals at times most accepted by the community and that there are not extensive time lapses between meals. This assures that the resident receives adequate and frequent meals.

§483.35(f)(1)(2)(3)(4)
Guidelines to Surveyors:

A "substantial evening meal" is defined as an offering of three or more menu items at one time, one of which includes a high-quality protein such as meat, fish, eggs, or cheese. The meal should represent no less than 20 percent of the day's total nutritional requirements.

"Nourishing snack" is defined as a verbal offering of items, single or in combination, from the basic food groups. Adequacy of the "nourishing snack" will be determined both by resident interviews and by evaluation of the overall nutritional status of residents in the facility (e.g., is the offered snack usually satisfying?).

§483.35(f)(1)(2)(3)(4)
Procedures:

Observe meal times and schedules and determine if there is a lapse in time between meals. Ask for resident input on meal service schedules, to verify if there are extensive lapses in time between meals.

F369 Assistive devices

§483.35(g)

(g) Assistive devices

The facility must provide special eating equipment and utensils for residents who need them.

§483.35(g)
Intent:

The intent of this regulation is to provide residents with assistive devices to maintain or improve their ability to eat independently. For example, improving poor grasp by enlarging silverware handles with foam padding, aiding residents with impaired coordination or tremor by installing plate guards, or providing postural supports for head, trunk, and arms.

§483.35(g)
Procedures:

Review sampled residents' comprehensive assessment for eating ability. Determine if recommendations were made for adaptive utensils and if they were, determine if these utensils are available and utilized by resident. If recommended but not used, determine if this is by resident's choice. If utensils are not being utilized, determine when these were recommended and how their use is being monitored by the facility and if the staff is developing alternative recommendations.

(Rev. 19, Issued: 06-01-06, Effective/Implementation: 06-01-06)

§483.35(h)

Paid Feeding Assistants-

(1) State-approved training course. A facility may use a paid feeding assistant, as defined in §488.301 of this chapter, if—

(i) The feeding assistant has successfully completed a State-approved training course that meets the requirements of §488.160 before feeding residents; and
(ii) The use of feeding assistants is consistent with State law.

(2) Supervision.

(iii) A feeding assistant must work under the supervision of a registered nurse (RN) or licensed practical nurse (LPN).
(iv) In an emergency, a feeding assistant must call a supervisory nurse for help on the resident call system.

(3) Resident Selection criteria.

(i) A facility must ensure that a feeding assistant feeds only residents who have no complicated feeding problems.
(ii) Complicated feeding problems include, but are not limited to, difficulty swallowing, recurrent lung aspirations, and tube or parenteral/IV feedings.
(iii) The facility must base resident selection on the charge nurse's assessment and the resident's latest assessment and plan of care.

F370 Food: procured from satisfactory sources

§483.35(i)(1)

(h) Sanitary conditions.

The facility must—

(1) Procure food from sources approved or considered satisfactory by Federal, State, or local authorities;

(Rev. 19, Issued: 06-01-06, Effective/Implementation: 06-01-06) i) Sanitary Conditions (Rev. 19, Issued: 06-01-06, Effective/Implementation: 06-01-06)

(i)(1) Procure food from sources approved or considered satisfactory by (Rev. 19, Issued: 06-01-06, Effective/Implementation: 06-01-06) i)(2) Store, prepare, distribute, and serve food under sanitary conditions; i)(2) i)(2)

§483.35(The facility must—

F371 Food: store, prepare, distribute, and serve under sanitary conditions

§483.35(i)(2)

(2) Store, prepare, distribute, and serve food under sanitary conditions; and

§483.35(i)(2)
Intent:

The intent of this regulation is to prevent the spread of foodborne illness and reduce those practices which result in food contamination and compromised food safety in nursing homes. Since foodborne illness is often fatal to nursing home residents, it can and must be avoided.

§483.35(i)(2)
Guidelines to Surveyors:

"Sanitary conditions" is defined as storing, preparing, distributing, and serving food properly to prevent food borne illness. Potentially hazardous foods must be subject to continuous time/temperature controls in order to prevent either the rapid and progressive growth of infections or toxigenic microorganisms such as Salmonella or the slower growth of *Clostridium Botulism* [sic: Botulinum]. In addition, foods of plant origin become potentially hazardous when the skin, husk, peel, or rind is breached, thereby possibly contaminating the fruit or vegetable with disease-causing micro-organisms. Potentially hazardous food tends to focus on animal products, including but not limited to milk, eggs, and poultry.

Improper holding temperature is a common contributing factor of food-borne illness. The facility must follow proper procedures in cooking, cooling, and storing food according to time, temperatures, and sanitary guidelines. Improper handling of food can cause salmonella and E-coli contamination. The 1993 FDA Food Code advises the following precautions:

Note: The 1993 FDA Food Code is not regulation and cannot be enforced as such. The food temperatures cited that are recommended in the 1993 FDA Food Code are target temperatures and give a margin of safety in temperature ranges and to avoid known harmful temperatures.

Refrigerator storage of food to prevent food-borne illness includes storing raw meat away from vegetables and other foods. Raw meat should be separated from cooked foods and other foods when refrigerated on its own tray on a bottom shelf so meat juices do not drip on other foods. Foods of both plant and animal origin must be cooked, maintained, and stored at appropriate temperatures.

- Foods of both plant and animal origin must be cooked, maintained, and stored at appropriate temperatures. These temperatures are better utilized as food hold temperatures rather than the food temperatures as residents receive the food.

- Hot foods which are potentially hazardous should leave the kitchen (or steam table) above 140° F, cold foods at or below 41° F, and freezer temperatures should be at 0° F or below. Refrigerator temperatures should be maintained at 41° F or below. The 1993 FDA Food Code can be used as an authoritative guide to clarify regulatory requirements on how to prepare and serve food to prevent food-borne illness. As the public becomes more informed and educated on how to prevent food-borne illness, this code will become the standard of practice the same as the 1976 Food Service Sanitation Manual did prior to 1993.

§483.35(i)(2)
Procedures:

Observe storage, cooling, and cooking of food. Record the time and date of all observations. If a problem is noted, conduct additional observations to verify findings.

Observe that employees are effectively cleaning their hands prior to preparing, serving, and distributing food. Observe that food is covered to maintain temperature and protected from other contaminants when transporting meals to residents.

Refrigerated storage:

- Check all refrigerators and freezers for temperatures. Use the facility's or the surveyor's own properly sanitized thermometer to evaluate the internal temperatures of potentially hazardous foods with a focus on the quantity of leftovers and the container sizes in which bulk leftovers are stored.

Food preparation:

- Use a sanitized thermometer to evaluate food temperatures.

In addition, how do kitchen staff process leftovers?

- Are they heated to the appropriate temperatures?
- How is frozen food thawed?
- How is potentially hazardous food handled during multi-step food preparation (e.g., chicken salad, egg salad)?
- Is hand contact with food minimized?

Food service:

- Using a properly sanitized thermometer, check the temperatures of hot and cold food prior to serving.
- How long is milk held without refrigeration prior to distribution?

Food distribution:

- Is the food protected from contamination as it is transported to the dining rooms and residents' rooms?

Pest free:

• Is the area pest free? (See §483.70(h)(4).) Look for signs of pests such as mice, roaches, rates, flies.

Preventing Contamination:

• Are handwashing facilities convenient and properly equipped for dietary services staff Use? (Staff uses good hygienic practices and staff with communicable disease or infected skin lesions do not have contact with food if that contact will transmit the disease.)

Hazard Free

• Are toxic items (such as insecticides, detergent, polishes) properly stored, labeled, and used separate from the food?

§483.35
Probes:

Observe food storage rooms and food storage in the kitchen.

• Are containers of food stored off the floor and on clean surfaces in a manner that protects it from contamination?
• Are other areas under storage shelves monitored for cleanliness to reduce attraction of pest.
• Are potentially hazardous foods stored at 41° F or below and frozen foods kept at 0° F or below?
• Do staff handle and cook potentially hazardous foods properly?
• Are potentially hazardous foods kept at an internal temperature of 41° F or below in cold food storage unit, or at an internal temperature of 140° F or above in a hot food storage unit during display and service?
• Is food transported in a way that protects against contamination (i.e., covered containers, wrapped, or packaged)?
• Is there any sign of rodent or insect infestation.

Dishwashing:

• The current 1993 Food Code, DHHS, FDA, PHS recommends the following water temperature and manual washing instructions:

Machine:

1. Hot Water:
    a. 140° F Wash (or according to the manufacturer's specifications or instructions).
    b. 180° F Rinse (180°, 160° or greater at the rack and dish/utensils surfaces.

2. Low Temperature:
   a. 120° F +25 ppm (parts per million) Hypochlorite (household bleach) on dish Surface.

Manual:

1. 3 Compartment Sink (wash, rinse and sanitize): Sanitizing solution used according to manufacturer's instructions.
   a. 75° F – 50 ppm Hypochlorite (household bleach) or equivalent, or 12.5 ppm of Iodine.
   b. Hot Water Immersion at 170° F for at least 30 seconds.

Are food preparation equipment, dishes, and utensils effectively sanitized and cleaned to destroy potential disease carrying organisms and stored in a protected manner?

F372 Proper disposal of garbage and refuse

§483.35(i)(3)

(3) Dispose of garbage and refuse properly.

§483.35(i)(3)
Guidelines:

The intent of this regulation is to assure that garbage, and refuse be properly disposed.

§483.35(i)(3)
Procedures:

(Garbage/refuse) Observe garbage and refuse container construction, and outside storage receptacles.

§483.35(i)(3)
Probes:

Are garbage and refuse containers in good condition (no leaks) and is waste properly contained in dumpsters or compactors with lids or otherwise covered? Are areas such as loading docks, hallways, and elevators used for both garbage disposal and clean food transport kept clean, free of debris, and free of foul odors and waste fat? Is the garbage storage area maintained in a sanitary condition to prevent the harborage and feeding of pests? Are garbage receptacles covered when being removed from the kitchen area to the dumpster?

---

§483.40 Physician Services   Tags 385 – 390

§483.40(a) Physician Supervision
§483.40(b) Physician Visits
§483.40(c) Frequency of Physician Visits
§483.40(d) Availability of Physicians for Emergency Care
§483.40(e) Physician Delegation of Tasks in SNFs
§483.40(f) Performance of Physician Tasks in NFs

F385 Physician services

§483.40(a)

§483.40 Physician services

A physician must personally approve in writing a recommendation that an individual be admitted to a facility. Each resident must remain under the care of a physician.

§483.40
Intent:

The intent of this regulation is to ensure the medical supervision of the care of nursing home residents by a personal physician.

§483.40
Guideline to Surveyors:

A physician's "personal approval" of an admission recommendation must be in written form. The physician's admission orders for the resident's immediate care as required in §483.20(a) will be accepted as "personal approval" of the admission.

"Supervising the medical care of residents" means participating in the resident's assessment and care planning, monitoring changes in resident's medical status, and providing consultation or treatment when called by the facility. It also includes, but is not limited to, prescribing new therapy, ordering a resident's transfer to the hospital, conducting required routine visits, or delegating and supervising follow-up visits to nurse practitioners or physician assistants. Each resident should be allowed to designate a personal physician. (See §483.10(d)((1).) The facility's responsibility in this situation is to simply assist the resident, when necessary, in his or her efforts to obtain those services. For example, the facility could put the resident in touch with the county medical society for the purpose of obtaining referrals to practicing physicians in the area.

Facilities should share MDS and other assessment data with the physician.

§483.40
Procedures:

If there is a deficiency in §483.10, Resident rights; §483.13, Resident behavior and facility practices; §483.15, Quality of life; or §483.25 Quality of care, fully review all of the tags under this requirement.

(a) Physician supervision.

The facility must ensure that—

(1) The medical care of each resident is supervised by a physician; and

(2) Another physician supervises the medical care of residents when their attending physician is unavailable.

§483.40(a)
Probes:

- How was the supervising physician involved in the resident's assessment and care planning?
- If staff reported a significant change in medical status to the supervising physician, did the physician respond?
- If the supervising physician was unavailable and could not respond, did the facility have a physician on call? Did this physician respond?
- Are residents sent to hospital emergency rooms routinely because the facility does not always have a physician on call?

F386 Physician review of total plan of care, other requirements

§483.40(b)

(b) Physician visits.

The physician must—

(1) Review the resident's total program of care, including medications and treatments, at each visit required by paragraph (c) of this section;

(2) Write, sign, and date progress notes at each visit; and

(3) Sign and date all orders with the exception of influenza and pneumococcal polysaccharide vaccines, which may be administered per physician approved facility policy after an assessment for contraindications. (Effective 11-19-2004)

§483.40(b)
Intent:

The intent of this regulation is to have the physician take an active role in supervising the care of residents. This should not be a superficial visit, but should include an evaluation of the resident's condition and a review of and decision about the continued appropriateness of the resident's current medical regime.

§483.40(b)
Guidelines to Surveyors:

Total program of care includes all care the facility provides residents to maintain or improve their highest practicable mental and physical functional status, as defined by the comprehensive assessment and plan of care. Care includes medical services and medication management; physical, occupational, and speech/language therapy; nursing care; nutritional interventions; social work; and activity services that maintain or improve psychosocial functioning.

The physician records residents' progress and problems in maintaining or improving their mental and physical functional status. The physician need not review the total plan of care at each visit, but must review the total plan of care at visits required by §483.40(c). There is no requirement for physician renewal of orders.

In cases where facilities have created the option for a resident's record to be maintained by computer, rather than hard copy, electronic signatures are acceptable. See Guidelines for §483.75(1)(1) for information on facility safeguards concerning electronic signatures.

Physician orders may be transmitted by facsimile machine if the following conditions are met:

- The physician should have signed and retained the original copy of the order from which the facsimile was transmitted and be able to provide it upon request. Alternatively, the original may be sent to the facility at a later time and substituted for the facsimile.
- The facility should photocopy the faxed order since some facsimiles fade over time. The facsimile copy can be discarded after facility photocopies it.
- A facility using such a system should establish adequate safeguards to assure that it is not subject to abuse.

It is not necessary for a physician to re-sign the facsimile order when he/she visits the facility.

When rubber stamp signatures are authorized by the facility's management, the individual whose signature the stamp represents shall place in the administrative offices of the facility a signed statement to the effect that he/she is the only one who has the stamp and uses it. A list of computer codes and written signatures must be readily available and maintained under adequate safeguards.

§483.40(b)
Probes:

- Do services ordered by a physician show a pattern of care to maintain or improve the resident's level of independent functioning? For example, how do physician orders reflect the resident's nutritional status and needs?

- Does documentation reflect continuity of care in maintaining or improving a resident's mental and physical functional status? For example, do the attending physician's rehabilitation services orders show a pattern of consistent restorative programming?

F387 Frequency of physician visits

§483.40(c)(1)(2)

(c) Frequency of physician visits

(1) The resident must be seen by a physician at least once every 30 days for the first 90 days after admission, and at least once every 60 days thereafter.

(2) A physician visit is considered timely if it occurs not later than 10 days after the date the visit was required.

F388 Physician visits: personal, permitted alternates

§483.40(c)(3)(4)

(3) Except as provided in paragraphs (c)(4) and (f) of this section, all required physician visits must be made by the physician personally.

(4) At the option of the physician, required visits in SNFs, after the initial visit, may alternate between personal visits by the physician and visits by a physician assistant, nurse practitioner or clinical nurse specialist in accordance with paragraph (e) of this section.

§483.40(c)
Guidelines to Surveyors:

"Must be seen" means that the physician must make actual face-to-face contact with the resident. There is no requirement for this type of contact at the time of admission, since the decision to admit an individual to a nursing facility (whether from a hospital or from the individual's own residence) generally involves physician contact during the period immediately preceding the admission.

After the initial physician visit in SNFs, where States allow their use, a qualified nurse practitioner (NP), clinical nurse specialist, or physician assistant (PA) may make every other required visit. (See §483.40(e) Physician delegation of tasks in SNFs.)

In a NF, the physician visit requirement, in accord with State law, may be satisfied by NP, clinical nurse specialist, or PA. (See §483.40(f).)

The timing of physician visits is based on the admission date of the resident. Visits will be made within the first 30 days, and then at 30 day intervals up until 90 days after the admission date. Visits will then be at 60 day intervals.

Permitting up to 10 days slippage of a due date will not affect the next due date. However, do not specifically look at the time tables for physician visits unless there is indication of inadequate medical care. The regulation states that the physician (or his/her delegate) must visit the resident at least every 30 days or 60 days. There is no provision for physicians to use discretion in visiting at intervals longer than those specified at §483.40(c).

Policy that allows a NP, clinical nurse specialist, or PA to make every other required visit, and that allows a 10-day slippage in the time of the visit, does not relieve the physician of the obligation to visit a resident when the resident's medical condition makes that visit necessary.

It is expected that visits will occur at the facility rather than the doctor's office unless office equipment is needed or a resident specifically requests an office visit. If the facility has an established policy that residents leave the grounds for medical care, the resident does not object, and this policy does not infringe on his/her rights, there is no prohibition to this practice. The facility should inform the resident of this practice, in accordance with §483.10(b).

§483.40(c)
Probes:

- How does the scheduling and frequency of physician visits relate to any identified quality of care problems?
- When a PA, clinical nurse specialist, or NP performs a delegated physician visit, and determines that the resident's condition warrants direct contact between the physician and the resident, does the physician follow up promptly with a personal visit?

F389 Availability of physicians for emergency care

§483.40(d)

(d) The facility must provide or arrange for the provision of physician services 24 hours a day, in case of an emergency.

§483.40(d)
Guidelines to Surveyors:

If a resident's own physician is unavailable, the facility should attempt to contact that physician's designated referral physician before assuming the responsibility of assigning a physician.

Arranging for physician services may include assuring resident transportation to a hospital emergency room/ward or other medical facility if the facility is unable to provide emergency medical care at the facility.

§483.40(d)
Probes:

Does the facility have a physician on call for medical emergencies? Does this physician respond?

For what reasons are residents sent to hospital emergency rooms?

Did medical management of the emergency affect the residents' maintaining or improving their functional abilities?

If the resident refused the physician's visit, what has the facility done to explain to the resident the results and alternatives that may be available?

F390 Physician delegation of tasks

§483.40(e)(f)

(e) Physician delegation of tasks in SNFs

(1) Except as specified in paragraph (e)(2) of this section, a physician may delegate tasks to a physician assistant, nurse practitioner, or clinical nurse specialist who—

(i) Meets the applicable definition in §491.2 of this chapter or, in the case of a clinical nurse specialist, is licensed as such by the State;

(ii) Is acting within the scope of practice as defined by State law; and

(iii) Is under the supervision of the physician.

(2) A physician may not delegate a task when the regulations specify that the physician must perform it personally, or when the delegation is prohibited under State law or by the facility's own policies.

§483.40(e)
Guidelines to Surveyors:

"Nurse practitioner" is a registered professional nurse now licensed to practice in the State and who meets the State's requirements governing the qualification of nurse practitioners.

"Clinical nurse specialist" is a registered professional nurse currently in practice in the State and who meets the State's requirements governing the qualification of clinical nurse specialists.

"Physician assistant" is a person who meets the applicable State requirements governing the qualifications for assistants of physicians.

When personal performance of a particular task by a physician is specified in the regulations, performance of that task cannot be delegated to anyone else. The tasks of examining the resident, reviewing the resident's total program of care, writing progress notes, and signing orders may be delegated according to State law. The extent to which physician services are delegated to physician extenders in SNFs will continue to be determined by the provisions of §483.40(e), while the extent to which these services are performed by physician extenders in NFs will be determined by the individual States under §483.40(f).

§483.40(e)
Probes:

- Do the facility's attending physicians delegate to NPs, clinical nurse specialists, or PAs?
- Do NP/clinical nurse specialist/PA progress notes and orders follow the scope of practice allowed by State law?
- What evidence is there of physician supervision of NPs or PAs? For example, do physicians countersign NP/PA orders, if required by State law?

(f) Performance of physician tasks in NFs

At the option of the State, any required physician task in a NF (including tasks which the regulations specify must be performed personally by the physician) may also be satisfied when performed by a nurse practitioner, clinical nurse specialist, or physician assistant who is not an employee of the facility but who is working in collaboration with a physician.

§483.40(f)
Guidelines to Surveyors:

If delegation of physician tasks is permitted in your State and the physician extender does not meet the qualifications listed here, cite F388.

§483.40(f)
Procedures:

If a nurse practitioner, clinical nurse specialist, or physician assistant is performing required physician tasks in a NF, is this allowed by the State? Is this person an employee of the facility? (Facility employees are prohibited from serving in this capacity.)

§483.40(f)
Probes:

Is this person working in collaboration with the physician?

---

§483.45 Specialized Rehabilitative Services   Tags 406–407

§483.45(a) Provision of Services
§483.45(b) Qualifications

F406 Specialized rehabilitative services

§483.45(a) Provision of Services

If specialized rehabilitative services such as, but not limited to physical therapy, speech-language pathology, occupational therapy, and mental health rehabilitative services for mental illness and mental retardation, are required in the resident's comprehensive plan of care, the facility must—

(1) Provide the required services; or

(2) Obtain the required services from an outside resource (in accordance with §483.75(h) of this part) from a provider of specialized rehabilitative services.

Intent §483.45(a)(1)(2)

The intent of this regulation is to assure that residents receive necessary specialized rehabilitative services as determined by the comprehensive assessment and care plan, to prevent avoidable physical and mental deterioration and to assist them in obtaining or maintaining their highest practicable level of functional and psychosocial well-being.

"Specialized rehabilitative services" are differentiated from restorative services which are provided by nursing staff. Specialized rehabilitative services are provided by or coordinated by qualified personnel.

Specialized rehabilitative services are considered a facility service and are, thus, included within the scope of facility services. They must be provided by or coordinated by qualified personnel. They must be provided to residents who need them even when the services are not specifically enumerated in the State plan. No fee can be charged a Medicaid recipient for specialized rehabilitative services because they are covered facility services.

A facility is not obligated to provide specialized rehabilitative services if it does not have residents who require these services. If a resident develops a need for these services after admission, the facility must either provide the services, or, where appropriate, obtain the services from an outside resource.

For a resident with mental illness (MI) or mental retardation (MR) to have his or her specialized needs met, the individual must receive all services necessary to assist the individual in maintaining or achieving as much independence and self-determination as possible. They are:

"Specialized services for MI or MR" refers to those services to be provided by the State which can only be delivered by personnel or programs other than those of the NF (e.g., outside the NF setting), because the overall level of NF services is not as intense as necessary to meet the individual's needs.

The Preadmission Screening and Annual Resident Review (PASARR) report indicates specialized services required by the resident. The State is required to list those services in the report, as well as provide or arrange for the provision of the services. If the State determines that the resident does not require specialized services, the facility is responsible to provide all services necessary to meet the resident's mental health or mental retardation needs.

"Mental health rehabilitative services for MI and MR" refers to those services of lesser frequency or intensity to be implemented by all levels of nursing facility staff who come into contact with the resident who is mentally ill or who has mental retardation. These services are necessary regardless of whether or not they are required to be subject to the PASARR process and whether or not they require additional services to be provided or arranged for by the State as specialized services.

The facility should provide interventions which complement, reinforce, and are consistent with any specialized services (as defined by the resident's PASARR) the individual is receiving or is required to receive by the State. The individual's plan of care should specify how the facility will integrate relevant activities throughout all hours of the individual's day at the NF to achieve this consistency and enhancement of PASARR goals. The surveyor should see competent interaction by staff at all times, in both formal and informal settings in accordance with the individual's needs.

Mental health rehabilitative services for MI and MR may include, but are not limited to:

- Consistent implementation during the resident's daily routine and across settings, of systematic plans which are designed to change inappropriate behaviors;
- Drug therapy and monitoring of the effectiveness and side effects of medications which have been prescribed to change inappropriate behavior or to alter manifestations of psychiatric illness;
- Provision of a structured environment for those individuals who are determined to need such structure (e.g., structured socialization activities to diminish tendencies toward isolation and withdrawal);
- Development, maintenance and consistent implementation across settings of those programs designed to teach individuals the daily living skills they need to be more independent and self-determining including, but not limited to, grooming, personal hygiene, mobility, nutrition, vocational skills, health, drug therapy, mental health education, money management, and maintenance of the living environment;

- Crisis intervention service;
- Individual, group, and family psychotherapy; and
- Development of appropriate personal support networks.

Probes §483.45(a)(1)(2)

1. For physical therapy

    a. What did the facility do to improve the resident's muscle strength? The resident's balance?

    b. What did the facility do to determine if an assistive device would enable the resident to reach or maintain his/her highest practicable level of physical function?

    c. If the resident has an assistive device, is he/she encouraged to use it on a regular basis?

    d. What did the facility do to increase the amount of physical activity the resident could do (for example, the number of repetitions of an exercise, the distance walked)?

    e. What did the facility do to prevent or minimize contractures, which could lead to decreased mobility and increased risk of pressure ulcer occurrence?

2. For occupational therapy

    a. What did the facility do to decrease the amount of assistance needed to perform a task?

    b. What did the facility do to decrease behavioral symptoms?

    c. What did the facility do to improve gross and fine motor coordination?

    d. What did the facility do to improve sensory awareness, visual-spatial awareness, and body integration?

    e. What did the facility do to improve memory, problem solving, attention span, and the ability to recognize safety hazards?

3. For speech-language pathology

    a. What did the facility do to improve auditory comprehension such as understanding common, functional words; concepts of time and place; and conversation?

    b. What did the facility do to improve speech production?

    c. What did the facility do to improve the expressive behavior such as the ability to name common, functional items?

    d. What did the facility do to improve the functional abilities of residents with moderate to severe hearing loss who have received an audiologic evaluation? For example, did the facility instruct the resident how to effectively and independently use environmental controls to compensate for hearing loss such as eye contact, preferential seating, use of the better ear?

    e. For the resident who cannot speak, did the facility assess for a communication board or an alternate means of communication?

4. For health rehabilitative services for MI and MR

    a. What did the facility do to decrease incidents of inappropriate behaviors, for individuals with MR, or behavioral symptoms for persons with MI? To increase appropriate behavior?

    b. What did the facility do to identify and treat the underlying factors behind tendencies toward isolation and withdrawal?

    c. What did the facility do to develop and maintain necessary daily living skills?

    d. How has the facility modified the training strategies it uses with its residents to account for the special learning needs of its residents with MI or MR?

    e. Questions to ask individuals with MI or MR:

        (1) Who do you talk to when you have a problem or need something?

        (2) What do you do when you feel happy? Feel sad? Can't sleep at night?

        (3) In what activities are you involved, and how often?

F407 Qualifications of specialized rehabilitative services personnel

§483.45(b) Qualifications

Specialized rehabilitative services must be provided under the written order of a physician by qualified personnel.

Intent §485.45(b)

The intent of this regulation is to assure that the rehabilitative services are medically necessary as prescribed by a physician and provided by qualified personnel to maximize potential outcomes.

Specialized rehabilitative services are provided for individual's under a physician's order by a qualified professional. Once the assessment for specialized rehabilitative services is completed, a care plan must be developed, followed, and monitored by a licensed professional. Once a resident has met his or her care plan goals, a licensed professional can either discontinue treatment or initiate a maintenance program which either nursing or restorative sides will follow to maintain functional and physical status.

Interpretive Guidelines §483.45(b)

"Qualified personnel" means that professional staff are licensed, certified, or registered to provide specialized therapy/rehabilitative services in accordance with applicable State laws.

Health rehabilitative services for MI and MR must be implemented consistently by all staff unless the nature of the services is such that they are designated or required to be implemented only by licensed or credentialed personnel.

Procedures §483.45(b)

Determine if there are any problems in quality of care related to maintaining or improving functional abilities. Determine if these problems are attributable in part to the qualifications of specialized rehabilitative services staff.

Probes §483.45(b)

If the facility does not employ professional staff who have experience working directly with or designing training or treatment programs to meet the needs of individuals with MI or MR, how has the facility arranged for the necessary direct or staff training services to be provided?

§483.55 Dental Services   Tags 411–412

§483.55(a) Skilled Nursing Facilities
§483.55(b) Nursing Facilities

F411 Dental services

§483.55(a)

§483.55 Dental services

The facility must assist residents in obtaining routine and 24-hour emergency dental care.

(a) Skilled nursing facilities

A facility

(1) Must provide or obtain from an outside resource, in accordance with §483.75(h) of this part, routine and emergency dental services to meet the needs of each resident;

(2) May charge a Medicare resident an additional amount for routine and emergency dental services;

(3) Must if necessary, assist the resident—

(i) In making appointments; and

(ii) By arranging for transportation to and from the dentist's office; and

(4) Promptly refer residents with loss of damaged dentures to a dentist.

§483.55
Intent:

The intent of this regulation is to ensure that the facility be responsible for assisting the resident in obtaining needed dental services, including routine dental services.

§483.55
Guidelines to Surveyors:

This requirement makes the facility directly responsible for the dental care needs of its residents. The facility must ensure that a dentist is available for residents, i.e., employ a staff dentist or have a contract (arrangement) with a dentist to provide services.

For Medicare and private pay residents, facilities are responsible for having the services available, but they may impose an additional charge for the services.

For all residents of the facility, if they are unable to pay for needed dental services, the facility should attempt to find alternative funding sources or alternative service delivery systems so that the resident is able to maintain his/her highest practicable level of well-being. (See §483.15(g).)

The facility is responsible for selecting a dentist who provides dental services in accordance with professional standards of quality and timeliness under §483.75(h)(2).

"Routine dental services" means an annual inspection of the oral cavity for signs of disease, diagnosis of dental disease, dental radiographs as needed, dental cleaning, fillings (new and repairs), minor dental plate adjustments, smoothing of broken teeth, and limited prosthodontic procedures, e.g., taking impressions for dentures and fitting dentures.

"Emergency dental services" includes services needed to treat an episode of acute pain in teeth, gums, or palate; broken, or otherwise damaged teeth; or any other problem of the oral cavity, appropriately treated by a dentist that requires immediate attention.

"Prompt referral" means, within reason, as soon as the dentures are lost or damaged. Referral does not mean that the resident must see the dentist at that time, but does mean that an appointment (referral) is made, or that the facility is aggressively working at replacing the dentures.

§483.55
Probes:

Do residents selected for comprehensive or focused reviews, as appropriate, with dentures use them? Are residents missing teeth and may be in need of dentures? Do sampled residents have problems eating and maintaining nutritional status because of poor oral health or oral hygiene? Are resident's dentures intact? Proper fit?

F412 Dental services required

§483.55(b)

(b) Nursing facilities

The facility

(1) Must provide or obtain from an outside resource, in accordance with §483.75(h) of this part, the following dental services to meet the needs of each resident:

(i) Routine dental services (to the extent covered under the State plan); and

(ii) Emergency dental services;

(2) Must, if necessary, assist the resident—

(i) In making appointments; and

(ii) By arranging for transportation to and from the dentist's office; and

(3) Must promptly refer residents with lost or damaged dentures to a dentist.

§483.55(b)(1)(i)
Guidelines to Surveyors:

For Medicaid residents, the facility must provide the resident, without charge, all emergency dental services, as well as those routine dental services that are covered under the State plan.

§483.60 Pharmacy Services   Tags 425 – 432

§483.60(a) Procedures
§483.60(b) Service Consultation
§483.60(c) Drug Regimen Review
§483.60(d) Labeling of Drugs and Biologicals
§483.60(e) Storage of Drugs and Biologicals

F425 Pharmacy services

§483.60

§483.60 Pharmacy services

The facility must provide routine and emergency drugs and biologicals to its residents, or obtain them under an agreement described in 483.75(h) of this part. The facility may permit unlicensed personnel to administer drugs if State law permits, but only under the supervision of a licensed nurse.

§483.60
Guideline to Surveyors:

The facility is responsible under §483.75(h) for the "timeliness of the services."

A drug, whether prescribed on a routine, emergency, or as needed basis, must be provided in a timely manner. If a failure to provide a prescribed drug in a timely manner causes the resident discomfort or endangers his or her health and safety, then this requirement is not met.

§483.60
Procedures:

During the surveyor's observation of the drug pass, are all ordered medications available?

F426 Pharmacy procedures

§483.60(a) Procedures

A facility must provide pharmaceutical services (including procedures that assure the accurate acquiring, receiving, dispensing, and administering of all drugs and biologicals) to meet the needs of each resident.

F427 Consultant pharmacist required

§483.60(b) Service Consultation

The facility must employ or obtain the services of a licensed pharmacist who—

(1) Provides consultation on all aspects of the provision of pharmacy services in the facility;

(2) Establishes a system of records of receipt and disposition of all controlled drugs in sufficient detail to enable an accurate reconciliation; and

(3) Determines that drug records are in order and that an account of all controlled drugs is maintained and periodically reconciled.

Interpretive Guidelines §483.60(b)(2) and (3)

A record of receipt and disposition of controlled drugs does not need to be proof of use sheets. The facility can use existing documentation such as the Medication Administration Record (MAR) to accomplish this record.

Periodic reconciliations should be monthly. If they reveal shortages, the pharmacist and the director of nursing may need to initiate more frequent reconciliations. In situations in which loss of controlled drugs is evident, the facility may have to utilize proof of use sheets on all controlled drugs for all shifts. However, when the source of shortage is located and remedied, the facility may go back to periodic reconciliation by the pharmacist.

Please note that the regulation does not prohibit shortages of controlled drugs — only that a record be kept and that it be periodically reconciled. If the survey reveals that all controlled drugs are not accounted for, refer the case to the State nursing home licensure authority, or to the State Board of Pharmacy.

F428 Drug regimen use

(Rev. 5, Issued: 11-19-04, Effective: 11-19-04, Implementation: 11-19-04)

§483.60(c) Drug Regimen Review

(1) The drug regimen of each resident must be reviewed at least once a month by a licensed pharmacist.

Interpretive Guidelines §483.60(c)(1)

It may be necessary to review more frequently (e.g., every week) depending on the residents' condition and the drugs they are taking.

F429 Pharmacist report of irregularities to physician and DON

(Rev. 12, Issued: 10-14-05, Effective: 10-14-05, Implementation: 10-14-05)

§483.60(c)(2) The pharmacist must report any irregularities to the attending physician, and the director of nursing.

Interpretive Guidelines 483.60(c)(2)

Miscellaneous Drugs That Are Potentially Inappropriate in the Elderly

The following list of drugs and diagnoses/drug combinations have been partially adapted from a paper entitled "Explicit Criteria for Determining Inappropriate Medication Use by the Elderly" by Mark H. Beers, MD. This paper was published in the "Archives of Internal Medicine," Volume 157, July 28, 1997. The paper lists numerous drugs and diagnosis/drug combinations that are judged to place a person over the age of 65 at greater risk of adverse drug outcomes (ADR). The judgments in this paper were arrived at through an extensive review of the literature by a panel of experts. There are two important quotations from the paper that the surveyor should keep in mind at all times:

1. "These criteria were developed to predict when the potential for adverse outcomes is greater than the potential for benefit."

2. "Without measuring outcomes, criteria cannot determine whether adverse outcomes have occurred; they can only determine that they are more likely to occur."

It should be noted that medication alterations may not be appropriate for some short-term residents. Many residents arrive in the long-term care setting already on medications that they have managed to tolerate for years or that have been prescribed in the hospital. For some short-stay residents, it is difficult to change these medications without a period of observation and information gathering. Therefore, review by the surveyor is not necessary for drug therapy given the first seven consecutive days upon admission/readmission, unless there is an immediate threat to health and safety.

List of Drug Combinations with High Potential for Less Severe Adverse Outcomes

1. Phenylbutazone (Butazolidin)

Risk: "May produce serious hematological side effects (blood disorders) and should not be used in elderly patients."

Blood disorders include bone marrow depression, aplastic anemia, agranulocytosis, leukopenia, pancytopenia, thrombocytopenia, macrocytic or megoblastic anemia.

2. Trimethobenzamide (Tigan)

Risk: "Trimethobenzamide is one of the least effective antiemetics, yet it can cause extrapyramidal side effects."

Extrapyramidal side effects may involve various combinations of tremors; postural unsteadiness; lack of or slowness of movement; cogwheel rigidity; expressionless face; drooling; infrequent blinking; shuffling gate; decreased arm swing; and rigidity of muscles in the limbs, neck, and trunk.

3. Indomethacin (Indocin, Indocin SR)

Risk: "Of all the nonsteroidal anti-inflammatory drugs, indomethacin produces the most central nervous system side effects and should therefore be avoided in the elderly." The most common side effects (in order of frequency of occurrence) are headache (10%); dizziness (3-9%); and vertigo, somnolence, depression, and fatigue (1-3%).

Exception: It is considered acceptable to use indomethacin for short-term (e.g., 1 week) treatment of an acute episode of gouty arthritis.

4. Dipyridamole (Persantine)

Risk: "Dipyridamole frequently cause orthostatic hypotension in the elderly. It has been proven beneficial only in patients with artificial heart valves. Whenever possible, its use in the elderly should be avoided."

5. Reserpine (Serpasil)

Combination products such as Ser-Ap-Es, Serathide, Hydropses, Unipres, Uni-serp, Diutensen-R, Metatensin #2 & #4, Diupres, Hydroserpine, Hydromox-R, Regroton, Renese-R, Salutensin.

Risk: "Reserpine imposes unnecessary risks in the elderly, inducing depression, impotence, sedation, and orthostatic hypotension. Safer alternatives exist."

6. Diphenhydramine (Benadryl)

Risk: "Diphenhydramine is potently anticholinergic and usually should not be used as a hypnotic in the elderly. When used to treat or prevent allergic reactions, it should be used in the smallest dose and with great caution." Anticholinergic side effects can include such symptoms as dry mouth, blurred vision, urinary retention, constipation, confusion, and sometimes, delirium or hallucinations.

Exception: For treatment of allergies, review by the surveyor is not necessary if these drugs are used periodically (once every three months) for a short duration (not over seven days) for symptoms of an acute, self-limiting illness.

7. Ergot Mesyloids (Hydergine), Cyclandelate (Cyclospasmol)

Risk: "Hydergine and the central vasodilators have not been shown to be effective, in the doses studied for treatment of dementia or any other condition."

8. Muscle Relaxants

Muscle Relaxants such as Methocarbamol (Robaxin), Carisoprodol (Soma), Chlorzoxazone (Paraflex), Metaxalone (Skelaxin), Cyclobenzaprine (Flexiril), Dantrolene (Dantrium), Orphenadrine (Norflex, Banflex, Myotrol).

Risk: "Most muscle relaxants are poorly tolerated by the elderly, leading to anticholinergic side effects, sedation, and weakness." Anticholinergic side effects include symptoms such as dry mouth, blurred vision, urinary retention, constipation, confusion, and sometimes, delirium or hallucinations.

Exception: Review by the surveyor is not necessary if these drugs are used periodically (once every three months) for a short duration (not over seven days) for symptoms of an acute, self-limiting illness.

9. Antihistamines

Chlorpheniramine (Chlor-Trimeton), Diphenhydramine (Benadryl), Hydroxyzine (Vistaril, Atarax), Cyproheptadine (Periactin), Promethazine (Phenergan), Tripelennamine (PBZ), Dexchlorpheniramine (Polarmine).

Risk: "All nonprescription and many prescription antihistamines have potent anticholinergic properties." Anticholinergic side effects can include such symptoms as dry mouth, blurred vision, urinary retention, constipation, confusion, and sometimes, delirium or hallucinations. When used to treat or prevent allergic reactions, antihistamines should be used in the smallest possible dose, and for the shortest period of time, and with great caution.

Diagnosis/Drug Combinations with High Potential for Less Severe Outcomes

1. Diabetes

Drugs: Corticosteriods such as Beclomethasone (beclovent, Vanceril), Betamethasone (Celestone), Cortisone Acetate (Cortone Acetate), Dexamethasone (Decadron, Dexone), Hydrocortisone (Cortef), Methyl prednisone (medrol), Prednisolone (many brands), Prednisone (many brands).

Risk: "May worsen diabetic control, if recently started."

If Recently Started: The panelists for the Beers' study believed that the severity of adverse reaction would be substantially greater when these drugs were recently started. In general, the greatest risk would be within about a 1-month period. If the surveyor encounters the use of this drug within the first month, they should pay close attention to obtaining a rationale for its use during that time. The surveyor should be responsible for in-depth investigation to determine when the drug was actually started. It should be noted that rapid withdrawal of these medicines in a steroid-dependent person can cause serious side effects.

2. Active or recurrent gastritis, peptic ulcer disease, or gastroesophageal reflux disease.

Drugs: Aspirin in excess of 325 mg per day.

Risk: "May exacerbate ulcer disease, gastritis, and gastroesophageal reflux disease (GERD)."

Note: The panelists did not believe that enteric coated aspirin would be beneficial since aspirin exacerbates these conditions primarily through its systemic effects rather than its local effects.

Potential Side Effects: Nausea, dyspepsia, vomiting, abdominal pain, heartburn, epigastric pain, diarrhea, flatulence.

Drugs: Potassium supplements such as Kaochlor, Klorvess, Kaon, K-Lor, K-Tab, K-Dur, K-Lyte, Slow K, Klotrix, Micro K, or Ten K. This includes liquid oral dosage forms which, if used, should be administered after meals with an optimal amount of water or fruit juice (depending on the resident's fluid restrictions) to decrease the potential of gastric distress or bad taste as much as possible.

Risk: "May cause gastric irritation with symptoms similar to ulcer disease."

Potential Side Effects: Nausea, dyspepsia, vomiting, abdominal pain, heartburn, epigastric pain, diarrhea, flatulence.

Exception: Use of these medications to treat low potassium levels until they return to normal range if determined by the prescriber that use of fresh fruits and vegetables or other dietary supplementation is not adequate or possible.

3. Seizures or Epilepsy

Drugs: Clozapine (Clozaril), Chlorpromazine (Thorazine), Thioridazine (Mellaril), Chlorpropthixene (Taractan), Metoclopramide (Reglan), Fluphenazine (Prolixin, Permitil), Perphenazine (Trilafon), Mesoridazine (Serentil), Prochlorperazine (Compazine), Promazine (Sparine), Trifluoperazine (Stelazine), Triflupromazine (Vesprin), Haloperidol (Haldol), Loxapine (Loxitane), Molindone (Moban), Olanzapine (Zyprexa), Pimozide (Orap), Risperidone (Risperdal), Thiothixene (Navane), Quetiapine (Seroquel).

Risk: "May lower seizure threshold."

Potential Side Effect: Increased risk of seizure activity.

4. Benign Prostatic Hypertrophy (BPH)

Drugs: Narcotic drugs such as Codeine (Empirin with Codeine, Tylenol with Codeine), Meperidine (Demerol), Fentanyl (Duragesic), Hydromorphone (Dilaudid), Morphine (many brands), Oxycodone (Percocet, Roxicodone, etc.), Propoxyphene (Darvon, Darvon Comp-65, Darvon-N, Darvocet-N, etc.).

Risk: "Anticholinergic drugs may impair micturition and cause obstruction in men with BPH."

Potential Side Effects: Urinary retention, urinary incontinence, reflux, pyelonephritis, nephritis, low grade temperature, low back pain.

Exception: Review by the surveyor is not necessary if these drugs are used periodically (once every three months) for a short duration (not over seven days) for symptoms of an acute, self-limiting illness.

Drugs: Flavoxate (Urispas), Oxybutynin (Ditropan), Bethanechol (Urecholine, Duvoid).

Risk: "Bladder relaxants may cause obstruction in persons with BPH."

Potential Side Effects: Urinary retention, incontinence, hesitancy, reflux, hydronephrosis.

5. Constipation

Drugs: Anticholinergic antihistamines such as Chlorpheniramine (Chlor-Trimeton), Diphenhydramine (Benadryl), Hydroxyzine (Vistaril & Atarax), Cyproheptadine (Periactin), Promethazine (Phenergan), Tripelennamine (PBZ), Dexchlorpheniramine (Polaramine).

Exception: Review by the surveyor is not necessary if these drugs are used periodically (once every three months) for a short duration (not over seven days) for symptoms of an acute, self-limiting illness.

Anti-Parkinson medications such as Benztropine (Cogentin), Trihexyphenidyl (Artane), Procyclidine (Kemadren), Biperiden (Akineton).

GI Antispasmodics such as Dicyclomine (Bentyl), Hyoscyamine (Levsin & Levsinex), Propantheline (Pro-Banthine), Belladonna Alkaloids (Donnatal), Clidinium containing products such as Librax.

Exception: Review by the surveyor is not necessary if these drugs are used periodically (once every three months) for a short duration (not over seven days) for symptoms of an acute, self-limiting illness.

Anticholinergic antidepressant drugs such as Amitriptyline (Elavil), Amoxapine (Asendin), Clomipramine (Anafranil), Desipramine (Pertofrane), Doxepin (Adapin, Sinequan), Imipramine (Tofranil), Maprotiline (Ludiomil), Nortriptyline (Aventyl, Pamelor), Protriptyline (Vivactil).

Narcotic Drugs such as Codeine (Empirin with Codeine, Tylenol with Codeine), Meperidine (Demerol), Fentanyl (Duragesic), Hydromorphone (Dilaudid), Morphine (many brands), Oxycodone (Percocet, Roxicodone, etc.), Propoxyphen (Darvon, Darvon Comp-65, Darvon-N, Darvocet-N, etc.).

Exception: Review by the surveyor is not necessary if these drugs are used periodically (once every three months) for a short duration (not over seven days) for symptoms of an acute, self-limiting illness.

6. Insomnia

Drugs:

- Decongestants such as Phenylephrine (Duo-Medihaler), Phenylpropanolamine (Genex), Pseudoephedrine (Novafed, Sudafed, Triaminic AM, Efidac/24);
- Theophylline (Elixophyllin Bronkodyl, Theo-Dur, Slo-Bid);
- Desipramine (Pertofrane, Norpramin);
- Selective Serotonin Reuptake Inhibitors such as Fluoxetine (Prozac), Paroxetine (Paxil), Sertraline (Zoloft);
- Methylphenidate (Ritalin);
- Monamine Oxidase Inhibitors (MAOIs) such as Phenelzine (Nardil), Tranylcypromine (Parnate); and
- Beta Agonists such as Isoproterenol (Isuprel), Albuterol (Proventil), Bitolterol (Tornalate), Terbutaline (Brethine).

Risk: "May cause or worsen insomnia."

(The surveyor should consider that insomnia is often a symptom of untreated depression and Chronic Obstructive Pulmonary Disease (COPD.))

F430 Action required on pharmacist reports

§483.60(c)(2)

These reports must be acted upon.

Interpretive Guidelines §483.60(c)(2)

The director of nursing and the attending physicians are not required to agree with the pharmacist's report, nor are they required to provide a rationale for their "acceptance" or "rejection" of the report. They must, however, act upon the report. This may be accomplished by indicating acceptance or rejection of the report and signing their names. The facility is encouraged to provide the medical director with a copy of drug regimen review reports and to involve the medical director in reports that have not been acted upon.

F431 Labeling of drugs and biologicals

§483.60(d) Labeling of Drugs and Biologicals

Drugs and biologicals used in the facility must be labeled in accordance with currently accepted professional principles, and include the appropriate accessory and cautionary instructions, and the expiration date when applicable.

Interpretive Guidelines §483.60(d)

This section imposes currently accepted labeling requirements on facilities, even though the pharmacies will be immediately responsible for accomplishing the task.

The critical elements of the drug label in a long-term care facility are the name of the drug and its strength.

The names of the resident and the physician do not have to be on the label of the package, but they must be identified with the package in such a manner as to assure that the drug is administered to the right patient.

All drugs approved by the Food and Drug Administration must have expiration dates on the manufacturer's container. "When applicable" means that expiration dates must be on the labels of drugs used in long-term care facilities unless State law stipulates otherwise.

F432 Storage of drugs and biologicals

§483.60(e) Storage of Drugs and Biologicals

(1) In accordance with State and Federal laws, the facility must store all drugs and biologicals in locked compartments under proper temperature controls, and permit only authorized personnel to have access to the keys.

(2) The facility must provide separately locked, permanently affixed compartments for storage of controlled drugs listed in Schedule II of the Comprehensive Drug Abuse Prevention and Control Act of 1976 and other drugs subject to abuse, except when the facility uses single unit

package drug distribution systems in which the quantity stored is minimal and a missing dose can be readily detected.

Interpretive Guidelines §483.60(e)

Compartments in the context of these regulations include but are not limited to drawers, cabinets, rooms, refrigerators, carts, and boxes. The provisions for authorized personnel to have access to keys must be determined by the facility management in accordance with Federal, State, and local laws and facility practices. "Separately locked" means that the key to the separately locked Schedule II drugs is not the same key that is used to gain access to the non-Schedule II drugs.

Probes §483.60(e)

Are all drugs and biologicals stored properly, locked, and at proper temperature?

§483.65 Infection Control   Tags 441–445

§483.65(a) Infection Control Program
§483.65(b) Preventing Spread of Infection
§483.65(c) Linens

F441 Infection control

§483.65 Infection Control

The facility must establish and maintain an infection control program designed to provide a safe, sanitary, and comfortable environment and to help prevent the development and transmission of disease and infection.

§483.65(a) Infection Control Program

The facility must establish an infection control program under which it—

(1) Investigates, controls, and prevents infections in the facility;

(2) Decides what procedures, such as isolation should be applied to an individual resident; and

(3) Maintains a record of incidents and corrective actions related to infections.

Intent §483.65(a)

The intent of this regulation is to assure that the facility has an infection control program which is effective for investigating, controlling, and preventing infections. If infection control has been identified as an area of concern during Phase 1 of the survey, investigate aspects of the program, as appropriate, during Phase 2.

Interpretive Guidelines §483.65(a)

The facility's infection control program must have a system to monitor and investigate causes of infection (nosocomial and community acquired) and manner of spread. A facility should, for example, maintain a separate record on infection that identifies each resident with an infection, states the date of infection, the causative agent, the origin or site of infection, and describes what cautionary measures were taken to prevent the spread of the infection within the facility. The system must enable the facility to analyze clusters, changes in prevalent organisms, or increases in the rate of infection in a timely manner.

Surveillance data should be routinely reviewed and recommendations made for the prevention and control of additional cases.

The written infection control program should be periodically reviewed by the facility and revised as indicated.

Current standards for infection control program address the following. The following are not regulatory requirements but provide guidance for evaluating the facility's program.

- Definition of nosocomial/facility acquired infections and communicable diseases.
- Risk assessment of occurrence of communicable diseases for both residents and staff that is reviewed annually, or more frequently if indicated.
- Methods for identifying, documenting, and investigating nosocomial infections and communicable diseases. The infection control program should be able to identify new infections quickly, paying particular attention to residents at high risk of infection (e.g., residents who are immobilized, have invasive devices or procedures, have pressure sores, have been recently discharged from a hospital to the long-term care facility, have MI or MR, have decreased mental status, are nutritionally compromised, or have altered immune systems).
- Early detection of residents who have signs and symptoms of tuberculosis (TB) and a referral protocol to a facility where TB can be evaluated and managed appropriately.
- Measures for prevention of infections, especially those associated with intravascular therapy, indwelling urinary catheters, tracheostomy care, stoma care, respiratory care, immunosuppression, pressures sores, bladder and bowel incontinence, and any other factors which compromise a resident's resistance to infections.
- Measures for the prevention of communicable disease outbreaks, including tuberculosis, flu, hepatitis, scabies, MRSA.
- Procedures to inform and involve a local or State epidemiologist, as required by the State for non-sporadic, facility-wide infections that are difficult to control.
- Isolation procedures and requirements for infected and at risk or immunosuppressed nursing home residents.
- Use of and inservice education regarding standard precautions (e.g., universal precautions/body substance isolation).
- Handwashing, respiratory protection, linen handling, housekeeping, needle and hazardous waste disposal, as well as other means for limiting the spread of communicable organisms.
- Authority, indications, and procedures for obtaining and acting upon microbiological cultures from residents and for isolating residents.
- Proper use of disinfectants, antiseptics, and germicides in accordance with the manufacturer's instructions and Environmental Protection Agency (EPA) or FDA label specifications to avoid harm to staff, residents, and visitors and to ensure its effectiveness.
- Orientation of all new facility personnel to the infection control program and periodic updates for all staff.
- Measures for the screening of the health care workers for communicable diseases, and for the evaluation of workers exposed to residents with communicable diseases including TB and bloodborne pathogens.
- Work restriction guidelines for an employee that is infected or ill with a communicable disease.

- Measures which address prevention of infection common to nursing home residents (e.g., vaccination for influenza and pneumococcal pneumonia as appropriate) TB screening and testing.
- Sanitization of tubs, whirlpools, and multiple use equipment to be performed according to manufacturer's recommendations.

Observe whether staff including direct care, housekeeping, and kitchen staff use gloves in accord with aseptic principles.

Determine if there is consistent use of aseptic technique for dressing changes.

If breaks in technique are observed, verify that the facility has a system in place for routine monitoring of staff infection control practices.

Ask direct care giver staff what do they do and who do they notify when an infection is noted.

Procedures §483.65(a)

Observe sanitation of tub, shower, multiple residents' whirlpool and care equipment, as necessary.

Identify all residents in the sample who are currently on antibiotic therapy and verify that these residents are reported on the facility's infection control logs/records to ensure that infections are being identified timely and that these residents are being adequately monitored for infection.

Review policies related to infection control if observation, record review, or staff interview indicate a problem with infection control.

- For sampled residents at high risk of infection, what has staff done to reduce residents' risk of infection?
- Do surveillance data show a significant increase in the rate of infection from month to month? Over several months? How is this being addressed?
- What infection control policies does the facility use for persons with AIDS, TB, or hepatitis B? Do these policies conform with Occupational Safety and Health Administration's requirements for protecting employees and current accepted standards of practice recommended by Centers for Disease Control and Prevention (CDC)? Does the staff follow its own procedures?
- How does the facility define and dispose of its infectious waste?

F442 Preventing spread of infection

§483.65(b)(1)

(b) Preventing the spread of infection

(1) When the infection control program determines that a resident needs isolation to prevent the spread of infection, the facility must isolate the resident.

Intent

To assure that the facility isolates residents appropriately to prevent the spread of infection. If infection control has been identified as an area of concern during Phase 1 of the survey, investigate aspects of the program, as appropriate, during Phase 2.

Procedures must be followed to prevent cross contamination, including handwashing, and/or changing gloves after providing personal care, or when performing tasks among individuals which provide the opportunity for cross-contamination to occur. Facilities for handwashing must exist and be available to staff. The facility should follow the CDC's Guidelines for Handwashing and Hospital Environmental control, 1985 for handwashing.

The facility should isolate infected residents only to the degree needed to isolate the infecting organism. The method used should be the least restrictive possible, while maintaining the integrity of the process. For example, the HIV virus is present in blood and other body fluids. The facility should take universal or standard blood and body fluid precautions related to HIV contamination for the following:

- Blood;
- Semen;
- Vaginal secretions;
- Cerebrospinal fluid;
- Synovial fluid;
- Pleural fluid;
- Peritoneal fluid;
- Pericardial fluid;
- Amniotic fluid; and/or
- Fluids with visible blood.

Residents, visitors, and employees should be protected from these fluids. Although the resident infected with HIV should not be isolated routinely, the resident should be isolated if he/she is in the communicable stages of an opportunistic infection, his/her body fluids cannot be contained, or he/she has very poor hygiene and the likelihood of spillage is high.

NOTE: TB isolation rooms are not needed if the facility does not provide care to active TB patients/residents.

"Universal precautions" or "Standard blood and body fluid precautions" is an approach to infection control where all human blood and certain human body fluids are treated as if known to be infectious for HIV, HBV, and other bloodborne pathogens.

Probes §483.65(b)

- For isolated residents, does the facility need to segregate them to control the infectious agent?

- For residents who have been isolated appropriately, does staff use correct procedures consistently? For example, if isolation procedures require wearing gowns, do all staff put on and dispose of the gown in a way that lessens the spread of infection?
- How does the facility control the spread of infection by persons who visit infectious residents? Is there a written protocol?
- Do persons with a communicable disease or infected skin lesions provide care to residents?
- Have any residents developed a communicable disease as defined by State law while in the facility? If so, have appropriate barrier or isolation precautions been followed to control further spread of infection?

Procedures §483.65(b)(1)

Verify that all residents who require isolation as determined by the infection control program are isolated. Observe residents that have been isolated. Determine what level of isolation they are required to have. Evaluate isolation procedures utilized by staff members. Determine if the facility has isolated the resident in the least restrictive environment possible.

F443 Employees with communicable disease or infected skin lesions

Intent §483.65(b)(2)

The intent of this regulation is to prevent the spread of communicable diseases from employees to residents when the employee has a communicable disease or an infected skin lesion.

Skin lesions should be considered infected if they have purulent drainage, or are red, hot, indurated without purulent drainage.

Procedures §483.65(b)(2)

Determine if the facility prohibits employees with diseases communicable through direct contact or infected skin lesions from having direct contact with residents. To make this determination, observe residents' condition and treatments provided, interview facility staff, and review relevant facility policies and procedures for preventing the spread of infection.

F444 Staff handwashing after direct resident contact

§483.65(b)(3)

The facility must require staff to wash their hands after each direct resident contact for which handwashing is indicated by accepted professional practice.

Intent §483.65(b)(3)

The intent of this regulation is to assure that staff use appropriate handwashing techniques to prevent the spread of infection from one resident to another.

Interpretive Guidelines §483.65(b)(3)

Procedures must be followed to prevent cross-contamination, including handwashing or changing gloves after providing personal care, or when performing tasks among individuals which provide the opportunity for cross-contamination to occur. Facilities for handwashing must exist and be readily available to staff. The facility should follow the CDC's "Guideline for Handwashing and Hospital Environmental Control, 1985," for handwashing.

Procedures §483.65(b)(3)

Verify that the facility has policy that requires staff to wash their hands after each direct resident contact when indicated. Observe handwashing by staff after direct contact with residents.

It is important for the surveyor to begin a thorough investigation of the facility's infection control program when poor resident outcomes and poor practices are observed.

Probes §483.65(b)(3)

- Does the facility have a written protocol describing handwashing practices and is it consistent with the latest published standards?
- Do staff follow the facility policy and protocol for handwashing?

F445 Linens

§483.65(c)

(c) Personnel must handle, store, process, and transport linens so as to prevent the spread of infection.

Intent §483.65(c)

The intent of this regulation is to prevent the spread of infection through linens.

Guidelines to Surveyors §483.65(c)

Soiled linens should be handled to contain and to minimize aerosolization and exposure to any waste products. Soiled linen storage areas should be well ventilated and maintained under a relative negative air pressure. The laundry should be designed to eliminate crossing of soiled and clean linen.

Probes §483.65(c)

- Do staff handle linens on the resident care floors and in the laundry areas to prevent the spread of infection?
- Do staff follow the facility's protocols for handling linens?
- Are linens processed, transported, stored, and handled properly?

§483.70 Physical Environment   Tags 454–469

§483.70(a) Life Safety from Fire
§483.70(b) Emergency Power
§483.70(c) Space and Equipment
§483.70(d) Resident Rooms
§483.70(e) Toilet Facilities
§483.70(f) Resident Call Systems
§483.70(g) Dining and Resident Activities
§483.70(h) Other Environmental Conditions

F454 Physical environment

The facility must be designed, constructed, equipped, and maintained to protect the health and safety of residents, personnel, and the public.

(Rev. 12, Issued: 10-14-05, Effective: 10-14-05, Implementation: 10-14-05)

§483.70(a)(1) Except as otherwise provided in this section—

§483.70(a)(1)(i) the facility must meet the applicable provisions of the 2000 edition. The Director of the Office of the Federal Register has approved the NFPA 101® 2000 edition of the Life Safety Code, issued January 14, 2000, for incorporation by reference in accordance with 5 U.S.C. 552(a) and 1 CFR Part 51. A copy of the Code is available for inspection at the CMS Information Resource Center, 7500 Security Boulevard, Baltimore, MD or at the National Archives and Records Administration (NARA). For information on the availability of this material at NARA, call 202-741-6030. Copies may be obtained from the National Fire Protection Association, 1 Batterymarch Park, Quincy, MA 02269. If any changes in this edition of the Code are incorporated by reference, CMS will publish notice in the FEDERAL REGISTER to announce the changes.

§483.70(a)(4) Beginning March 13, 2006, a long-term care facility must be in compliance with Chapter 19.2.9, Emergency Lighting.

§483.70(a)(5) Beginning March 13, 2006, Chapter 19.3.6.3.2, exception number 2 does not apply to long-term care facilities.

§483.70(a)(6) Notwithstanding any provisions of the 2000 edition of the Life Safety Code (LSC) to the contrary, a long-term care facility may install alcohol-based hand rub dispensers in its facility if—

§483.70(a)(6)(i) Use of alcohol-based hand rub dispensers does not conflict with any State or local codes that prohibit or otherwise restrict the placement of alcohol-based hand rub dispensers in health care facilities;

§483.70(a)(6)(ii) The dispensers are installed in a manner that minimizes leaks and spills that could lead to falls;

§483.70(a)(6)(iii) The dispensers are installed in a manner that adequately protects against access by vulnerable populations; and

§483.70(a)(1)(ii) Chapter 19.3.6.3.2, exception number 2 of the adopted edition of the LSC does not apply to long-term care facilities.

§483.70(a)(6)(iv) The dispensers are installed in accordance with chapter 18.3.2.7 or chapter 19.3.2.7 of the 2000 edition of the Life Safety Code, as amended by NFPA Temporary Interim Amendment 00-1(101), issued by the Standards Council of the National Fire Protection Association on April 15, 2004. The Director of the Office of the Federal Register has approved NFPA temporary interim Amendment 00-1(101) for incorporation by reference in accordance with 5 U.S.C. 552(a) and 1 CFR part 51. A copy of the amendment is available for inspection at CMS Information Resource Center, 7500 Security Boulevard, Baltimore, MD and at the Office of the Federal Register, 800 North Capitol Street NW, Suite 700, Washington, DC. Copies may be obtained from the National Fire Protection Association, 1 Batterymarch Park, Quincy, MA 02269. If any additional changes are made to this amendment, CMS will publish notice in the Federal Register to announce the changes.

§483.70(a)(7) A long-term care facility must:

§483.70(a)(7)(i) Install battery-operated smoke detectors in resident sleeping rooms and public areas by May 24, 2006.

§483.70(a)(7)(ii) Have a program for testing, maintenance, and battery replacement to insure the reliability of the smoke detectors.

§483.70(a)(7)(iii) Exception:

§483.70(a)(7)(iii)(A) The facility has a hard-wired AC smoke detection system in patient rooms and public areas that is installed, tested, and maintained in accordance with NFPA 72, National Fire Alarm Code, for hard-wired AC systems; or

§483.70(a)(7)(iii)(B) The facility has a sprinkler system throughout that is installed, tested, and maintained in accordance with NFPA 13, Automatic Sprinklers.

Interpretive Guidelines §483.70(a)

A waiver of specific provisions of the Life Safety Code is reviewed each time a facility is certified. The State fire authority will determine if the waiver continues to be justified, in that compliance with the requirement would result in an unreasonable hardship upon the facility and does not adversely affect the health and safety of residents or personnel. The State fire authority will forward its findings and recommendation as soon as possible to the State survey agency which will forward it to the CMS RO for a decision on granting a waiver.

Procedures §483.70(a)

The survey for safety from fire is normally conducted by the designated State fire authority. The State agency must establish a procedure for the State fire authority to notify them whether the facility is or is not in compliance with the requirement. If the survey team observes fire hazards or possible deficiencies in life safety from fire, they must notify the designated State fire authority or the RO.

§483.70(a)(4) A long-term care facility must be in compliance with the following provisions on March 13, 2006:

(i) Chapter 19.3.6.3.2, exception number 2

(ii) Chapter 19.2.9

F455 Emergency power

(1) An emergency electrical power system must supply power adequate at least for lighting all entrances and exits; equipment to maintain the fire detection, alarm, and extinguishing systems; and life support systems in the event the normal electrical supply is interrupted.

Interpretive Guidelines §483.70(b)(1)

§483.70(b) Emergency Power: "Emergency electrical power system" includes, at a minimum, battery-operated lighting for all entrances and exits, fire detection and alarm systems, and extinguishing systems. An "exit" is defined as a means of egress which is lighted and has three components: an exit access (corridor leading to the exit), an exit (a door), and an exit discharge (door to the street or public way). We define an entrance as any door through which people enter the facility. Furthermore, when an entrance also serves as an exit, its components (exit access, exit, and exit discharge) must be lighted. A waiver of lighting required for both exits and entrances is not permitted.

Procedures §483.70(b)(1)

Review results of inspections by the designated State fire safety authority that the emergency power system has been tested periodically and is functioning in accordance with the Life Safety Code.

Check placement of lighting system to ensure proper coverage of the listed areas. Test all batteries to ensure they work.

Probes §483.70(b)(1)

Is emergency electrical service adequate?

Additional guidance is available in the National Fire Protection Association's Life Safety Code 99 and 101 (NFPA 99 and NFPA 101), 12-5.1.3 which is surveyed in Tags K105 and K106 of the Life Safety Code survey.

§483.70(b)(2) When life support systems are used, the facility must provide emergency electrical power with an emergency generator (as defined in NFPA 99, Health Care Facilities) that is located on the premises.

Interpretive Guidelines §483.70(b)(2)

"Life support systems" is defined as one or more Electro-mechanical device(s) necessary to sustain life, without which the resident will have a likelihood of dying (e.g., ventilators, suction machines if necessary to maintain an open airway). The determination of whether a piece of equipment is life support is a medical determination dependent upon the condition of the individual residents of the facility (e.g., suction machine maybe required "life support equipment" in a facility, depending on the needs of its residents).

If life support systems are used, determine if there is a working emergency generator at the facility. A generator is not required if a facility does not use life support systems. Check that the emergency generator starts and transfers power under load conditions within 10 seconds after interruption of normal power. Where residents are on life support equipment, do not test transfer switches by shutting off the power unless there is an uninterruptible power supply available.

Probes §483.70(b)(2)

Is there a working generator if the facility is using life support systems?

§483.70(c) Space and Equipment

The facility must—

(1) Provide sufficient space and equipment in dining, health services, recreation, and program areas to enable staff to provide residents with needed services as required by these standards and as identified in each resident's plan of care.

Intent §483.70 (c)(1)

The intent of this regulation is to ensure that dining, health services, recreation, and activities and programs areas are large enough to comfortably accommodate the needs of the residents who usually occupy this space.

Dining, health services, recreation, and program areas should be large enough to comfortably accommodate the persons who usually occupy that space, including the wheelchairs, walkers, and other ambulating aids used by the many residents who require more than standard movement spaces. "Sufficient space" means the resident can access the area, it is not functionally off-limits, and the resident's functioning is not restricted once access to the space is gained.

(Rev. 12, Issued: 10-14-05, Effective: 10-14-05, Implementation: 10-14-05)

Program areas where residents receive physical therapy should have sufficient space and equipment to meet the needs of the resident's therapy requirement.

Procedures §483.70(c)(1)

In the use of space, consider if available space allows residents to pursue activities and receive health services and programs as identified in their care plan.

Program areas where resident groups engage in activities focused on manipulative skills and hand-eye coordination should have sufficient space for storage of their supplies and "works in progress."

Recreation/activities area means any area where residents can participate in those activities identified in their plan of care.

F456 Maintain all essential mechanical, electrical, and patient care equipment in safe operating condition

§483.70(c)(2)

Maintain all essential mechanical, electrical, and patient care equipment in safe operating condition.

Probes §483.70(c)(2)

Is essential equipment (e.g., boiler room equipment, nursing unit/medication room refrigerators, kitchen refrigerator/freezer, and laundry equipment) in safe operating condition?

Is equipment maintained according to manufacturer's recommendations?

(Rev. 12, Issued: 10-14-05, Effective: 10-14-05, Implementation: 10-14-05)

§483.70(d) Resident Rooms

Resident rooms must be designed and equipped for adequate nursing care, comfort, and privacy of residents.

F457 Bedroom limited to four residents

§483.70(d)(1) Bedrooms must—

§483.70(d)(1)(i) Accommodate no more than four residents;

Probes §483.70(d)(1)(i)

Unless a variation has been applied for and approved under §483.70(d)(3), do the residents' bedrooms accommodate no more than four residents?

F458 80 square feet per resident in multiple rooms, 100 square feet in single rooms

§483.70(d)(1)(ii) Measure at least 80 square feet per resident in multiple resident bedrooms, and at least 100 square feet in single resident rooms;

Interpretive Guidelines §483.70(d)(1)(ii)

The measurement of the square footage should be based upon the useable living space of the room. Therefore, the minimum square footage in resident rooms should be measured based upon the floor's measurements exclusive of toilets and bath areas, closets, lockers, wardrobes, alcoves, or vestibules. However, if the height of the alcoves or vestibules reasonably provides useful living area, then the corresponding floor area may be included in the calculation.

The space occupied by movable wardrobes should be excluded from the useable square footage in a room unless it is an item of the resident's own choice and it is in addition to the individual closet space in the resident's room. Non-permanent items of the resident's own choice should have no effect in the calculation of useable living space.

Protrusions such as columns, radiators, ventilation systems for heating and/or cooling should be ignored in computing the useable square footage of the room if the area involved is minimal (e.g., a baseboard heating or air conditioning system or ductwork that does not protrude more than 6 to 8 inches from the wall, or a column that is not more than 6 to 8 inches on each side) and does not have an adverse effect on the resident's health and safety or does not impede the ability of any resident in that room to attain his or her highest practicable well-being. If these protrusions are not minimal they would be deducted from useable square footage computed in determining compliance with this requirement.

The swing or arc of any door which opens directly into the resident's room should not be excluded from the calculations of useable square footage in a room.

Procedures §483.70(1)(ii)

The facility layout may give square footage measurements. Carry a tape measure and take measurements if the room appears small.

Probe

Unless a variation has been applied for and approved under §483.70(d)(3), are there at least 80 square feet per resident in multiple resident rooms and at least 100 square feet for single resident rooms?

F459 Direct access to an exit corridor for resident rooms

§483.70(d)(1)(iii) Have direct access to an exit corridor;

Interpretive Guidelines §483.70(d)(1)(iii)

There is no authority under current regulations to approve a variation to this requirement.

Additional guidance is available in the National Fire Protection Association's Life Safety Code 101 (NFPA 101), 12-2.5.1, which is Tag K41 of the Life Safety Code Survey.

F460 Full visual privacy for each resident

§483.70(d)(1)(iv) Be designed or equipped to assure full visual privacy for each resident;

Interpretive Guidelines §483.70(d)(1)(iv)

"Full visual privacy" means that residents have a means of completely withdrawing from public view while occupying their bed (e.g., curtain, moveable screens, private room). The guidelines do not intend to limit the provisions of privacy to solely one or more curtains, movable screens, or a private room. Facility operators are free to use other means to provide full visual privacy, with those means varying according to the needs and requests of residents. However, the requirement explicitly states that bedrooms must "be designed or equipped to assure full visual privacy for each resident." For example, a resident with a bed by the window cannot be required to remain out of his or her room while his/her roommate is having a dressing change. Room design or equipment must provide privacy. Surveyors will assess whether the means the facility is using to assure full visual privacy meets this requirement without negatively affecting any other resident rights.

Procedures §483.70(d)(1)(iv)

There are no provisions for physician statements to be used as a basis for variation of the requirements for full visual privacy.

Probes §483.70(d)(1)(iv)

Observe whether each resident selected for a comprehensive or focused review has a means to achieve full visual privacy.

§483.70(d)(1)(v) In facilities initially certified after March 31, 1992, except in private rooms, each bed must have ceiling suspended curtains, which extend around the bed to provide total visual privacy in combination with adjacent walls and curtains.

Interpretive Guidelines §483.70(d)(1)(v)

The term "**initially certified**" is defined as all newly certified nursing facilities (NFs) or SNFs as well as NFs and SNFs after March 31, 1992, which re-enter the Medicare or Medicaid programs, whether they voluntarily or involuntarily left the program. It is not necessary for the bed to be accessible from both sides when the privacy curtain is pulled.

Additional guidance is available in the National Fire Protection Association's Life Safety Code 101 (NFPA 101), 31-1.4.1, 31-4.5, which is Tag K74 of the Life Safety Code Survey.

F461 Resident room window to the outside

§483.70(d)(1)(vi) Have at least one window to the outside; and

Interpretive Guidelines §483.70(d)(1)(vi)

A facility with resident room windows, as defined by section 13-3.8.1 of the 1985 edition of the Life Safety Code, that open to an atrium in accordance with Life Safety Code 6-2.2.3.5 can meet this requirement for a window to the outside.

In addition to conforming with the Life Safety Code, this requirement was included to assist the resident's orientation to day and night, weather, and general awareness of space outside the facility. The facility is required to provide for a "safe, clean, comfortable, and homelike environment" by deemphasizing the institutional character of the setting, to the extent possible. Windows are an important aspect in assuring the homelike environment of a facility.

Probes §483.70(d)(1)(vi)

Is there at least one window to the outside?

§483.70(d)(1)(vii) Have a floor at or above grade level.

Interpretive Guidelines §483.70(d)(1)(vii)

"At or above grade level" is defined as a room in which the floor is at or above ground level.

Probes §483.70(d)(1)(vii)

Are the bedrooms at or above ground level?

Additional guidance is available in the National Fire Protection Association's Life Safety Code 101 (NFPA 101), 12-2.5.1, 12-2.5.7, which is Tag K41 of the Life Safety Code survey.

§483.70(d)(2) The facility must provide each resident with—

(i) A separate bed of proper size and height for the convenience of the resident;

(ii) A clean, comfortable mattress;

(iii) Bedding appropriate to the weather and climate; and

Probes §483.70(d)(2)(i), (ii), and (iii)

Are mattresses clean and comfortable?

Is bedding appropriate to weather and climate?

§483.70(d)(2)(iv) Functional furniture appropriate to the resident's needs, and individual closet space in the resident's bedroom with clothes racks and shelves accessible to the resident.

Interpretive Guidelines §483.70(d)(2)(iv)

"Functional furniture appropriate to the residents' needs" means that the furniture in each resident's room contributes to the resident attaining or maintaining his or her highest practicable level of independence and well-being. In general, furnishings include a place to put clothing away in an organized manner that will let it remain clean, free of wrinkles, and accessible to the resident while protecting it from casual access by others; a place to put personal effects such as pictures and a bedside clock, and furniture suitable for the comfort of the resident and visitors (e.g., a chair). There may be instances in which individual residents determine that certain items are not necessary or will impede their ability to maintain or attain their highest practicable well-being (e.g., Both the resident and spouse use wheelchairs. They visit more easily without another chair in the room.). In this case, the resident's wishes should determine the furniture needs.

"Shelves accessible to the resident" means that the resident, if able, or a staff person at the direction of the resident, can get to their clothes whenever they choose.

Probes §483.70(d)(2)(iv)

Functional furniture: Is there functional furniture, appropriate to residents' needs?

Closet space: Is there individual closet space with accessible clothes racks and shelves?

§483.70(d)(3) CMS, or in the case of a nursing facility the survey agency, may permit variations in requirements specified in paragraphs (d)(1)(i) and (ii) of this section relating to rooms in individual cases when the facility demonstrates in writing that the variations—

(i) Are in accordance with the special needs of the residents; and

(ii) Will not adversely affect residents' health and safety.

Interpretive Guidelines §483.70(d)(3)

A variation must be in accordance with the special needs of the residents and must not adversely affect the health or safety of residents. Facility hardship is not part of the basis for granting a variation. Since the special needs of residents may change periodically, or different residents may be transferred into a room that has been granted a variation, variations must be reviewed and considered for renewal whenever the facility is certified. If the needs of the residents within the room have not changed since the last annual inspection, the variance should continue if the facility so desires.

Interpretive Guidelines §483.70(d)(1)(i)

As residents are transferred or discharged from rooms with more than four residents, beds should be removed from the variance until the number of residents occupying the room does not exceed four.

F462 Toilet facilities

§483.70(e) Toilet Facilities

Each resident room must be equipped with or located near toilet facilities.

Interpretive Guidelines §483.70(e)

"Toilet facilities" is defined as a space that contains a lavatory and a toilet. If the resident's room is not equipped with an adjoining toilet facility, then "located near" means residents who are independent in the use of a toilet, including chairbound residents, can routinely use a toilet in the unit.

Probes §483.70(e)

Are resident rooms equipped with or located near toilet and bathing facilities?

F463 Resident call systems

§483.70(f) Resident Call System

The nurses' station must be equipped to receive resident calls through a communication system from—

(1) Resident rooms; and

(2) Toilet and bathing facilities.

Interpretive Guidelines §483.70(f)

This requirement is met only if all portions of the system are functioning (e.g., system is not turned off at the nurses' station, the volume too low to be heard, the light above a room or rooms is not working).

Probes §483.70(f)

Is there a functioning communication system from rooms, toilets, and bathing facilities?

F464 Resident dining and activities area

(Rev. 12, Issued: 10-14-05, Effective: 10-14-05, Implementation: 10-14-05)

§483.70(g) Dining and Resident Activities

The facility must provide one or more rooms designated for resident dining and activities.

These rooms must—

§483.70(g)(1) Be well lighted;

Interpretive Guidelines §483.70(g)(1)

"Well lighted" is defined as levels of illumination that are suitable to tasks performed by a resident.

Probes §483.70(g)(1)

Are there adequate and comfortable lighting levels?

Are illumination levels appropriate to tasks with little glare?

Does lighting support maintenance of independent functioning and task performance?

§483.70(g)(2) Be well ventilated, with nonsmoking areas identified;

Interpretive Guidelines §483.70(g)(2)

"Well ventilated" is defined as good air circulation, avoidance of drafts at floor level, and adequate smoke exhaust removal.

"Nonsmoking areas identified" is defined as signs posted in accordance with State law regulating indoor smoking policy and facility policy.

Probes §483.70(g)(2)

How well is the space ventilated?

Is there good air movement?

Are temperature, humidity, and odor levels all acceptable?

Are non-smoking areas identified?

§483.70(g)(3) Be adequately furnished; and

Interpretive Guidelines §483.70(g)(3)

An "adequately furnished" dining area accommodates different residents' physical and social needs. An adequately furnished organized activities area accommodates the specific activities offered by the facility.

Probes §483.70(g)(3)

How adequate are furnishings?

Are furnishings structurally sound and functional (e.g., chairs of varying sizes to meet varying needs of residents, wheelchairs can fit under the dining room table)?

§483.70(g)(4) Have sufficient space to accommodate all activities.

Probes §483.70(g)(4)

How sufficient is space in dining, health services, recreation and program areas to accommodate all activities?

Are spaces adaptable for all intended uses?

Is resident access to space limited?

(Rev. 12, Issued: 10-14-05, Effective: 10-14-05, Implementation: 10-14-05)

Do residents and staff have maximum flexibility in arranging furniture to accommodate residents who use walkers, wheelchairs, and other mobility aids?

Is there resident crowding?

F465 Other environmental conditions

(Rev. 12, Issued: 10-14-05, Effective: 10-14-05, Implementation: 10-14-05)

§483.70(h) Other Environmental Conditions

The facility must provide a safe, functional, sanitary, and comfortable environment for residents, staff, and the public.

F466 Water available at all times

§483.70(h)(1) The facility must—

Establish procedures to ensure that water is available to essential areas when there is a loss of normal water supply;

F467 Adequate outside ventilation

§483.70(h)(2)

Have adequate outside ventilation by means of windows, or mechanical ventilation, or a combination of the two;

F468 Firmly secured handrails in corridors

§483.70(h)(3) Equip corridors with firmly secured handrails on each side;

"Secured handrails" means handrails that are firmly affixed to the wall.

Probes §483.70(h)(3)

Are handrails secure?

F469 Pest control

§483.70(h)(4) Maintain an effective pest control program so that the facility is free of pests and rodents.

Interpretive Guidelines §483.70(h)(4)

An "effective pest control program" is defined as measures to eradicate and contain common household pests (e.g., roaches, ants, mosquitoes, flies, mice, and rats).

Procedures §483.70(h)(4)

As part of the overall review of the facility, look for signs of vermin. Evidence of pest infestation in a particular space is an indicator of noncompliance.

Probes §483.70(h)(4)

Is area pest free?

---

§483.75 Administration   Tags 490 – 522

§483.75(a) Licensure
§483.75(b) Compliance with Federal, State, and Local Laws and Professional Standards
§483.75(c) Relationship to Other HHS Regulations
§483.75(d) Governing Body
§483.75(e) Required Training of Nursing Aides
§483.75(f) Proficiency of Nurse Aides
§483.75(g) Staff Qualifications
§483.75(h) Use of Outside Resources
§483.75(i) Medical Director
§483.75(j) Laboratory Services
§483.75(k) Radiology and Other Diagnostic Services
§483.75(l) Clinical Records
§483.75(m) Disaster and Emergency Preparedness
§483.75(n) Transfer Agreement
§483.75(o) Quality Assessment and Assurance
§483.75(p) Disclosure of Ownership

F490 Administration

§483.75 Administration

A facility must be administered in a manner that enables it to use its resources effectively and efficiently to attain or maintain the highest practicable physical, mental, and psychosocial well-being of each resident.

Procedures §483.75

If there is a deficiency in §483.13, Resident behavior and facility practices; §483.15, Quality of life; or §483.25, Quality of care, which has the scope and/or severity to be defined as sub-standard quality of care, fully review for compliance all the tags within this section (§483.75).

F491 Licensure: facility

§483.75(a) Licensure: A facility must be licensed under applicable State and local law.

Interpretive Guidelines §483.75(a)

Applicable licenses, permits, and approvals must be available to you for inspection upon request.

Procedures §483.75(a)

If there are problems with care provided or supervised by licensed personnel, verify applicable licenses, permits, and approvals.

F492 Comply with federal, state, local laws and professional standards

§483.75(b) Compliance with Federal, State, and Local Laws and Professional Standards

The facility must operate and provide services in compliance with all applicable Federal, State, and local laws, regulations, and codes, and with accepted professional standards and principles that apply to professionals providing services in such a facility.

Intent §483.75(b)

The intent of this regulation is to ensure that a facility is in compliance with Federal, State, and local laws, regulations, and codes relating to health, safety, and sanitation.

Interpretive Guidelines §483.75(b)

The State is responsible for making decisions about whether there are violations of State laws and regulations. Licenses, permits, and approvals of the facility must be available to you upon request. Current reports of inspections by State and/or local health authorities are on file, and notations are made of action taken by the facility to correct deficiencies.

§483.75(c) Relationship to Other HHS Regulations

In addition to compliance with the regulations set forth in this subpart, facilities are obliged to meet the applicable provisions of other HHS regulations, including but not limited to those pertaining to nondiscrimination on the basis of race, color, or national origin (45 CFR part 80); nondiscrimination on the basis of handicap (45 CFR part 84); nondiscrimination on the basis of age (45 CFR part 91); protection of human subjects of research (45 CFR part 46); and fraud and abuse (42 CFR part 455). Although these regulations are not in themselves considered requirements under this part, their violation may result in the termination or suspension of, or the refusal to grant or continue payment with Federal funds.

Procedures §483.75(b)

If resident/family interviews reveal possible problems with admission contracts, review these contracts for violations of requirements at §§483.10 and 483.12. As appropriate, refer problems to an ombudsman or other agencies, e.g., Office for Civil Rights. Some State or local laws are more stringent than the Federal requirement on the same issue. Failure of the facility to meet a

Federal, State, or local law may be cited at this tag only when the authority having jurisdiction has **both** made a determination of non-compliance and has taken a final adverse action as a result. Accepted professional standards and principles include the various practice acts and scope of practice regulations in each State, and current, commonly accepted health standards established by national organizations, boards, and councils. If interviews with residents suggest that the facility may have required deposits from Medicare residents at admission, review the facility's admissions documents.

Procedures §483.75(c)

If during the survey you identify problems relating to one or more of these requirements, which are under the purview of another Federal agency, forward the information to the RO, who will forward it to the appropriate Federal agency.

F493 Governing Body

483.75(d) Governing Body

(1) The facility must have a governing body, or designated persons functioning as a governing body, that is legally responsible for establishing and implementing policies regarding the management and operation of the facility; and

(2) The governing body appoints the administrator who is—

(i) Licensed by the State where licensing is required; and (ii) Responsible for the management of the facility.

Interpretive Guidelines §483.75(d)(2)(1)

The administrator must be licensed where required by the State.

F494 Training of nurses aides

§483.75(e) Required Training of Nursing Aides

(1) Definitions "Licensed health professional" means a physician; physician assistant; nurse practitioner; physical, speech, or occupational therapist; physical or occupational therapy assistant; registered professional nurse; licensed practical nurse; or licensed or certified social worker. "Nurse aide" means any individual providing nursing or nursing-related services to residents in a facility who is not a licensed health professional, a registered dietitian, or someone who volunteers to provide such services without pay.

Interpretive Guidelines §483.75(e)

Volunteers are not nurse aides and do not come under the nurse aide training provisions of these requirements. Unpaid students in nursing education programs who use facilities as clinical practice sites under the direct supervision of an RN are considered volunteers. Private duty nurse aides who are not employed or utilized by the facility on a contract, per diem, leased, or other basis, do not come under the nurse aide training provisions

§483.75(e)(2) General rule

A facility must not use any individual working in the facility as a nurse aide for more than 4 months, on a full-time basis, unless:

(i) That individual is competent to provide nursing and nursing-related services; and

(ii)(A) That individual has completed a training and competency evaluation program, or a competency evaluation program approved by the State as meeting the requirements of §§483.151-483.154 of this part; or (B) That individual has been deemed or determined competent as provided in §483.150(a) and (b).

§483.75(e)(3) Non-permanent employees

A facility must not use on a temporary, per diem, leased, or any basis other than a permanent employee any individual who does not meet the requirements in paragraphs (e)(2)(i) and (ii) of this section. (See tag F495 for guidelines, probes, and procedures for §483.75(e)(2-4).)

F495 Competency

(4) Competency

A facility must not use any individual who has worked less than 4 months as a nurse aide in that facility unless the individual—

(i) Is a full-time employee in a State-approved training and competency evaluation program;

(ii) Has demonstrated competence through satisfactory participation in a State-approved nurse aide training and competency evaluation program or competency evaluation program; or

(iii) Has been deemed or determined competent as provided in §483.150(a) and (b).

Interpretive Guidelines §483.75(e)(2–4)

Facilities may use, as nurse aides, any individuals who have successfully completed either a nurse aide training and competency evaluation program or a competency evaluation program.

However, if an individual has not completed a program at the time of employment, a facility may only use that individual as a nurse aide if the individual is in a nurse aide training and competency evaluation program (not a competency evaluation program alone) and that individual is a permanent employee in his or her first four months of employment in the facility.

Facilities may not use non-permanent employees as nurse aides unless they have either completed a training and competency evaluation program, or a competency evaluation program.

Probes §483.75(e)(2 - 4)

During an extended or partial extended survey:

- Have all nurse aides completed a nurse aide training and competency evaluation program or a competency evaluation program? If not, are those nurse aides permanent employees enrolled in a training and competency evaluation program who have worked in the facility for 4 months or less?
- Ask nurse aides where they received their training, how long the training was, and how long they have worked in the facility as a nurse aide.

During all surveys:

- If incorrect nurse aide work performance is observed during the survey, check to see if the nurse aide received training and licensed nurse supervision to correctly carry out the task. A "**permanent employee**" is defined as any employee you expect to continue working on an ongoing basis.

Procedures §483.75(e)(2-4)

Review competency requirements for nurse aides if you identify potential deficient care practices in quality of care, resident rights, resident behavior, and facility practice or quality of life which may be related to nurse aide competency. Is there evidence that the nurse aide has successfully completed the competency evaluation program, or has the individual been grandfathered in by the State? If you identify deficient care practices by nurse aides who do not have evidence of having successfully completed a competency evaluation program, determine:

- If the aide is currently receiving training in a State approved Nurse Aide Training Program;
- If the aide is under the supervision of a licensed nurse; and
- If the aide has been trained and determined to be proficient for the tasks to which he or she is assigned.

See §483.152 for specific training that the aide is to receive. This training includes:

- At least 16 hours of training in the following subjects **before** any direct contact with the resident:

✦ Communication and interpersonal skills;

✦ Infection control;

✦ Safety and emergency procedures, including the Heimlich Maneuver;

✦ Promoting resident's independence; and

✦ Respecting resident's rights.

- Basic nursing skills;
- Personal care skills;
- Mental health and social services of residents;
- Care of cognitively impaired residents;
- Basic restorative services; and
- Resident's rights.

F496 Registry verification

§483.75(e)(5) Registry verification

Before allowing an individual to serve as a nurse aide, a facility must receive registry verification that the individual has met competency evaluation requirements unless —

(i) The individual is a full-time employee in a training and competency evaluation program approved by the State; or

(ii) The individual can prove that he or she has recently successfully completed a training and competency evaluation program or competency evaluation program approved by the State and has not yet been included in the registry. Facilities must follow up to ensure that such an individual actually becomes registered.

§483.75(e)(6) Multi-State registry verification

Before allowing an individual to serve as a nurse aide, a facility must seek information from every State registry established under sections 1819(e)(2)(A) or 1919(e)(2)(A) of the Act the facility believes will include information on the individual.

§483.75(e)(7) Required retraining

If, since an individual's most recent completion of a training and competency evaluation program, there has been a continuous period of 24 consecutive months during none of which the individual provided nursing or nursing-related services for monetary compensation, the individual must complete a new training and competency evaluation program or a new competency evaluation program.

Interpretive Guidelines §483.75(e)(7)

If an individual does not wish to be retrained, the individual must establish that he or she performed nursing or nursing-related services for monetary compensation for at least one documented day (i.e., 8 consecutive hours) during the previous 24 months. The State is required to remove the individual's name from the registry if the services are not provided for monetary compensation during the 24-month period. Thus, in the absence of any evidence to the contrary, you can assume that the retraining requirement does not apply to an individual whose name appears on the registry.

F497 Regular in-service education

§483.75(e)(8) Regular In-Service Education

The facility must complete a performance review of every nurse aide at least once every 12 months, and must provide regular in-service education based on the outcome of these reviews. The in-service training must —

(i) Be sufficient to ensure the continuing competence of nurse aides, but must be no less than 12 hours per year;

(ii) Address areas of weakness as determined in nurse aides' performance reviews and may address the special needs of residents as determined by the facility staff; and

(iii) For nurse aides providing services to individuals with cognitive impairments, also address the care of the cognitively impaired.

Interpretive Guidelines §483.75(e)(8)

The adequacy of the in-service education program is measured not only by documentation of hours of completed in-service education, but also by demonstrated competencies of nurse aide staff in consistently applying the interventions necessary to meet residents' needs. If there has been deficient care practices identified during Phase 1 of the survey, review as appropriate training received by nurse aides in that corresponding subject area. For example, if the facility has deficiencies in infection control, review the infection control unit in the facility's in-service nurse aide training program. Each nurse aide must have no less than 12 hours of in-service education per year. Calculate the date by which a nurse aide must receive annual in-service education by the employment date rather than the calendar year.

Probes §483.75(e)(8)

During an extended or partial extended survey, or during any survey in which nurse aide performance is questioned. (See §483.75(f).)

- Does the facility review the performance of its nurse aides?
- How has in-service education addressed areas of weakness identified in performance reviews, special resident needs, and needs of residents with cognitive impairments?

- How has in-service education addressed quality of care problems including those of special care needs and resident rights?

F498 Proficiency of nurse aides

§483.75(f) Proficiency of Nurse Aides

The facility must ensure that nurse aides are able to demonstrate competency in skills and techniques necessary to care for residents' needs, as identified through resident assessments, and described in the plan of care.

Interpretive Guidelines §483.75(f)

"Competency in skills and techniques necessary to care for residents' needs" includes competencies in areas such as communication and personal skills, basic nursing skills, personal care skills, mental health and social service needs, basic restorative services, and resident rights.

Procedures §483.75(f)

During the Resident Review, observe nurse aides.

Probes §483.75(f)

Do nurse aides show competency in skills necessary to:

Maintain or improve the resident's independent functioning, e.g.:

Performing range of motion exercises,

Assisting the resident to transfer from the bed to a wheelchair,

Reinforcing appropriate developmental behavior for persons with MR, or

Psychotherapeutic behavior for persons with MI;

Observe and describe resident behavior and status and report to charge nurse;

Follow instructions; and

Carry out appropriate infection control precautions and safety procedures.

F499 Staff qualifications

§483.75(g) Staff Qualifications

(1) The facility must employ on a full-time, part-time, or consultant basis those professionals necessary to carry out the provisions of these requirements.

(2) Professional staff must be licensed, certified, or registered in accordance with applicable State laws.

If there is reason to doubt the qualifications of temporary agency personnel working in the facility, check with the appropriate registry or professional licensing board.

F500 Use of outside resources

§483.75(h)

Use of Outside Resources

(1) If the facility does not employ a qualified professional person to furnish a specific service to be provided by the facility, the facility must have that service furnished to residents by a person or agency outside the facility under an arrangement described in section 1861(w) of the Act or an agreement described in paragraph (h)(2) of this section.

(2) Arrangements as described in section 1861(w) of the Act or agreements pertaining to services furnished by outside resources must specify in writing that the facility assumes responsibility for —

(i) Obtaining services that meet professional standards and principles that apply to professionals providing services in such a facility; and

(ii) The timeliness of the services.

F501 Medical Director

(Rev. 15, Issued: 11-28-05; Effective/Implementation: 11-25-05)

§483.75(i) Medical Director

(1) The facility must designate a physician to serve as medical director.

(2) The medical director is responsible for—

(i) Implementation of resident care policies; and

(ii) The coordination of medical care in the facility.

INTENT:

The intent of this requirement is that:

- The facility has a licensed physician who serves as the medical director to coordinate medical care in the facility and provide clinical guidance and oversight regarding the implementation of resident care policies;
- The medical director collaborates with the facility leadership, staff, and other practitioners and consultants to help develop, implement and evaluate resident care policies and procedures that reflect current standards of practice; and
- The medical director helps the facility identify, evaluate, and address/resolve medical and clinical concerns and issues that:

  ◇ Affect resident care, medical care or quality of life; or
  ◇ Are related to the provision of services by physicians and other licensed health care practitioners.

NOTE: While many medical directors also serve as attending physicians, the roles and functions of a medical director are separate from those of an attending physician. The medical director's role involves the coordination of facility-wide medical care while the attending physician's role involves primary responsibility for the medical care of individual residents.[1]

DEFINITIONS

Definitions are provided to clarify terms related to the provision of medical director services.

- "Attending Physician" refers to the physician who has the primary responsibility for the medical care of a resident.
- "Current standards of practice" refers to approaches to care, procedures, techniques, treatments, etc., that are based on research and/or expert consensus and that are contained in current manuals, textbooks, or publications, or that are accepted, adopted or promulgated by recognized professional organizations or national accrediting bodies.
- "Medical care" refers to the practice of medicine as consistent with State laws and regulations.
- "Medical director" refers to a physician who oversees the medical care and other designated care and services in a health care organization or facility. Under these regulations, the medical director is responsible for coordinating medical care and helping to develop, implement and evaluate resident care policies and procedures that reflect current standards of practice.
- "Resident care policies and procedures"—Resident care policies are the facility's overall goals, directives, and governing Statements that direct the delivery of care and services to

residents. Resident care procedures describe the processes by which the facility provides care to residents that is consistent with current standards of practice and facility policies.

OVERVIEW

The medical director has an important leadership role in actively helping long term care facilities provide quality care. The regulation requires each facility to have a medical director who is responsible for the implementation of resident care policies and the coordination of medical care. These two roles provide the basis for the functions and tasks discussed in this guidance. The medical director's roles and functions require the physician serving in that capacity to be knowledgeable about current standards of practice in caring for long term care residents, and about how to coordinate and oversee related practitioners. As a clinician, the medical director plays a pivotal role in providing clinical leadership regarding application of current standards of practice for resident care and new or proposed treatments, practices, and approaches to care. The medical director's input promotes the attainment of optimal resident outcomes which may also be influenced by many other factors, such as resident characteristics and preferences, individual attending physician actions, and facility support. The 2001 Institute of Medicine report, "Improving the Quality of Long Term Care," urged facilities to give medical directors greater authority for medical services and care. The report states, "nursing homes should develop structures and processes that enable and require a more focused and dedicated medical staff responsible for patient care."[2]

The medical director is in a position, because of his/her roles and functions, to provide input to surveyors on physician issues, individual resident's clinical issues, and the facility's clinical practices. The text "Medical Direction in Long Term Care"[3] asserts that:

> "The Medical Director has an important role in helping the facility deal with regulatory and survey issues . . . the medical director can help ensure that appropriate systems exist to facilitate good medical care, establish and apply good monitoring systems and effective documentation and follow up of findings, and help improve physician compliance with regulations, including required visits. During and after the survey process, the medical director can clarify for the surveyors clinical questions or information about the care of specific residents, request surveyor clarification of citations on clinical care, attend the exit conference to demonstrate physician interest and help in understanding the nature and scope of the facility's deficiencies, and help the facility draft corrective actions."

Nationally accepted statements concerning the roles, responsibilities and functions of a medical director can be found at the American Medical Directors Association Web site at www.amda.com.

NOTE: References to non-CMS sources or sites on the Internet are provided as a service and do not constitute or imply endorsement of these organizations or their programs by CMS or the U.S. Department of Health and Human Services. CMS is not responsible for the content of pages found at these sites. URL addresses were current as of the date of this publication.

MEDICAL DIRECTION

The facility is responsible for designating a medical director, who is currently licensed as a physician in the State(s) in which the facility(ies) he/she serves is (are) located. The facility may provide for this service through any of several methods, such as direct employment, contractual arrangements, or another type of agreement. Whatever the arrangement or method employed, the facility and the medical director should identify the expectations for how the medical director will work with the facility to effectively implement resident care policies and coordinate medical care.

NOTE: While the roles of medical directors who work for multi-facility organizations with corporate or regional offices may vary for policy development, the medical directors, nonetheless, should be involved in facility level issues such as application of those policies to the care of the facility's residents.

Implementation of Resident Care Policies and Procedures

The facility is responsible for obtaining the medical director's ongoing guidance in the development and implementation of resident care policies, including review and revision of existing policies. The medical director's role involves collaborating with the facility regarding the policies and protocols that guide clinical decision making (for example, interpretation of clinical information, treatment selection, and monitoring of risks and benefits of interventions) by any of the following: facility staff; licensed physicians; nurse practitioners; physician assistants; clinical nurse specialists; licensed, certified, or registered health care professionals such as nurses, therapists, dieticians, pharmacists, social workers, and other health care workers.

The medical director has a key role in helping the facility to incorporate current standards of practice into resident care policies and procedures/guidelines to help assure that they address the needs of the residents. Although regulations do not require the medical director to sign the policies or procedures, the facility should be able to show that its development, review, and approval of resident care policies included the medical director's input.

This requirement does not imply that the medical director must carry out the policies and procedures or supervise staff performance directly, but rather must guide, approve, and help oversee the implementation of the policies and procedures. Examples of resident care policies include, but are not limited to:

- Admission policies and care practices that address the types of residents that may be admitted and retained based upon the ability of the facility to provide the services and care to meet their needs;
- The integrated delivery of care and services, such as medical, nursing, pharmacy, social, rehabilitative and dietary services, which includes clinical assessments, analysis of assessment findings, care planning including preventive care, care plan monitoring and modification, infection control (including isolation or special care), transfers to other settings, and discharge planning;
- The use and availability of ancillary services such as x-ray and laboratory;
- The availability, qualifications, and clinical functions of staff necessary to meet resident care needs;
- Resident formulation and facility implementation of advance directives (in accordance with State law) and end-of-life care;

- Provisions that enhance resident decision making, including choice regarding medical care options;
- Mechanisms for communicating and resolving issues related to medical care;
- Conduct of research, if allowed, within the facility;
- Provision of physician services, including (but not limited to):

  ✦ Availability of physician services 24 hours a day in case of emergency;
  ✦ Review of the resident's overall condition and program of care at each visit, including medications and treatments;
  ✦ Documentation of progress notes with signatures;
  ✦ Frequency of visits, as required;
  ✦ Signing and dating all orders, such as medications, admission orders, and re-admission orders; and
  ✦ Review of and response to consultant recommendations.

- Systems to ensure that other licensed practitioners (e.g., nurse practitioners) who may perform physician-delegated tasks act within the regulatory requirements and within the scope of practice as defined by State law; and
- Procedures and general clinical guidance for facility staff regarding when to contact a practitioner, including information that should be gathered prior to contacting the practitioner regarding a clinical issue/question or change in condition.

Coordination of Medical Care

The medical director is responsible for the coordination of medical care in the facility. The coordination of medical care means that the medical director helps the facility obtain and maintain timely and appropriate medical care that supports the healthcare needs of the residents, is consistent with current standards of practice, and helps the facility meet its regulatory requirements. In light of the extensive medical needs of the long term care population, physicians have an important role both in providing direct care and in influencing care quality. The medical director helps coordinate and evaluate the medical care within the facility by reviewing and evaluating aspects of physician care and practitioner services, and helping the facility identify, evaluate, and address health care issues related to the quality of care and quality of life of residents. "A medical director should establish a framework for physician participation, and physicians should believe that they are accountable for their actions and their care."[4]

The medical director addresses issues related to the coordination of medical care identified through the facility's quality assessment and assurance committee and quality assurance program, and other activities related to the coordination of care. This includes, but is not limited to, helping the facility:

- Ensure that residents have primary attending and backup physician coverage;
- Ensure that physician and health care practitioner services are available to help residents attain and maintain their highest practicable level of functioning, consistent with regulatory requirements;

- Develop a process to review basic physician and health care practitioner credentials (e.g., licensure and pertinent background);
- Address and resolve concerns and issues between the physicians, health care practitioners and facility staff; and
- Resolve issues related to continuity of care and transfer of medical information between the facility and other care settings.

Throughout this guidance, a response from a physician implies appropriate communication, review, and resident management, but does not imply that the physician must necessarily order tests or treatments recommended or requested by the staff, unless the physician agrees that those are medically valid and indicated.

In addition, other areas for medical director input to the facility may include:

- Facilitating feedback to physicians and other health care practitioners about their performance and practices;
- Reviewing individual resident cases as requested or as indicated;
- Reviewing consultant recommendations;
- Discussing and intervening (as appropriate) with a health care practitioner about medical care that is inconsistent with applicable current standards of care;
- Assuring that a system exists to monitor the performance of the health care practitioners;
- Guiding physicians regarding specific performance expectations;
- Identifying facility or practitioner educational and informational needs;
- Providing information to the facility practitioners from sources such as nationally recognized medical care societies and organizations where current clinical information can be obtained; and
- Helping educate and provide information to staff, practitioners, residents, families and others.

NOTE: This does not imply that the medical director must personally present educational programs.

REFERENCES

1. Pattee JJ, Otteson OJ. (1991). Medical direction in the nursing home (p.5). Minneapolis, MN: Northridge Press.

2. Institute of Medicine (2001). Improving The Quality Of Long-Term Care (pp. 201). Washington, DC: National Academy Press.

3. Levenson, S. A. (1993). Medical Direction In Long-Term Care. A Guidebook For The Future (2nd ed., pp. 135). Durham, NC: Carolina Academic Press.

4. Levenson, SA. Medical Director and Attending Physicians Policy and Procedure Manual for Long-term Care. Dayton, Ohio: MedPass. 2005.

INVESTIGATIVE PROTOCOL
MEDICAL DIRECTOR

Objective

- To determine whether the facility has designated a licensed physician to serve as medical director; and
- To determine whether the medical director, in collaboration with the facility, coordinates medical care and the implementation of resident care policies.

Use

Use this protocol for all initial and extended surveys or, as indicated, during any other type of survey. Use this protocol if the survey team has identified:

- That the facility does not have a licensed physician serving as medical director; and/or
- That the facility has designated a licensed physician to serve as medical director; however, concerns or noncompliance identified indicate that:

  ◇ The facility has failed to involve the medical director in his/her roles and functions related to coordination of medical care and/or the implementation of resident care policies; and/or
  ◇ The medical director may not have performed his/her roles and functions related to coordination of medical care and/or the implementation of resident care policies.

Procedures

The investigation involves interviews, review of pertinent policies and procedures, and may involve additional review of resident care.

Provision of a Medical Director

Determine whether the medical director is available during the survey to respond to surveyor questions about resident care policies, medical care, and physician issues.

Interview the facility leadership (e.g., Administrator, Director of Nursing [DON], others as appropriate) about how it has identified and reviewed with the medical director his/her roles and functions as a medical director, including those related to coordination of medical care and the facility's clinical practices and care.

Interview the medical director about his/her understanding and performance of the medical director roles and functions, and about the extent of facility support for performing his/her roles and functions.

If the survey team has identified that the facility lacks a medical director, collect information from the facility administrator to:

- Determine the duration and possible reasons for this problem; and
- Identify what the facility has been doing to try to retain a medical director.

Facility/Medical Director Responsibility for Resident Care Policies

After identifying actual or potential noncompliance with the provision of resident care or medical care:

- Review related policies/procedures;
- Interview facility leadership (e.g., Administrator, DON) to determine how or if they involved the medical director in developing, reviewing, and implementing policies and procedures regarding clinical care of residents (especially where these involve medical and clinical issues; for example, management of causes of delirium, falling, and weight loss) to ensure that they are clinically valid and consistent with current standards of care;
- Interview the medical director regarding his/her input into:

  ◇ Scope of services the facility has chosen to provide;
  ◇ The facility's capacity to care for its residents with complex or special care needs, such as dialysis, hospice or end-of-life care, respiratory support with ventilators, intravenous medications/fluids, dementia and/or related conditions, or problematic behaviors or complex mood disorders;
  ◇ The following areas of concern:

    – Appropriateness of care as it relates to clinical services (for example, following orders correctly, communicating important information to physicians in a timely fashion, etc.);
    – Processes for accurate assessment, care planning, treatment implementation, and monitoring of care and services to meet resident needs; and
    – The review and update of policies and procedures to reflect current standards of practice for resident care (e.g., pressure ulcer prevention and treatment and management of incontinence, pain, fall risk, restraint reduction, and hydration risks) and quality of life.

Coordination of Medical Care/Physician Leadership

If the survey team has identified issues or concerns related to the provision of medical care:

- Interview appropriate facility staff and management as well as the medical director to determine what happens when a physician (or other healthcare practitioner) has a pattern of inadequate or inappropriate performance or acts contrary to established rules and procedures of the facility; for example, repeatedly late in making visits, fails to take time to discuss resident problems with staff, does not adequately address or document key medical issues when making resident visits, etc;

- If concerns are identified for any of the following physician services, determine how the facility obtained the medical director's input in evaluating and coordinating the provision of medical care:

  ◇ Assuring that provisions are in place for physician services 24 hours a day and in case of emergency (§483.40(b));

  ◇ Assuring that physicians visit residents, provide medical orders, and review a resident's medical condition as required (§483.40(b)&(c));

  ◇ Assuring that other practitioners who may perform physician delegated tasks, act within the regulatory requirements and within their scope of practice as defined by State law (§483.40(e)&(f));

  ◇ Clarifying that staff know when to contact the medical director; for example, if an attending or covering physician fails to respond to a facility's request to evaluate or discuss a resident with an acute change of condition;

  ◇ Clarifying how the medical director is expected to respond when informed that the staff is having difficulty obtaining needed consultations or other medical services; or

  ◇ Addressing other concerns between the attending physician and the facility, such as issues identified on medication regimen review, or the problematic use of restraints.

In addition, determine how the facility and medical director assure that physicians are informed of expectations and facility policies, and how the medical director reviews the medical care and provides guidance and feedback regarding practitioner performance, as necessary.

Regardless of whether the medical director is the physician member of the quality assurance committee, determine how the facility and medical director exchange information regarding the quality of resident care, medical care, and how the facility disseminates information from the committee to the medical director and attending physicians regarding clinical aspects of care and quality such as infection control, medication and pharmacy issues, incidents and accidents, and other emergency medical issues (§483.75(o)).

DETERMINATION OF COMPLIANCE (Task 6, Appendix P)

Synopsis of Regulation (F501)

This requirement has 3 aspects: Having a physician to serve as medical director, implementing resident care policies, and coordinating medical care. As with all other long term care requirements, the citation of a deficiency at F501, Medical Director, is a deficiency regarding the facility's failure to comply with this regulation. The facility is responsible for designating a physician to serve as medical director and is responsible for oversight of, and collaboration with, the medical director to implement resident care policies and to coordinate medical care.

Criteria for Compliance

The facility is in compliance if:

- They have designated a medical director who is a licensed physician;
- The physician is performing the functions of the position;

- The medical director provides input and helps the facility develop, review and implement resident care policies, based on current clinical standards; and
- The medical director assists the facility in the coordination of medical care and services in the facility.

If not, cite F501.

Noncompliance for F501

After completing the Investigative Protocol, analyze the data in order to determine whether or not noncompliance with the regulation exists. The survey team must identify whether the noncompliance cited at other tags relates to the medical director's roles and responsibilities. In order to cite at F501 when noncompliance has been identified at another tag, the team must demonstrate an association between the identified deficiency and a failure of medical direction. Noncompliance for F501 may include (but is not limited to) the **facility's** failure to:

- Designate a licensed physician to serve as medical director; or
- Obtain the medical director's input for timely and ongoing development, review and approval of resident care policies;

Noncompliance for F501 may also include (but is not limited to) the **facility** and **medical director** failure to:

- Coordinate and evaluate the medical care within the facility, including the review and evaluation of aspects of physician care and practitioner services;
- Identify, evaluate, and address health care issues related to the quality of care and quality of life of residents;
- Assure that residents have primary attending and backup physician coverage;
- Assure that physician and health care practitioner services reflect current standards of care and are consistent with regulatory requirements;
- Address and resolve concerns and issues between the physicians, health care practitioners and facility staff;
- Resolve issues related to continuity of care and transfer of medical information between the facility and other care settings;
- Review individual resident cases, as warranted, to evaluate quality of care or quality of life concerns or other problematic situations and take appropriate steps to resolve the situation as necessary and as requested;
- Review, consider and/or act upon consultant recommendations that affect the facility's resident care policies and procedures or the care of an individual resident, when appropriate;
- Discuss and intervene (as appropriate) with the health care practitioner about medical care that is inconsistent with applicable current standards of care; or
- Assure that a system exists to monitor the performance and practices of the health care practitioners.

This does not presume that a facility's noncompliance with the requirements for the delivery of care necessarily reflects on the performance of the medical director.

V. DEFICIENCY CATEGORIZATION (Part V, Appendix P)

Once the survey team has completed its investigation, analyzed the data, reviewed the regulatory requirements, and determined that noncompliance exists, the team must determine the severity of each deficiency, based on the resultant effect or potential for harm to the resident.

The key elements for severity determination for F501 are as follows:

1. **Presence of harm/negative outcome(s) or potential for negative outcomes because of lack of resident care policies and/or medical care.**

Deficient practices related to actual or potential harm/negative outcome for F501 may include but are not limited to:

- Lack of medical director involvement in the development, review and/or implementation of resident care policies that address the types of residents receiving care and services, such as a resident with end-stage renal disease, pressure ulcers, dementia, or that address practices such as restraint use;
- Lack of medical director involvement in coordinating medical care regarding problems with physician coverage or availability; or
- Lack of medical director response when the facility requests intervention with an attending physician regarding medical care of a resident.

2. **Degree of harm (actual or potential) related to the noncompliance.**

Identify how the facility practices caused, resulted in, allowed or contributed to the actual or potential for harm:

- If harm has occurred, determine if the harm is at the level of serious injury, impairment, death, compromise, or discomfort; and
- If harm has not yet occurred, determine the potential for serious injury, impairment, death, compromise, or discomfort to occur to the resident.

3. **The immediacy of correction required.**

Determine whether the noncompliance requires immediate correction in order to prevent serious injury, harm, impairment, or death to one or more residents.

The survey team must evaluate the harm or potential for harm based upon the following levels of severity for F501. First, the team must rule out whether Severity Level 4, Immediate Jeopardy, to a resident's health or safety exists by evaluating the deficient practice in relation to immediacy, culpability, and severity. (Follow the guidance in Appendix Q.)

Severity Level 4 Considerations: Immediate Jeopardy to Resident Health or Safety

Immediate Jeopardy is a situation in which the facility's noncompliance with one or more requirements of participation:

- Has allowed/caused/resulted in, or is likely to allow/cause/result in serious injury, harm, impairment, or death to a resident; and
- Requires immediate correction, as the facility either created the situation or allowed the situation to continue by failing to implement preventative or corrective measures.

NOTE: The death or transfer of a resident who was harmed or injured as a result of facility noncompliance does not remove a finding of immediate jeopardy. The facility is required to implement specific actions to correct the noncompliance which allowed or caused the immediate jeopardy.

In order to cite immediate jeopardy at this tag, the surveyor must be able to identify the relationship between noncompliance cited as immediate jeopardy at other regulatory tags, and the failure of the medical care and systems associated with the roles and responsibilities of the medical director. **In order to select severity level 4 at F501, both of the following must be present:**

1. Findings of noncompliance at Severity Level 4 at another tag:

    - Must have allowed, caused or resulted in, or is likely to allow, cause or result in serious injury, harm, impairment or death and require immediate correction. The findings of noncompliance associated with immediate jeopardy are written at tags that also show evidence of process failures with respect to the medical director's responsibilities; and

2. There is no medical director or the facility failed to involve the medical director in resident care policies or resident care or medical care as appropriate, or the medical director had knowledge of a problem with care, or physician services, or lack of resident care policies and practices that meet current standards of practice and failed:

    - To get involved or to intercede with the attending physician in order to facilitate and/or coordinate medical care; and/or
    - To provide guidance and/or oversight for relevant resident care policies.

NOTE: If immediate jeopardy has been ruled out based upon the evidence, then evaluate whether actual harm that is not immediate jeopardy exists at Severity Level 3.

Severity Level 3 Considerations: Actual Harm that is not Immediate Jeopardy

Level 3 indicates noncompliance that results in actual harm, and may include, but is not limited to, clinical compromise, decline, or the resident's inability to maintain and/or reach his/her highest practicable well-being.

In order to cite actual harm at this tag, the surveyor must be able to identify a relationship between noncompliance cited at other regulatory tags and failure of medical care or processes and practices associated with roles and responsibilities of the medical director, such as:

1. Findings of noncompliance at Severity Level 3 at another tag must have caused actual harm:

- The findings of noncompliance associated with actual harm are written at tags that show evidence of process failures with respect to the medical director's responsibilities; and

2. There is no medical director or the facility failed to involve the medical director in resident care policies or resident care or medical care as appropriate or the medical director had knowledge of a problem with care, or physician services, or lack of resident care policies and practices that meet current standards of practice and failed:

- To get involved or intercede with the attending physician in order to facilitate and/or coordinate medical care (medical care and systems associated with roles and responsibilities of the medical director show evidence of breakdown); or
- To provide guidance and/or oversight for resident care policies.

NOTE: If Severity Level 3 (actual harm that is not immediate jeopardy) has been ruled out based upon the evidence, then evaluate as to whether Level 2 (no actual harm with the potential for more than minimal harm) exists.

Severity Level 2 Considerations: No Actual Harm with Potential for More than Minimal Harm that is not Immediate Jeopardy

In order to cite no actual harm with potential for more than minimal harm at this tag, the surveyor must be able to identify a relationship between noncompliance cited at other regulatory tags and the failure of medical care, processes and practices associated with roles and responsibilities of the medical director, such as:

1. Findings of noncompliance at Severity Level 2 at another tag:

- Must have caused no actual harm with potential for more than minimal harm (Level 2). Level 2 indicates noncompliance that results in a resident outcome of no more than minimal discomfort and/or has the potential to compromise the resident's ability to maintain or reach his or her highest practicable level of well being. The potential exists for greater harm to occur if interventions are not provided; and

2. There is no medical director or the facility failed to involve the medical director in resident care policies or resident care as appropriate or the medical director had knowledge of an issue with care or physician services, and failed:

- To get involved with or intercede with attending physicians in order to facilitate and/or coordinate medical care; or
- To provide guidance and/or oversight for resident care policies.

Severity Level 1 Considerations: No Actual Harm with Potential for Minimal Harm

In order to cite no actual harm with potential for minimal harm at this tag, the survey team must have identified that:

- There is no medical director; and

    - There are no negative resident outcomes that are the result of deficient practice; and
    - Medical care and systems associated with roles and responsibilities of the medical director are in place; and
    - There has been a relatively short duration of time without a medical director; and
    - The facility is actively seeking a new medical director.

F502 Laboratory services

§483.75(j) Laboratory Services

(1) The facility must provide or obtain laboratory services to meet the needs of its residents. The facility is responsible for the quality and timeliness of the services.

Intent §483.75(j)(1)

The intent of this regulation is to assure that laboratory services are accurate and timely so that the utility of laboratory testing for diagnosis, treatment, prevention, or assessment is maximized. The facility is responsible for quality and timely laboratory services whether or not services are provided by the facility or an outside agency.

Interpretive Guidelines §483.75(j)(1)

A "laboratory service or test" is defined as any examination or analysis of materials derived from the human body for purposes of providing information for the diagnosis, prevention, or treatment of any disease or impairment of, or the assessment of the health of human beings.

Services provided must be both accurate and timely. Timely means that laboratory tests are completed and results are provided to the facility (or resident's physician) within time frames normal for appropriate intervention. All laboratories providing services for facility residents must meet applicable requirements of 42 CFR Part 493. The purpose of this requirement is to assist in assuring quality of laboratory services.

Procedures §483.75(j)(1)

Verify that laboratory services are provided to meet the needs of the residents. If a problem in quality of care leads you to suspect a problem in laboratory services, timeliness, or quality, refer to the interpretive guidelines for laboratory testing found in Appendix C.

Probes §483.75(j)(1)

Are problems attributable to:

- An inability to order laboratory tests in a timely manner, including delays in transporting the resident to and from the source of service, if needed?
- A delay of treatment due to untimely receipt of lab results?
- A large lag time between an order for a test and the recording of the results that may have resulted in poor care?

F503 Requirement if facility does own lab work

§483.75(j)(1)(i) If the facility provides its own laboratory services, the services must meet the applicable requirements for laboratories specified in Part 493 of this chapter.

§483.75(j)(1)(ii) If the facility provides blood bank and transfusion services, it must meet the applicable requirements for laboratories specified in Part 493 of this chapter.

§483.75(j)(1)(iii) If the laboratory chooses to refer specimens for testing to another laboratory, the referral laboratory must be certified in the appropriate specialties and subspecialties of services in accordance with the requirements of Part 493 of this chapter.

§483.75(j)(1)(iv) If the facility does not provide laboratory services on site, it must have an agreement to obtain these services from a laboratory that meets the applicable requirements of Part 493 of this chapter.

Intent §483.75(j)(1)(i) - (iv)

The intent of this regulation is to assure that laboratory services, blood bank, and transfusion services are obtained from an entity that meets the requirements of 42 CFR Part 493 in order to provide a standard of quality for laboratory and transfusion services. If the long-term care facility does not provide laboratory services on site, there must be an agreement to obtain these services from a laboratory that meets the same requirements.

Interpretive Guidelines §483.75(j)(1)(i) - (iv)

If a facility provides its own laboratory services, the provisions of 42 CFR Part 493 apply. The facility must have a Clinical Laboratory Improvement Amendments (CLIA) certificate appropriate for the level of testing performed. An application for a certificate of waiver may be made if the facility performs only those tests categorized as waived under CLIA. Direct questions concerning the application of these requirements to your State laboratory consultant or the CMS RO.

Procedures §483.75(j)(1)(i) - (iv)

Determine if all laboratory services provided for the facility are provided by a laboratory that meets the requirements of 42 CFR Part 493. The surveyor should determine if the facility has an arrangement in writing to assume responsibility for (a) obtaining services that meet professional standards and principles that apply to professionals providing services in such a facility; and (b) the timeliness of the services.

Probes §483.75(j)(1)(i) - (iv)

Are problems attributable to:

- Lack of an arrangement to provide or obtain clinical laboratory services from a source that meets the applicable conditions for coverage of the services?
- Delays in interpreting the results of laboratory tests?

F504 Lab work only when ordered by the attending physician

§483.75(j)(2) The facility must —

§483.75(j)(2)(i) Provide or obtain laboratory services only when ordered by the attending physician.

Intent §483.75(j)(2)(i)

The intent of this regulation is to assure that only medically necessary laboratory services are ordered.

Procedures §483.75(j)(2)(i)

Verify that all laboratory services received were ordered by the attending physician.

F505 Prompt notification to physicians of laboratory results received back

§483.75(j)(2)(ii) Promptly notify the attending physician of the findings;

Intent §483.75(j)(2)(ii)

The intent of this regulation is to assure that the physician is notified of all lab results so that prompt, appropriate action may be taken if indicated for the resident's care.

Procedures §483.75(j)(2)(ii)

If you have reason to believe that a physician(s) may not have been notified of laboratory results in a timely manner, determine if the facility has a policy/procedure for routine notification of physician and if the procedure is implemented.

Probes §483.75(j)(2)(ii)

• Are any problems identified as relating to lack of prompt notification of the attending physician, contributing to delays in changing the course of treatment or care plan?

F506 Assist resident to laboratory work if needed

§483.75(j)(2)(iii) Assist the resident in making transportation arrangements to and from the source of service, if the resident needs assistance; and

Intent §483.75(j)(2)(iii)

The intent of this regulation is to assure that residents are able to get to and receive necessary laboratory testing when the testing is conducted outside of the facility.

Probes §483.75(j)(2)(iii)

• Does the resident ever have to cancel lab service appointments due to difficulties with transportation?

F507 File laboratory reports in resident's clinical record

§483.75(j)(2)(iv)

File in the resident's clinical record laboratory reports that are dated and contain the name and address of the testing laboratory.

Intent §483.75(j)(2)(iv)

The intent of this regulation is to assure that the laboratory performing the tests is Medicare approved, and that test results are accurate and are available for clinical management.

F508 Facility responsibility for radiology and other diagnostic services

§483.75(k) Radiology and Other Diagnostic Services

(1) The facility must provide or obtain radiology and other diagnostic services to meet the needs of its residents. The facility is responsible for the quality and timeliness of the services.

Intent §483.75(k)(1)

The intent of this regulation is to assure that the resident receives quality radiologic and diagnostic services in a timely manner to meet his/her needs for diagnosis, treatment, and prevention.

Probes §483.75(k)(1)

If problems are identified in radiology or other diagnostic services, are problems attributable to:

- An inability to order radiological and diagnostic services in a timely manner, including delays in transporting the resident for these services?
- Delays in interpreting the results of x-rays and other tests?
- Lack of prompt notification, in writing, of test results to the attending physician, contributing to delays in changing care plans or the course of treatment?

F509 Approval, if facility does own diagnostic services

§483.75(k)(1)(i) If the facility provides its own diagnostic services, the services must meet the applicable conditions of participation for hospitals contained in §482.26 of this subchapter.

§483.75(k)(1)(ii) If the facility does not provide it's own diagnostic services, it must have an agreement to obtain these services from a provider or supplier that is approved to provide these services under Medicare.

F510 Radiology and other diagnostic services only on order of a physician

§483.75(k)(2) The Facility must—

(i) Provide or obtain radiology and other diagnostic services only when ordered by the attending physician;

F511 Notify attending physician of radiological results

§483.75(k)(2)(ii) Promptly notify the attending physician of the findings;

F512 Assist resident with radiological services transportation

§483.75(k)(2)(iii) Assist the resident in making transportation arrangements to and from the source of service, if the resident needs assistance; and

F513 File radiological work results in patient's clinical file

§483.75(k)(2)(iv) File in the resident's clinical record signed and dated reports of x-ray and other diagnostic services.

F514 Clinical records

(Rev. 5, Issued: 11-19-04, Effective: 11-19-04, Implementation: 11-19-04)

§483.75(l) Clinical Records

(1) The facility must maintain clinical records on each resident in accordance with accepted professional standards and practices that are—

(i) Complete;

(ii) Accurately documented;

(iii) Readily accessible; and

(iv) Systematically organized.

Intent §483.75(l)(1)

To assure that the facility maintains accurate, complete, and organized clinical information about each resident that is readily accessible for resident care.

Interpretive Guidelines §483.75(l)(1)

A complete clinical record contains an accurate and functional representation of the actual experience of the individual in the facility. It must contain enough information to show that the facility knows the status of the individual, has adequate plans of care, and provides sufficient evidence of the effects of the care provided. Documentation should provide a picture of the resident's progress, including response to treatment, change in condition, and changes in treatment.

The facility determines how frequently documentation of an individual's progress takes place apart from the annual comprehensive assessment, periodic reassessments when a significant change in status occurs, and quarterly monitoring assessments. Good practice indicates that for functional and behavioral objectives, the clinical record should document change toward achieving care plan goals. Thus, while there is no "right" frequency or format for "reporting" progress, there is a unique reporting schedule to chart each resident's progress in maintaining or improving functional abilities and mental and psychosocial status. Be more concerned with whether the staff has sufficient progress information to work with the resident and less with how often that information is gathered. In cases in which facilities have created the option for an individual's record to be maintained by computer, rather than hard copy, electronic signatures are acceptable.

In cases when such attestation is done on computer records, safeguards to prevent unauthorized access, and reconstruction of information must be in place. The following guideline is an example of how such a system may be set up:

- There is a written policy, at the health care facility, describing the attestation policy(ies) in force at the facility.
- The computer has built-in safeguards to minimize the possibility of fraud.
- Each person responsible for an attestation has an individualized identifier.
- The date and time is recorded from the computer's internal clock at the time of entry.
- An entry is not to be changed after it has been recorded.
- The computer program controls what sections/areas any individual can access or enter data, based on the individual's personal identifier (and, therefore his/her level of professional qualifications).

Procedures §483.75(l)(1)

In reviewing sampled residents' clinical records:

- Is there enough record documentation for staff to conduct care programs and to revise the program, as necessary, to respond to the changing status of the resident as a result of interventions?
- How is the clinical record used in managing the resident's progress in maintaining or improving functional abilities and mental and psychosocial status?

§483.75(l)(5) the clinical record must contain—

(i) Sufficient information to identify the resident;

(ii) A record of the resident's assessments;

(iii) The plan of care and services provided;

(iv) The results of any preadmission screening conducted by the State; and

(v) Progress notes.

F515 Retention of clinical records

§483.75(l)(2) Clinical records must be retained for—

(i) The period of time required by State law; or

(ii) Five years from the date of discharge when there is no requirement in State law; or,

(iii) For a minor, three years after a resident reaches legal age under State law.

F516 Safeguards of patient's clinical record

(Rev. 5, Issued: 11-19-04, Effective: 11-19-04, Implementation: 11-19-04)

Automated Resident Assessment Instrument (RAI) data are part of a resident's clinical record and as such are protected from improper disclosure by facilities under current law.

§483.20(f)(5)

(5) Resident-identifiable information.

(i) A facility may not release information that is resident-identifiable to the public.

(ii) The facility may release information that is resident-identifiable to an agent only in accordance with a contract under which the agent agrees not to use or disclose the information except to the extent the facility itself is permitted to do so.

Interpretive Guidelines §483.20(f)(5)

Facilities are required by §§1819(c)(1)(A)(iv) and 1919(c)(1)(A)(iv) of the Act and 42 CFR Part 483.75(l)(3) and (l)(4), to keep confidential all information contained in the resident's record and to maintain safeguards against the unauthorized use of a resident's clinical record information, regardless of the storage method of the records.

§483.75(l) (3) The facility must safeguard clinical record information against loss, destruction, or unauthorized use.

Intent §483.75(l)(3)

To maintain the safety and confidentiality of the resident's record.

Procedures §483.75(l)(3)

Determine through observations and interviews with staff, the policy and implementation of that policy, for maintaining confidentiality of residents' records.

Probes §483.75(1)(3)

- How does the facility ensure confidentiality of resident records?
- If there is a problem with confidentiality, is it systematic, that is, does the problem lie in the recordkeeping system, or with a staff person's use of records, e.g., leaving records in a place easily accessible to residents, visitors, or other unauthorized persons?

F517 Disaster and emergency preparedness

§483.75(m) Disaster and Emergency Preparedness

§483.75(m)(1) The facility must have detailed written plans and procedures to meet all potential emergencies and disasters, such as fire, severe weather, and missing residents.

F518 Training for all employees in emergency procedures

§483.75(m)(2)

The facilities must train all employees in emergency procedures when they begin to work in the facility, periodically review the procedures with existing staff, and carry out unannounced staff drills using those procedures.

Interpretive Guidelines §483.75(m)

The facility should tailor its disaster plan to its geographic location and the types of residents it serves. "Periodic review" is a judgment made by the facility based on its unique circumstances, changes in physical plant, or changes external to the facility that can cause a review of the disaster review plan. The purpose of a "staff drill" is to test the efficiency, knowledge, and response of institutional personnel in the event of an emergency. Unannounced staff drills are directed at the responsiveness of staff, and care should be taken not to disturb or excite residents.

Procedures §483.75(m)

Review disaster and emergency preparedness plan, including plans for natural or man made disasters.

Probes §483.75(m)

Ask two staff persons separately (e.g., nurse aide, housekeeper, maintenance person) and the charge nurse:

- If the fire alarm goes off, what do you do?
- If you discover that a resident is missing, what do you do?
- What would you do if you discovered a fire in a resident's room?
- Where are fire alarms and fire extinguisher(s) located on this unit?
- How do you use the fire extinguisher?

NOTE: Also, construct probes relevant to geographically specific natural emergencies (e.g., for areas prone to hurricanes, tornadoes, earthquakes, or floods, each of which may require a different response). Are the answers to these questions correct (staff answers predict competency in assuring resident safety)?

Are the answers to these questions correct (staff answers predict competency in assuring resident safety)?

F519 Transfer agreement

§483.75(n) Transfer Agreement

(1) In accordance with section 1861(1) of the Act, the facility (other than a nursing facility which is located in a State on an Indian reservation) must have in effect a written transfer agreement with one or more hospitals approved for participation under the Medicare and Medicaid programs that reasonably assures that —

(i) Residents will be transferred from the facility to the hospital, and ensured of timely admission to the hospital when transfer is medically appropriate, as determined by the attending physician; and

(ii) Medical and other information needed for care and treatment of residents, and, when the transferring facility deems it appropriate, for determining whether such residents can be adequately cared for in a less expensive setting than either the facility or the hospital, will be exchanged between the institutions.

(2) The facility is considered to have a transfer agreement in effect if the facility has attempted in good faith to enter into an agreement with a hospital sufficiently close to the facility to make transfer feasible.

F520 Quality assessment and assurance

(Rev. 19, Issued: 06-01-06, Effective/Implementation: 06-01-06)

483.75(o) Quality Assessment and Assurance

(1) A facility must maintain a quality assessment and assurance committee consisting of—

(i) The director of nursing services;

(ii) A physician designated by the facility; and

(iii) At least 3 other members of the facility's staff.

(2) The quality assessment and assurance committee—

(i) Meets at least quarterly to identify issues with respect to which quality assessment and assurance activities are necessary; and

(ii) Develops and implements appropriate plans of action to correct identified quality deficiencies.

(3) State or the Secretary may not require disclosure of the records of such committee except insofar as such disclosure is related to the compliance of such committee with the requirements of this section.

(4) Good faith attempts by the committee to identify and correct quality deficiencies will not be used as a basis for sanctions.

Intent: 483.75(o) Quality Assurance and Assessment

The intent of this requirement is that:

- The facility has an ongoing quality assessment and assurance (QAA) committee that includes designated key members and that meets at least quarterly; and
- The committee identifies quality deficiencies and develops and implements plans of action to correct these quality deficiencies, including monitoring the effect of implemented changes and making needed revisions to the action plans.

Definitions

Definitions are provided to clarify terms related to the requirement for a quality assessment and assurance committee.

- "Quality Assessment" is an evaluation of a process and/or outcomes of a process to determine if a defined standard of quality is being achieved.
- "Quality Assurance" is the organizational structure, processes, and procedures designed to ensure that care practices are consistently applied and the facility meets or exceeds an expected standard of quality. Quality assurance includes the implementation of principles of continuous quality improvement.
- "Quality Deficiencies" are potential markers of quality that the facility considers to be in need of investigating and which, after investigation, may or may not represent a deviation from quality that results in a potential or actual undesirable outcome. The term "quality deficiency" in this regulation is meant to describe a deficit or an area for improvement. This term is not synonymous with a deficiency cited by surveyors.
- "Quality Improvement (QI)" is an ongoing interdisciplinary process that is designed to improve the delivery of services and resident outcomes.

NOTE: Many facilities have changed their terminology for the QAA processes to "quality improvement (QI)." However, in these guidelines, we will continue to use the designation of QAA, as specified in the requirement. The elements are comparable regardless of the terminology.

Overview

QAA is a management process that is ongoing, multi-level, and facility-wide. It encompasses all managerial, administrative, clinical, and environmental services, as well as the performance of outside (contracted or arranged) providers and suppliers of care and services. Its purpose is continuous evaluation of facility systems with the objectives of:

- Keeping systems functioning satisfactorily and consistently including maintaining current practice standards;
- Preventing deviation from care processes from arising, to the extent possible;
- Discerning issues and concerns, if any, with facility systems and determining if issues/concerns are identified; and
- Correcting inappropriate care processes.

Several studies conducted under the auspices of the U.S. Department of Health and Human Services have examined quality of care and quality of life in nursing homes.[1,2] These studies have concluded that QAA committees provide an important point of accountability for ensuring both quality of care and quality of life in nursing homes. The QAA committees represent key internal mechanisms that allow nursing homes opportunities to deal with quality deficiencies in a confidential manner.

Resources are available that recommend processes and standards to develop and enhance quality improvement programs. Some Web site resources include:

- American Medical Directors Association (www.amda.com);
- American Health Care Association (www.ahca.org);
- American College of Physicians Quality Indicators for Assessing Care of Vulnerable Elders (www.acponline.org/sci-policy/acove/);
- American Geriatric Society (www.americangeriatrics.org);
- Agency for Healthcare Research and Quality (www.ahrq.gov);
- Medicare Quality Improvement Community (www.Medqic.org);
- American Association of Homes and Services for the Aging (www.aahsa.org); and
- The American Health Quality Association (www.ahqa.org).

NOTE: References to non-CMS sources or sites on the Internet are provided as a service and do not constitute or imply endorsement of these organizations or their programs by CMS or the U.S. Department of Health and Human Services. CMS is not responsible for the content of pages found at these sites. The URL addresses were current as of the date of this publication.

The guidance below includes sections that describe facility responsibilities to meet the various aspects of the QAA requirement, including:

- The composition of the QAA committee and the minimum frequency of committee meetings;
- The committee's monitoring of systems and identification of concerns with the quality of facility systems; and
- Modification and correction of facility systems, when needed, including monitoring the effect of action plans.

QAA COMMITTEE FUNCTIONS

Key aspects of the QAA requirements include the specifications that the facility must have a QAA committee, that this committee must include certain staff members, and that the committee must meet at least quarterly. The QAA committee is responsible for identifying whether quality deficiencies are present (potential or actual deviations from appropriate care processes or facility procedures) that require action. If there are quality deficiencies, the committee is responsible for developing plans of action to correct them and for monitoring the effect of these corrections. These functions of the QAA committee are described below.

Committee Composition and Frequency of Meetings

The regulation states that the QAA committee must include the director of nursing, a physician, and three other staff. These additional members may include:

- The administrator (facilities with effective QAA committees include members who have knowledge of facility systems and the authority to change those systems, including the administrator or assistant administrator due to their responsibility to manage the facility, and make changes to facility systems);
- The medical director (part of the medical director's responsibility (see F501)) is to guide the facility's development and implementation of resident care policies and coordination

of medical care. If the medical director is not a committee member, exchange of information with the medical director enhances the functioning of the QAA committee);

- Staff with responsibility for direct resident care and services, such as nursing aides, therapists, staff nurses, social workers, activities staff members; and
- Staff with responsibility for the physical plant, such as maintenance, housekeeping, and laundry staff.

NOTE: Facilities may have a larger committee than required by the regulation. Consideration should be given as to how committee information is provided to consultants who may not be members of the committee, but whose responsibilities include oversight of departments or services.

Meetings of the QAA committee must be held at least quarterly or more often as the facility deems necessary to fulfill committee functions and operate effectively.
The Committee should maintain a record of the dates of all meetings and the names/titles of those attending each meeting.

Identification of Quality Deficiencies

Facilities can collect and analyze data about their performance from various sources that may help them to identify quality deficiencies. These may include information from reports such as open and closed record audits, facility logs and tracking forms, incident reports, consultants' reports, and other reports as part of the QAA function. Quality deficiencies related to facility operations and practices are not only related to those that cause negative outcomes, but also may be directed toward enhancing quality of care and quality of life for residents. The committee responds to quality deficiencies and serves a preventative function by reviewing and improving systems.

Records of the committee meetings identifying quality deficiencies, by statute, may not be reviewed by surveyors unless the facility chooses to provide them. However, the documents the committee used to determine quality deficiencies are subject to review by the surveyors.

NOTE: A State or the Secretary may not require disclosure of the records of the QAA committee except insofar as such disclosure is related to the compliance of the QAA committee with the regulations. If concerns, especially repeat survey deficiencies, have not been identified by the facility's QAA committee, this may be an indication that the committee is not performing the functions required by this regulation.

Development of Action Plans

In order to fulfill the regulatory mandate, the facility's Q committee, having identified the root causes which led to their confirmed quality deficiencies, must develop appropriate corrective plans of action. Action plans may include, but are not limited to, the development or revision of clinical protocols based on current standards of practice, revision of policies and procedures, training for staff concerning changes, plans to purchase or repair equipment and/or improve the physical plant, and standards for evaluating staff performance.

Implementation of Action Plans and Correction of Identified Quality Deficiencies

The facility's action plans to address quality deficiencies may be implemented in a variety of ways, including: staff training and deployment of changes to procedures; monitoring and feedback mechanisms; and processes to revise plans that are not achieving or sustaining desired outcomes. The committee may delegate the implementation of action plans to various facility staff and/or outside consultants.

ENDNOTES

1. Institute of Medicine (2001). Improving the Quality of Long-Term Care. Washington, DC: National Academy Press
2. Office of Inspector General (2003) Quality Assurance Committees in Nursing Homes, Baltimore, MD: U.S. Department of Health and Human Services (OEI-01-01-00090).

INVESTIGATIVE PROTOCOL QUALITY ASSESSMENT AND ASSURANCE (Rev. XX)

Objectives

- To determine if the facility has a QAA committee consisting of the director of nursing, a physician designated by the facility, and at least three other staff members; and
- To determine if the QAA committee:

  - ✧ Meets at least quarterly (or more often, as necessary);
  - ✧ Identifies quality deficiencies; and
  - ✧ Develops and implements appropriate plans of action to address identified quality deficiencies.

Use

Use this protocol for all initial and standard surveys. Also, use it as necessary on revisits and abbreviated standard surveys (complaint investigations).

Procedures During Offsite Survey Preparation (see Appendix P, Task 1)

The survey team must review information about the facility prior to the survey. Sources include, at a minimum:

- Quality Measure/Quality Indicator Reports;
- The OSCAR 3 Report (includes a 4-year history of the facility's deficiencies from standard surveys, revisits, and complaint surveys). The survey team should determine if the facility has had repeat deficiencies as well as recent serious deficiencies (Levels F and H and above); and
- Information from the State ombudsman.

The regulation states that good faith attempts by the committee to identify and correct quality deficiencies will not be used as a basis for sanctions. The facility is not required to release the records of the QAA committee to the surveyors to review, and the facility is not required to disclose records of the QAA committee beyond those that demonstrate compliance with the regulation (F520). However the facility may choose such disclosure if it is the facility's only means of showing the composition and functioning of the QAA committee. If the facility has provided the records for surveyor review, this information may not be used to cite deficiencies unrelated to the QAA committee requirement. It is recommended that surveyors not review QAA records (if provided) until after they complete their investigations of other tags.

If the survey team's review of the QAA committee records reveals that the committee is making good faith efforts to identify quality deficiencies and to develop action plans to correct quality deficiencies, this requirement (F520) should not be cited. However, if the survey team had already independently (not through use of the records) identified noncompliance in the same areas as those that have been selected by the QAA committee, the team is expected to cite the noncompliance for the other requirements.

Throughout the survey, the survey team may become aware of other concerns regarding the delivery of care and services that may reflect that the QAA committee is not functioning in identifying ongoing and current quality deficiencies.

During the daily meetings, the team discusses concerns about facility compliance that they are identifying through observations, interviews, and record reviews. The information from the entrance conference about the composition and meetings of the QAA committee is reviewed and relayed to the team.

The team coordinator assigns a surveyor to obtain information from the person the facility has designated as responsible for the QAA committee. The surveyor should interview this designated person to determine:

- How the committee identifies current and ongoing issues for committee action. This could include how they monitor the provision of care and services on an ongoing basis, and how they ascertain from residents and/or their families information regarding the facility's provision of care and services, in addition to facility staff throughout the various departments, and outside consultants and/or suppliers and providers of care;
- The methods the committee uses to develop action plans; and
- How current action plans are being implemented, including: staff training; deployment of changes to procedures; monitoring and feedback mechanisms that have been established; and, for any plans that are not achieving or sustaining desired outcomes to correct the deficiencies, the process underway for revision to these plans.

The assigned surveyor should interview staff in various departments to determine if they know how to bring an issue to the attention of the QAA committee.

If, during the course of the survey, the survey team identifies noncompliance at a particular requirement, the assigned surveyor should interview the designated person responsible for the QAA committee to determine whether the committee knew of or should have known of the issues related to the noncompliance. The assigned surveyor should determine if the committee had considered the quality deficiency and if it was determined that an action plan was needed. If so, the surveyor determines whether the committee developed and implemented any action plans to address these concerns. The survey team should verify that the action plans that are described are actually implemented, and that staff are providing care and services according to the directives of these action plans.

DETERMINATION OF COMPLIANCE (Task 6, Appendix P)

NOTE: Although the literature of QAA and QI provides various definitions of the facility's achievement of quality, surveyors will need to determine the facility's compliance based on the language of this regulation.

Synopsis of Regulation (F520)

This requirement has two aspects: the facility must have a committee composed of certain key members that meets at least quarterly (or more often, as necessary); and the committee functions to develop and implement appropriate plans of actions to correct identified quality deficiencies.

Criteria for Compliance

The facility is in compliance if:

- It has a functioning QAA committee, consisting of the director of nursing, a physician, and at least three other staff members, that meets at least quarterly; and
- The committee:

    ✧ Identifies quality deficiencies; and
    ✧ Develops and implements appropriate plans of actions

If not, cite F520.

Noncompliance for F520

After completing the investigative protocol, the survey team determines whether or not compliance with the regulation exists. Examples of noncompliance may include, but are not limited to, the following:

- Lack of a physician member of the committee;
- The committee met only twice during the previous year;
- The action plan to correct a quality deficiency regarding food temperatures was not being followed by staff in the dietary department, and food was not being served at proper temperatures; or
- An action plan was developed to correct a problem with inadequate assessment of root causes of falls. Staff did not implement the plan, and residents continued to experience serious falls.

- An action plan that was developed to correct the issue of resident falls did not take account of the root cause of the falls being overuse of sedative type medications. The plan was to increase the use of restraints which was an inappropriate action plan.

DEFICIENCY CATEGORIZATION (Part V, Appendix P)

Once the survey team has determined that noncompliance exists, the team will select the appropriate level of severity for the deficiency using the guidance below.

The survey team must identify a relationship between noncompliance at other regulatory requirements and the facility's failure to have a functional QAA committee. The key elements for severity determination for F520 are as follows:

1. Presence of harm/negative outcome(s) or potential for negative outcomes because of a failure of the QAA committee structure or function

   Actual or potential harm/negative outcome for F520 may include, but is not limited to:

   - Failure of the QAA committee to identify and implement an action plan to reduce of medication errors committed by agency staff, resulting in the noncompliance for medication errors based on the resident receiving the wrong medication, which resulted in the resident experiencing insulin shock; or

   - Failure of the QAA committee to develop an action plan to address assessment of the cause of a pattern of recent falls of several residents, resulting in noncompliance at the accident requirement based on several residents sustaining avoidable falls with bruises but no fractures.

2. Degree of harm (actual or potential) related to the noncompliance

   Identify how the facility practices caused, resulted in, allowed, or contributed to the actual or potential for harm:

   - If harm has occurred, determine if the harm is at the level of serious injury, impairment, death, compromise, or discomfort; and
   - If harm has not yet occurred, determine how likely is the potential for serious injury, impairment, death, compromise, or discomfort to occur to the resident.

3. The immediacy of correction required

   Determine whether the noncompliance requires immediate correction in order to prevent serious injury, harm, impairment, or death to one or more residents.

The survey team must evaluate the harm or potential for harm based upon the following levels of severity for Tag F520. First, the team must rule out whether Severity Level 4, Immediate Jeopardy to a resident's health or safety, exists by evaluating the deficient practice in relation to immediacy, culpability, and severity. (Follow the guidance in Appendix Q.)

Severity Level 4 Considerations: Immediate Jeopardy to Resident Health or Safety

Immediate Jeopardy is a situation in which the facility's noncompliance with one or more requirements of participation:

- Has caused, or is likely to cause, serious injury, harm, impairment, or death to a resident; and
- Requires immediate correction, as the facility either created the situation or allowed the situation to continue by failing to implement preventive or corrective measures.

NOTE: The death or transfer of a resident who was harmed or injured as a result of facility noncompliance does not remove a finding of immediate jeopardy. The facility is required to implement specific actions to correct the noncompliance which allowed or caused the immediate jeopardy.

In order to select Severity Level 4 for this regulation, the surveyor must be able to identify the relationship between the facility's noncompliance cited at Severity Level 4 at other regulatory tags, and the failure of the QAA Committee to function effectively. In order to select Severity Level 4 at F520, both of the following must be present:

- Deficiency(ies) has been cited at Severity Level 4 in other tags that are related to QAA committee failure; and
- The facility does not have a QAA committee, or the facility's QAA committee failed to develop and implement appropriate plans of action to correct identified quality deficiencies.

Severity Level 3: Actual Harm that is Not Immediate Jeopardy

In order to select Severity Level 3 for this regulation, the surveyor must be able to identify the relationship between the facility's noncompliance cited at Severity Level 3 at other regulatory tags, and the failure of the QAA Committee to function effectively. In order to select Severity Level 3 at F520, both of the following must be present:

- Deficiency(ies) has been cited at Severity Level 3 in other tags that are related to QAA committee failure; and
- The facility does not have a QAA committee, or the facility's QAA committee failed to develop and implement appropriate plans of action to correct identified quality deficiencies.

Severity Level 2: No Actual Harm with Potential for More than Minimal Harm that is Not Immediate Jeopardy

In order to select Severity Level 2 for this regulation, the surveyor must be able to identify the relationship between the facility's noncompliance cited at Severity Level 2 at other regulatory tags, and the failure of the QAA Committee to function effectively. In order to select Severity Level 2 at F520, both of the following must be present:

- Deficiency(ies) has been cited at Severity Level 2 in other tags that are related to QAA committee failure; and
- The facility does not have a QAA committee, or the facility's QAA committee failed to develop and implement appropriate plans of action to correct identified quality deficiencies.

Severity Level 1: No Actual Harm with Potential for Minimal Harm

Severity Level 1 should be selected if any of the following circumstances are present:

- The facility does not have a QAA committee, and there have been no other deficiencies cited above Severity Level 1; or
- The facility has a QAA committee that has failed to meet the regulatory specifications for the composition of the committee and/or the frequency of committee meetings, and there have been no deficiencies cited above Severity Level 1; or
- The facility's QAA committee meets regulatory specifications for committee membership and frequency of meetings, and deficiencies have been cited at Severity Level 1 in other tags. In order to select Severity Level 1 in this case, the surveyor must be able to identify the relationship between the facility's noncompliance cited at Severity Level 1 at other tags, and the failure of the QAA committee to function effectively.

F521 Quarterly meeting of quality assessment and assurance committee

(2) The quality assessment and assurance committee—

(i) Meets at least quarterly to identify issues with respect to which quality assessment and assurance activities are necessary; and

(ii) Develops and implements appropriate plans of action to correct identified quality deficiencies.

(3) A State or the Secretary may not require disclosure of the records of such committee except insofar as such disclosure is related to the compliance of such committee with the requirements of this section.

(4) Good faith attempts by the committee to identify and correct quality deficiencies will not be used as a basis for sanctions.

F522 Disclosure of ownership

§483.75(p) Disclosure of Ownership

(1) The facility must comply with the disclosure requirements of §§420.206 and 455.104 of this chapter.

(2) The facility must provide written notice to the State agency responsible for licensing the facility at the time of change, if a change occurs in—

(i) Persons with an ownership or control interest, as defined in §§420.201 and 455.101 of this chapter;

(ii) The officers, directors, agents, or managing employees;

(iii) The corporation, association, or other company responsible for the management of the facility; or

(iv) The facility's administrator or director of nursing.

(3) The notice specified in the paragraph (p)(2) of this section must include the identity of each new individual or company.

State Operations Manual

Appendix P — Survey Protocol for Long-term Care Facilities — Part I

INDEX

(Rev. 9, 08-05-05)

VI. Information Transfer
VII. Additional Procedures for Medicare-Participating Long-term Care Facilities

I. Introduction

Skilled nursing facilities (SNFs) and nursing facilities (NFs) are required to be in compliance with the requirements at 42 CFR Part 483, Subpart B, to receive payment under the Medicare or Medicaid programs. To certify a SNF or NF, complete at least a:

- Life Safety Code (LSC) survey; and
- Standard Survey. There are two types of Standard Surveys:

    ✧ The Quality Indicators Survey (QIS), which uses the QIS procedures and forms as contained in the QIS Surveyor Training Manual. The QIS is only used by a State Survey Agency upon approval by the Centers for Medicare and Medicaid (CMS), and only by the surveyors who have received QIS training; and
    ✧ The Traditional Survey, which uses Forms CMS-670, CMS-671, CMS-672, CMS-677, and CMS-801 through CMS-807 (see Exhibits 85, 86, and 88 thru 95).

NOTE: CMS is beginning the process of a staged implementation of a revised survey process, the Quality Indicators Survey (QIS), as a replacement for the current (Traditional) survey process. The QIS is a two-staged, computer-assisted survey process with Stage 1 consisting of both computer analysis of offsite data from the Minimum Data Set (MDS) system as well as data collected by surveyors onsite from observations, interviews, and record reviews of large computer-selected resident samples. The information collected throughout Stage 1 is analyzed by computer to derive a set of approximately 160 Quality of Care Indicators (QCIs) that are used to compare the facility being surveyed to national norms. QCIs that score beyond a statistical threshold are computer-selected for Stage 2 review, and the relevant residents are also computer selected. Stage 2 consists of systematic surveyor investigations of triggered issues and residents using a set of detailed investigative tools known as critical elements protocols. In addition to the Stage 1 and Stage 2 sample-based investigations, the QIS also contains several facility-level tasks that are unstaged and are completed either on every survey or when triggered as areas of concern.

During this period, as CMS conducts pilot implementation, CMS deems both the QIS and Traditional Survey as surveys-of-record to evaluate compliance of nursing homes with the requirements at 42 CFR 483.5–483.75.

II. The Survey Process

Do not announce SNF/NF surveys to the facility. Conduct standard surveys and complete them on consecutive workdays, whenever possible. They may be conducted at any time including weekends, 24 hours a day. When standard surveys begin at times beyond the business hours of 8:00 a.m. to 6:00 p.m., or begin on a Saturday or Sunday, the entrance conference and initial tour should be modified in recognition of the residents' activity (e.g., sleep, religious services) and types and numbers of staff available upon entry.

Use the standard survey procedure discussed in this section for all standard surveys of SNFs and NFs, whether freestanding, distinct parts, or dually participating. For surveys of facilities predominantly serving short stay residents, modifications of offsite survey preparation and sampling procedures will be necessary.

NOTE: Do not use this process for surveys of intermediate care facilities for the mentally retarded (ICFs/MR), swing-bed hospitals, or skilled nursing sections of hospitals that are not separately certified as SNF distinct parts. Survey Protocols and Interpretive Guidelines for these surveys are found in Appendix J (ICFs/MR) and Appendix T (swing-bed hospitals and hospitals with non-distinct part SNFs).

When the survey team suspects substandard quality of care (SQC), expand the standard (or abbreviated) survey sample as necessary to determine scope. If the existence of SQC is verified, then inform the Administrator that the facility has SQC and an extended (or partial extended) survey will be conducted.

Surveys

If a possible noncompliant situation related to any requirement is identified while conducting the information gathering tasks of the survey, investigate the situation to determine whether the facility is in compliance with the requirements.

Standard Survey

The QIS Standard Survey is composed of Tasks 1 – 9 and the Traditional Standard Survey is composed of Tasks 1 – 7. Both versions of the survey process are resident-centered, outcome-oriented inspections that rely on a case-mix stratified sample of residents to gather information about the facility's compliance with participation requirements. Outcomes include both actual and potential negative outcomes, as well as failure of a facility to help residents achieve their highest practicable level of well-being. Based on the specific procedures detailed in this Appendix, a standard survey assesses:

- Compliance with residents' rights and quality of life requirements;
- The accuracy of residents' comprehensive assessments and the adequacy of care plans based on these assessments;

- The quality of care and services furnished, as measured by indicators of medical, nursing, rehabilitative care and drug therapy; dietary and nutrition services; activities and social participation; sanitation and infection control; and
- The effectiveness of the physical environment to empower residents, accommodate resident needs, and maintain resident safety, including whether requested room variances meet health, safety, and quality of life needs for the affected residents.

Extended Survey

The extended survey is conducted after substandard quality of care is determined during a standard survey. If, based on performing the resident-centered tasks of the standard survey it is determined that the facility has provided substandard quality of care in 42 CFR 483.13, Resident Behavior and Facility Practices; 42 CFR 483.15, Quality of Life; and/or 42 CFR 483.25, Quality of Care, conduct an extended survey within 14 days after completion of the standard survey. (See Section II.A.2. for further information about the QIS extended survey and Section III for further information about the Traditional Extended Survey.)

Abbreviated Standard Survey

This survey focuses on particular tasks that relate, for example, to complaints received or a change of ownership, management, or director of nursing. The abbreviated standard survey does not cover all aspects covered in the standard survey, but rather concentrates on a particular area of concern(s). For example, an abbreviated standard survey may be conducted to substantiate a complaint. The survey team can expand the abbreviated standard survey to cover additional areas, or to a *Traditional Standard Survey* if, during the Abbreviated Standard Survey, evidence is found that warrants a more extensive review. (See also Chapter 5 of this manual for additional administrative procedures related to complaints.) *At this time, the QIS is not used to conduct an abbreviated standard survey. See §II.A.4. below for investigation of complaints during the QIS standard survey.*

Partial Extended Survey

A partial extended survey is always conducted after substandard quality of care is found during an abbreviated standard survey or during a revisit, when substandard quality of care was not previously identified. If, based on performing the abbreviated standard survey or revisit, it is determined that the facility has provided substandard quality of care in 42 CFR 483.13, Resident Behavior and Facility Practices; 42 CFR 483.15, Quality of Life; and/or 42 CFR 483.25, Quality of Care, conduct a partial extended survey. (See Section III for further information about the partial extended survey.) *At this time, the QIS is not used for partial extended surveys.*

Post-Survey Revisit (Follow-up)

The post-survey revisit is an onsite visit intended to verify correction of deficiencies cited in a prior survey. See §2732 and Appendix P, Part I, Section III, "Writing the Statement of Deficiencies." *(See Section II.A.3. for further information about the QIS revisit and Section II.B.3 for further information about the Traditional revisit.)* If substandard quality of care is determined during a revisit, complete a partial extended survey, if a partial extended or extended survey had not been conducted as the result of the prior standard or abbreviated standard survey.

Initial Certification Survey

In a survey for initial certification of SNFs or NFs, perform the tasks of both the Traditional Standard and Extended Surveys. During the initial survey, focus both on residents and the structural requirements that relate to qualification standards and resident rights notification, whether or not problems are identified during the information gathering tasks. Gather additional information to verify compliance with every tag number. For example, during an initial survey, verify the qualifications of the social worker, dietitian, and activities professional. Also, review the rights notification statements on admissions contracts. Complete the "Statement of Deficiencies and Plan of Correction" (Form CMS-2567) in Exhibit 7.

Specialty Surveyors

All members of a survey team need not be onsite for the entire survey. Specialty surveyors participating in surveys (e.g., a pharmacist, physician, or registered dietitian) may be onsite only during that portion of the survey dealing with their area of expertise. However, they must conduct that portion while the rest of the team is present. All members of the survey team should enter the facility at the same time, if possible. Before leaving the facility, at the completion of his/her portion of the survey, the specialty surveyor must meet with the team or team coordinator to discuss his/her findings and to provide supporting documentation. The specialty surveyor should also share any information he/she obtained that may be useful to other team members. If he/she is not present at the information analysis for deficiency determination, the specialty surveyor should be available by telephone at that time and during the exit conference.

Team Communication

Throughout the survey process, the team (including specialty surveyors onsite at the time) should discuss among themselves, on a daily basis, observations made and information obtained in order to focus on the concerns of each team member, to facilitate information gathering and to facilitate decision making at the completion of the standard survey.

II.A. – The Quality Indicators Survey (QIS)

The QIS survey is used as the survey-of-record only for states that have received CMS approval, and only by surveyors who have completed QIS training. Sections II.A.1.-4. below describe the use of the QIS for standard surveys, extended surveys, post-survey revisits, and complaint investigations.

1. The QIS Standard Survey

The QIS standard survey consists of the following Tasks (details are contained in the QIS Surveyor Training Manual, which is incorporated by reference):

Introduction

Task 1: Offsite Survey Preparation:

- Offsite Survey Preparation and Initial Sampling

Task 2: Onsite Preparatory Activities and Entrance Conference

- Prior to the Entrance Conference
- Entrance Conference
- Possible Off Hours Activities

Task 3: Initial Tour

- Tour

Task 4: Stage I Survey Tasks

- Finalize Sample Selection

    ✧ Stage I Sample Selection Procedures

- Stage I Team Meetings (first meeting)
- Stage I Information Gathering
- Stage I Admission Sample Review

    ✧ Medical Record Review

- Stage I Census Sample Review

    ✧ Resident Interviews
    ✧ Resident Unavailable for Interviews
    ✧ Resident Observations
    ✧ Staff Interviews
    ✧ Medical Record Review
    ✧ Family Interviews

Task 5: Non-Staged Survey Tasks

- Resident Council President/Representative Interview
- Dining Observation

- Kitchen/Food Service Observation
- Infection Control Policies and Practices
- Demand Billing Review
- Abuse Prohibition Review
- Quality Assessment and Assurance (QA&A Review)

Task 6: Transition from Stage I to Stage II

- Update the Resident Pool
- Review Completion of Stage I
- Review Surveyor-Initiated Residents and/or Care Areas
- Import All Data into the Primary Laptop
- Review the Relevant Findings Report
- Review the QCI Results Report

Task 7: Stage II Survey Tasks

- Introduction
- Team Meetings
- Stage II Sample Selection

    ✧ Substituting Residents
    ✧ Supplementing the Sample

- Staff Assignments
- Stage II Information Gathering

    ✧ Stage II Critical Element Pathways
    ✧ Medication Administration Observation and Unnecessary Drug Review

- Facility-Level Investigations

    ✧ Environmental Observation
    ✧ Resident Funds
    ✧ Admission, Transfer, and Discharge Review
    ✧ Sufficient Staff

Task 8: Analysis and Decision-Making: Integration of Information

- Integration of Facility-Level Information
- Integration of Critical Element Pathways
- Analysis of Information Gained
- Analysis of Scope and Severity and Team Decision-Making

Task 9: Exit Conference

- Exit Conference

2. The QIS Extended Survey

When the survey team is conducting a QIS standard survey and they have determined there is substandard quality of care, they will conduct QIS extended survey procedures. Substandard quality of care is defined as one or more deficiencies with scope/severity levels of F, H, I, J, K, or L in any of the following regulatory groupings:

- 42 CFR 483.13, Resident Behavior and Facility Practices;
- 42 CFR 483.15, Quality of Life; and/or
- 42 CFR 483.25, Quality of Care.

The purpose of the QIS extended survey is to gather further information (unless already gathered during the standard survey) concerning the facility's nursing and medical services and administration, in order to evaluate systemic issues with the facility's provision of services and management that may be non-compliant with the long-term care requirements, and may have contributed to problems cited in the substandard quality of care deficiency(ies). When conducting the QIS extended survey, the survey team coordinator will surveyor-initiate all Tags within the following regulatory groupings into the QIS survey software: 42 CFR 483.30, Nursing Services; 42 CFR 483.40, Physician Services; and 42 CFR 483.75, Administration. There are no specific QIS forms to assist this review. The survey team shall document their findings about these Tags on Surveyor Notes Worksheets (Form CMS-807) and shall input their findings into the QIS software. If the QIS Staffing Review protocol was not already completed during the standard survey, the survey team will complete this protocol.

At the discretion of the State Survey Agency, the QIS extended survey can be conducted either:

- Prior to the exit conference, in which case the facility will be provided with findings from the standard and extended survey; or
- Subsequent to the standard survey, but no longer than 2 weeks after the completion of the standard survey, if the survey team is unable to complete the extended survey prior to the exit conference.

3. The QIS Post-Survey Revisit (Follow-up)

A QIS post-survey revisit is conducted in accordance with §7317 to confirm that the facility is in compliance and has the ability to remain in compliance. The purpose of the revisit is to reevaluate the specific care and services that were cited as noncompliant during the QIS standard and/or extended survey. The specific procedures for each revisit depend on the deficiencies that were cited during the QIS standard survey. Detailed procedures are found in the QIS Surveyor Training Manual. For each QIS revisit, the surveyor(s) will use portions of the QIS standard survey, only as applicable to their need to evaluate the facility's return to compliance for requirements cited as deficiencies. For all QIS revisits, the surveyor(s) will review offsite the Statement of Deficiencies and conduct a focused review of the summary information from the QIS standard survey. Once onsite, the surveyor(s) will ask the facility to provide a roster of residents. The surveyor(s) will use the QIS software as well as information from the QIS standard survey (such as residents investigated) to surveyor-initiate the Care Areas and/or Tags and residents to be investigated. The surveyor(s) will use Stage 2 Critical Element Pathways (CEs) protocols as applicable to the Tags that have been cited, or the general CE for aspects of care not covered by the other CEs. For example, if deficiencies were cited for pressure ulcers and medication errors, the surveyor(s) would use the pressure ulcer CE and the QIS Medication Administration and Unnecessary Drug Review form to conduct these investigations. The surveyor(s) will input findings into the QIS software and proceed through QIS deficiency decision making, and scoring of scope and severity for any deficiencies that are cited.

4. The QIS Complaint Survey Procedures

The QIS is used for investigation of complaints during a QIS standard survey. The survey team coordinator will surveyor-select the complaint area(s) of concern and the resident(s) involved in the complaint and add them to the list of issues and residents evaluated during the QIS standard survey. The QIS Surveyor Training Manual contains further details concerning the manner in which these surveyor-selected concerns and issues are added to the standard survey for investigation, determination of whether they are substantiated or unsubstantiated, and conveying of findings into the CMS ASPEN data system.

At this time, the QIS is not used for investigation of complaints during an abbreviated standard survey. Surveyors should use the procedures contained in §VII.A. below for these investigations.

II.B. – The Traditional Survey

II.B.1 – Traditional Standard Survey Tasks

Task 1 – Offsite Survey Preparation

A. General Objectives

The objectives of offsite survey preparation are to analyze various sources of information available about the facility in order to:

- Identify and pre-select concerns for Phase 1 of the survey, based on the Facility Quality *Measure/Indicator Report* (see description below at B.3.a.). This pre-selection is subject to amendment based on the results of the tour;
- Pre-select potential residents for Phase I of the survey based on the Resident Level *Quality Measure/Indicator Reports* (see description below at B.3.a.). This pre-selection is subject to amendment based on the results gathered during the tour, entrance conference, and facility Roster/Sample Matrix;
- Note concerns based on other sources of information listed below and note other potential residents who could be selected for the sample; and
- Determine if the areas of potential concerns or special features of the facility require the addition to the team of any specialty surveyors.

B. Information Sources for Offsite Survey Preparation

The following sources of information (1–8) are used during the offsite team meeting to focus the survey.

1. **Quality Measure/Indicator Reports**

    QM/QIs are to be used as indicators of potential problems or concerns that warrant further investigation. They are not determinations of facility compliance with the long term care requirements. There are three QM/QI reports which *should* be downloaded from the State database:

    • Facility Characteristics Report (Exhibit 268)

    This report provides demographic information about the resident population (in percentages) for a selected facility compared to all the facilities in the State. It includes information in the following domains: Gender, age, payment source, diagnostic characteristics, type of assessment, stability of conditions, and discharge potential.

    • Facility Quality Measure/Indicator Report (Exhibit 269)

    This report provides facility status for each of the MDS-based QM/QIs (quality measures and quality indicators) as compared to State and national averages. Listed are the individual QM/QIs (grouped by domains). This report begins with a set of 12 domains and a total of 31 QM/QIs for the chronic (long-stay) resident population, followed by three additional QM/QIs for the post-acute care (PAC) resident population. For each QM/QI, (reading across a row *from left to right*) are:

    ✧ The numerator — the number of residents in the facility who have the condition;
    ✧ The denominator — the number of residents in the facility who could have the condition;
    ✧ The *facility observed percentage* of residents who have the condition;
    ✧ The *facility adjusted percentage* of residents who have the condition;
    ✧ The *State average percentage* of residents who have the condition;
    ✧ The *national average percentage* of residents who have the condition; and
    ✧ The *State percentile* ranking of the facility on the QM/QI – a descriptor of how the facility compares (ranks) with other facilities in the state. The higher the percentile rank, the greater potential there is for a care concern in the facility.
    ✧ An asterisk is present in any row in which the facility flagged on a QM/QI, which means that the facility is at or above the 90th percentile; and any of the three sentinel event rows if any resident has the condition (see D. below for more information on sentinel events).

    • Resident Level Quality Measure/Indicator Reports (Exhibit 270)

    The resident level reports are divided into Chronic Care and PAC samples, to correspond to the division of residents in the Facility Quality Measure/Indicator Report described above. Both reports provide resident-specific information generated using current records from the CMS Minimum Data Set (MDS) data base. An *X* appears in a QM/QI column for a resident who has that condition. If a QM/QI is risk adjusted, this *X* is in either the high or low risk subcolumn, indicating whether this resident was at high or low risk to develop the condition. The Chronic Care version contains the following columns for each long-stay resident, reading from left to right:

- Resident identification number;
- Resident name in alphabetical order;
- MDS type of assessment (1 = admission, 2 = annual, 3 = significant change, 4 = significant correction, and 5 = quarterly);
- Columns for each QM/QI for the chronic care resident in the same order and under the same domains as on the Facility Quality Measure/Indicator Report; and
- A column that counts how many QM/QIs the resident triggered.

The PAC version contains the following columns for each PAC resident, reading from left to right:

- Resident identification number;
- Resident name in alphabetical order;
- Columns for the three PAC QM/QIs; and
- A column that counts how many QM/QIs the resident triggered.

NOTE: Resident-specific information in the Resident Level *reports* must be kept confidential in accordance with the Privacy Act. *These reports are* only for the use of the State agency, CMS representatives, and the facility.

2. **Statements of Deficiencies (CMS-2567) and Statements of Isolated Deficiencies Which Cause No Actual Harm with Only Potential for Minimal Harm (Form A)**

Statements of deficiencies from the previous survey should be reviewed, along with the sample resident identifiers list. Review the specific information under each deficiency and note any special areas of concern. For example, a deficiency was cited for comprehensive care planning last year. Share with the team the specific care planning problems that were listed as the reasons for this deficiency. For resident-centered requirements, determine if any residents identified in the deficiency might be good candidates for the sample. For example, a deficiency was cited for abuse partly based on surveyor observation of a staff member striking a resident who was combative. Identify this resident by name and add the name to the Offsite Preparation Worksheet. During the Initial Tour, evaluate this resident for inclusion in the sample.

3. **OSCAR Report 3, History Facility Profile, and OSCAR Report 4, Full Facility Profile from CMS' OSCAR Computer System**

(Refer to Exhibit 96 for sample copies of Reports 3 and 4.) **Report 3** contains the compliance history of the facility over the past 4 surveys. Use it to determine if the facility has patterns of repeat deficiencies in particular tags or related tags. This report also lists the dates of any complaint investigations and Federal monitoring surveys during the 4-year time period.

Report 4 contains information provided by the facility during the previous survey on the Resident Census (Form CMS-672). This report compares facility population characteristics with State, CMS region, and national averages.

4. Results of Complaint Investigations

Review information from both complaints investigated since the previous standard survey and complaints filed with the survey agency, but not yet investigated. Note resident and staff names related to the complaints and note patterns of problems relating to specific wings or shifts.

5. Information about Waivers or Variances

If the facility has, or has requested any staffing waiver or room variances, note these for onsite review. The team will determine onsite if these should be granted, continued, or revoked due to a negative effect on resident care or quality of life.

6. Information from the State Ombudsman Office

Note any potential areas of concern reported by the ombudsman office and note resident names reported as potential sample residents, residents for closed record review, or family members for family interviews and the reasons for their recommendation by the ombudsman.

7. Preadmission Screening and Resident Review Reports (PASRR)

Some States may have formal mechanisms to share with the survey agency the results of PASRR screens for residents with mental illness or mental retardation. If this information is available, evaluate if there are any potential concerns and note names of residents for possible inclusion in the sample.

8. Other Pertinent Information

At times, the survey agency may be aware of special potential areas of concern that were reported in the news media or through other sources. Evaluate this information to determine if there are potential areas of concern that should be investigated onsite.

C. Team Coordinator Responsibilities

The team coordinator and/or designee is responsible for completing the following tasks:

1. Contact the ombudsman office in accordance with the policy developed between the State survey agency and State ombudsman agency. The purposes of this contact are to

notify the ombudsman of the proposed day of entrance into the facility and to obtain any information the ombudsman wishes to share with the survey team. Ascertain whether the ombudsman will be available if residents participating in the group or individual interviews wish her/him to be present.

2. Obtain all information sources listed in B. above for presentation at the offsite team meeting. (See Section B. for descriptive information about these reports.) They are as follows:

- Specified QI/QM Reports:

  ✧ Facility Characteristics Report;
  ✧ Facility Quality Measure/Indicator Report; and
  ✧ The two resident level reports:
    - Resident Level Quality Measure/Indicator Report: Chronic Care Sample; and
    - Resident Level Quality Measure/Indicator Report: Post Acute Care Sample

  NOTE: It is important that the QM/QI reports be generated as close to the date of survey as possible, preferably no more than a few days prior to the survey.

- Form CMS-2567 and Statement of Isolated Deficiencies Which Cause No Actual Harm With Only Potential For Minimal Harm;
- Standard OSCAR Report 3 and 4;
- Results of complaint investigations;
- Information about waivers or variances;
- Information from the State Ombudsman office;
- Preadmission Screening and Resident Review Reports; and
- Other pertinent information.

3. Complete the following additional duties:

- Copy and distribute to the team the facility's floor plan if the team is unfamiliar with the facility's layout;
- Make extra copies of the OSCAR Reports 3 and 4, and the QM/QI reports to be given to the facility's administrator;
- Obtain an extra copy of the group interview worksheet (see Form CMS-806B, Exhibit 94) to give to the council president.

D. Offsite Survey Preparation Team Meeting

Present copies of the information obtained to the survey team members for review at a team meeting **offsite**. The team must prepare for the survey offsite, so that they are ready to begin the Entrance Conference and Initial Tour immediately after they enter the facility. The team should:

1. Review the Facility Characteristics Report to note the facility's demographics. This report can be used to identify whether the facility's population is unusual, e.g., high preva-

lence of young or male residents, high prevalence of residents with psychiatric diagnosis, high percentage of significant change assessments, etc.;

2. Use a copy of the Roster/Sample Matrix (Form CMS-802, Exhibit 90) to highlight concerns the team identifies for Phase 1 of the survey, and to list residents pre-selected and the QM/QI conditions for which each was selected. Mark the offsite block on this form to distinguish it from the Phase 1 version that will be completed in Task 4, "Sample Selection;"

The Facility Quality Measure/Indicator Report divides the QM/QIs into a set for the chronic care residents, followed by three post acute measures, which are based on MDS information for short-stay residents. The three PAC QM/QI items include two that are the same topics as the chronic care residents (13.2, Short-stay residents who had moderate to severe pain, and 13.3, Short-stay residents with pressure ulcers) and one unique item (13.1, Short-stay residents with delirium). Use this report to select concerns based on the following:

- Any sentinel health event QM/QI that is flagged. For the chronic care sample, a "sentinel health event" is a QM/QI that represents a significant occurrence that should be selected as a concern, even if it applies to only one or a few residents. The sentinel event QM/QIs are 5.4, Prevalence of fecal impaction; 7.3, Prevalence of dehydration; and 12.2, Low-risk residents with pressure ulcers. This means that even if one resident has any of these conditions, this QM/QI will flag and the care area must be selected as a concern and the resident with the problem must be selected for the sample. If there are multiple residents who flag on a sentinel event QM/QI, it is not necessary to select all of them;
- Any other QM/QI that is flagged at the 90th percentile; and
- Any unflagged QM/QI in which the facility is at the 75th percentile or greater.

For the items that are duplicated between the chronic care and PAC residents (pain and pressure ulcers), note whether the area of concern was selected based on only chronic or PAC samples, or both. The survey team may also wish to select as concerns any other QM/QIs that are of interest to them because they are related to QM/QIs that have been selected.

3. Begin selection of potential residents for the Phase 1 survey sample with the chronic care sample residents to represent the concerns that have been selected, including selecting residents who have sentinel event QM/QI conditions; if multiple residents have a sentinel event QM/QI condition, it is not necessary to select all of them. Use Table 1 in this section and the number of the total resident census to determine the sample size for the Phase 1 sample. Most if not all residents from the PAC sample are likely to have been discharged. The survey team may use this sample of residents from which to select potential closed records for review. (If some PAC residents that triggered a selected QM/QI are still at the facility, the team may select some of these residents in order to investigate issues of concern).

- In any facility in which the team has noted concerns with weight loss, dehydration, and/or pressure sores, select approximately one-half of the pre-selected sample as residents who have one or more of these conditions.

For the condition of hydration, select a resident who has flagged for the sentinel event QM/QI 7.3 (Prevalence of dehydration) and residents may be selected who have any of the following related QM/QI conditions: *5.4* – Prevalence of fecal impaction; *6.1* – Residents with a urinary tract infection; *7.1* – Residents who lose too much weight; *7.2* – Prevalence of tube feeding; and *9.1* – Residents whose need for help with daily activities has increased. The best residents to select will be those who also have multiple care areas that have been selected as concerns. For any facility in which these concerns were not identified, the team should still select some residents who have these QM/QI conditions, if any, on the Resident Level Quality Measure/Indicator Reports, but this need not be 50% of the Phase 1 sample size.

- For the remaining half of the Phase 1 preliminary sample, select residents to represent the remaining areas of concern.

NOTE: If there are no other QM/QIs that have been selected as concerns, the team may select residents based on other sources of information, e.g., complaints or a report from the ombudsman, or may wait to select the remaining Phase 1 residents based on Initial Tour findings.

If the average length of stay for the facility's population is less than 14 days, there may be little information available. Pre-selection of QM/QI-based concerns and/or the full sample may not be possible. Selection of some or all concerns and residents may need to be totally conducted onsite.

- The survey team should be alert to inconsistencies on the Facility Quality Measure/Indicator Report that may indicate facility error in completing and/or transmitting its Minimum Data Set (MDS) records, or a problem with State's software or CMS' database. The following are some possible indicators of data quality problems:

  ✧ The denominator for QM/QIs that use "all residents" substantially exceeds or is substantially smaller than the facility bed size;
  ✧ The number of residents with a QM/QI condition, i.e., the numerator, exceeds the resident population; or,
  ✧ The numerator for a particular QM/QI is zero although other information sources indicate otherwise. For example, the QM/QI report shows zero residents in restraints, but the ombudsman notified the team that she/he verified complaints about restraints. The most common reason for this type of inconsistency is incorrect MDS coding by the facility.

If these or other potential accuracy concerns are noted, the team should add resident assessment accuracy as a concern for the survey.

NOTE: This review need not be done for "short-stay" facilities, which will often have unusual values in the numerator and denominator due to rapid turnover of residents.

The Facility Quality Measure/Indicator Report is generated using the current MDS records in the State database at the time the report was generated. However, it excludes residents who have only an initial MDS record in the system. This was done so that the report reflects the care residents have received while residing in the facility, as opposed to the conditions of residents at the time of admission to the facility. The Resident Level reports are calculated using the most recently transmitted MDS record, e.g., annual, significant change, quarterly, or initial MDS record. Differences could be seen between the Facility Quality Measure/Indicator Report and the Resident Level reports since the former does not use the admission MDS data. For example, a Resident Level report may indicate a resident had a catheter but the Facility Quality Measure/Indicator Report might show a "0." This is not an accuracy problem, it only reflects the use of different data to generate each report.

4. Review the OSCAR reports after the review of the QM/QI reports to add corroborative information to the QM/QI information, e.g., a pattern of repeat deficiencies in a requirement related to a flagged QM/QI, and/or to point out areas of large discrepancies between the QM/QI numerators and the OSCAR Reports, e.g., the OSCAR 4 report lists the facility as having triple the average number of residents in restraints, but the QM/QI for restraints shows the facility has less restraints than most facilities). The team coordinator may wish to discuss such discrepancies with the administrator on entrance to determine the reason for them.

Relate information between Reports 3 and 4 such as a pattern of repeat deficiencies in range of motion and a lower than average percentage of residents receiving rehabilitative services. Also, note any special resident characteristics not contained in the QM/QI reports.

NOTE: Both the OSCAR reports and the QM/QI reports can alert surveyors to the acuity and characteristics of the facility's residents at the time the information for these reports was determined. This information may not represent the current condition of residents in the facility at the time of the survey. Keep in mind that the OSCAR information is approximately 1 year old, and the QM/QI information may be from 2–6 months old. Resident characteristics that were reported by the facility during the last survey may have changed significantly and may be the source of some discrepancies between OSCAR and QM/QI information.

5. Review all other sources of information and record additional information on the Offsite Preparation Worksheet (Form CMS-801, Exhibit 89), for example, residents' names for possible inclusion in the Phase 2 sample based on non-QM/QI sources of information (B. 2 through 8 above), special features of the facility, or special resident populations. Identify any outstanding complaints needing investigation. At this meeting, establish preliminary surveyor assignments and projections of which days team members will enter early and/or stay late to make observations of resident care and quality of life.

Task 2 – Entrance Conference/Onsite Preparatory Activities

A. Entrance Conference

1. The team coordinator informs the facility's administrator about the survey and introduces team members.
2. After the introduction to the administrator, the other team members should proceed to the initial tour (Task 3), while the team coordinator conducts the entrance conference.
3. The team coordinator should:

*   Request a copy of the actual working schedules for licensed and registered nursing staff for this time period by the end of the tour or earlier if possible.
*   Inform facility staff that the survey team will be communicating with them throughout the survey and will ask for facility assistance when needed. (See §2713.A for further information about facility staff accompanying surveyors.) Advise them that they have the opportunity to provide the team with any information that would clarify an issue brought to their attention.
*   Explain the survey process and answer any questions from facility staff.
*   Give the Administrator copies of the QM/QI reports and the OSCAR 3 and 4 reports that are being used for the survey. Briefly explain these reports and how they were used by the survey team in Task 1. If there are discrepancies between the OSCAR information and the QM/QI Facility Characteristics report, ask the administrator, or person designated by the administrator, to explain the discrepancies.
*   Ask the administrator to describe any special features of the facility's care and treatment programs, organization, and resident case-mix. For example, does the facility have a special care unit for residents with dementia? Are residents with heavy care needs placed in particular units? If so, which ones?
*   Inform the administrator that there will be interviews with individual residents, groups of residents, family members, friends, and legal representatives, and that these interviews are conducted privately, unless the interviewees request the presence of a staff member. Ask the administrator to ensure that there are times during the survey when residents can contact the survey team without facility staff present and without having to ask facility staff to leave or to allow access to the team.
*   Ask the administrator to provide the following information within 1 hour of the conclusion of the entrance conference (or later at the survey team's option):

    1. List of key facility personnel and their locations, e.g., the Administrator; directors of finance, nursing services, social services, and activities; dietitian or food supervisor; rehabilitation services staff; charge nurses; pharmacy consultant; plant engineer; housekeeping supervisor; persons responsible for infection control and quality assurance; health information management professional; and the medical director;
    2. A copy of the written information that is provided to residents regarding their rights;

3. Meal times, dining locations, copies of all menus, including therapeutic menus, that will be served for the duration of the survey;
4. Medication pass times (by unit, if variable);
5. List of admissions during the past month, and a list of residents transferred or discharged during the past 3 months with destinations;
6. A copy of the facility's layout, indicating the location of nurses' stations, individual resident rooms, and common areas, if not obtained in Task 1;
7. A copy of the facility admission contract(s) for all residents, i.e., Medicare, Medicaid, other payment sources;
8. Facility policies and procedures to prohibit and investigate allegations of abuse and the name of a person the administrator designates to answer questions about what the facility does to prevent abuse. (See Task 5G, Abuse Prohibition Review, for further information);
9. Evidence that the facility, on a routine basis, monitors accidents and other incidents, records these in the clinical or other record; and has in place a system to prevent and/or minimize further accidents and incidents;

NOTE: At the discretion of the facility, this evidence could include or be a record of accident and incident reports.

10. The names of any residents age 55 and under; and
11. The names of any residents who communicate with non-oral communication devices, sign language, or who speak a language other than the dominant language of the facility.

- Ask the facility to complete, to the best of their ability, the Roster/Sample Matrix (Form CMS-802), including all residents on bed-hold, by the end of the initial tour, or to provide this information in some other format, e.g., computer-generated list.

NOTE: This is an important source of resident information, which is crucial for the team to have for their sample selection meetings. Stress to the facility that this form should be completed first and given to the team coordinator by the end of the initial tour. After the Roster/Sample Matrix is delivered to the team, the facility may make modifications for accuracy or add additional information within 24 hours.

- Ask the facility to provide the following within 24 hours of the Entrance Conference:

1. A completed Long Term Care Facility Application for Medicare and Medicaid (Form CMS-671) (see Exhibit 85) and a Resident Census and Conditions of Residents (Form CMS-672) (see Exhibit 86); and
2. A list of Medicare residents who requested demand bills in the last 6 months (SNFs or dually-participating SNF/NFs only).

- Also, ask the administrator the following questions:

1. Which, if any, rooms have less square footage than required? Do you have a variance in effect and are you prepared to continue to request a variance for any such rooms? (F458)

2. Which, if any, rooms are occupied by more than four residents? Do you have a variance in effect and are you prepared to continue to request a variance for any such rooms? (F457)
3. Is there at least one window to the outside in each room? (F461)
4. Which, if any, bedrooms are not at or above ground level? (F461)
5. Do all bedrooms have access to an exit corridor? (F459)
6. What are the procedures to ensure water is available to essential areas when there is a loss of normal supply? (F466)

NOTE: If the survey is commencing at times beyond the business hours of 8:00 a.m. to 6:00 p.m., or on a Saturday or Sunday, once onsite, announce the survey, ascertain who is in charge, ask the person to notify the administrator that a survey has begun. Modify the entrance conference in accordance with staff available and complete the task and the onsite preparatory activity as appropriate within the context of the survey.

B. Onsite Preparatory Activities

1. In areas easily observable by residents and visitors, post, or ask the facility to post, signs announcing that a survey is being performed and that surveyors are available to meet with residents in private.
2. The team coordinator or designee should contact the resident council president after the Entrance Conference to introduce her/himself and to announce the survey. Provide the president with a copy of the group interview questions. Request the assistance of the president for arranging the group interview and to solicit any comments or concerns. Ask the council president for permission to review council minutes for the past 3 months (see Task 5D, Section 3B, for further information). If there is not an active resident council, or if the council does not have officers, ask for a list of residents who attend group meetings, if any, and select a resident representative to assist in arranging the group interview. If the ombudsman has indicated interest in attending the group interview, ask the president if that is acceptable to the group; if it is, notify the ombudsman of the time/place of the meeting.
3. The team coordinator, the surveyor assigned to conduct the group interview, or a designee should arrange for date, time, and private meeting space for the interview. Advise the facility staff that non-interviewable residents are not part of this meeting. (See Task 5D for further guidance.)

Task 3 – Initial Tour

A. General Objectives

The Initial Tour is designed to:

*   Provide an initial review of the facility, the residents, and the staff;
*   Obtain an initial evaluation of the environment of the facility, including the facility kitchen; and

- Confirm or invalidate the pre-selected concerns, if any, and add concerns discovered onsite.

B. General Procedures

The initial tour is used to gather information about concerns which have been pre-selected, new concerns discovered onsite, and whether residents pre-selected for the Phase 1 sample off-site are still present in the facility. In addition, attempt to meet and talk with as many residents as possible during the tour in order to identify other candidates for the sample, to get an initial overview of facility care and services, to observe staff/resident interactions, and to evaluate the impact of the facility environment on the residents. The tour also includes a first brief look at the facility's kitchen.

Document tour information, on either the Roster/Sample Matrix (Form CMS-802) or the Surveyor Notes Worksheet (Form CMS-807). Document any concerns regarding the general environment on the General Observations of the Facility Worksheet (Form CMS-803) or Surveyor Notes Worksheets (Form CMS-807). (See Task 5A for further information.) Surveyors may also document notes on the facility's Roster/Sample Matrix or other list of residents provided by the facility. Document any concerns noted in the brief tour of the facility kitchen on the Kitchen/Food Service Observation worksheet (Form CMS-804, Exhibit 92). (See Task 5B for information regarding observations to make during this brief tour.)

C. Protocol

Surveyors should tour individually as assigned by the team coordinator. It is desirable for team members to have a facility staff person who is familiar with the residents accompany them during the tour to answer questions and provide introductions to residents or family. However, do not delay the beginning of the Initial Tour if facility staff are not available. Begin the tour as soon as possible after entering the facility.

NOTE: When standard surveys begin at times beyond the business hours of 8:00 a.m. to 6:00 p.m., or begin on a Saturday or Sunday, the initial tour will need to be modified in recognition of the residents' activity, e.g., sleep, religious services, and types and numbers of staff available upon entry. The tour may focus on specific care and quality of life issues, e.g., restraint use, meal service, use of foam or paper meal service products rather than regular dinnerware, adherence to the planned menu; sufficiency of staff; whether enteral/parenteral fluids are being administered as ordered; whether incontinent residents are being checked, toileted, changed; etc., as appropriate. The tour should not be delayed for lack of staff to accompany the surveyor and/or survey team.

Phase 1—Pre-selected Concerns and Potential Residents:

During the tour, determine whether each resident pre-selected offsite for the Phase 1 sample is still there. Determine which, if any, of the pre-selected Phase 1 sample residents are interviewable residents who can be selected to participate in a Quality of Life Assessment Resident Interview or Group Interview. (See Task 5D.) This can be accomplished by talking with residents and asking questions. Examples of questions that can be asked are: What is your name? What are you planning to do today?

NOTE: Do not rely solely on the information that the facility provides concerning which residents are interviewable. The survey team should determine the residents who are able to participate in a Quality of Life Assessment interview.

If possible, determine if there are family members of non-interviewable residents in the pre-selected Phase 1 sample who can be selected for a Quality of Life Assessment family interview. Also note other non-interviewable residents among the facility population whose family members could be selected for interviews.

Observations of All Residents During the Tour

Ask staff to identify those residents who have no family or significant others. The team may include one or more of these residents in the Phase 2 sample for investigation of quality of life issues.

Have staff identify newly admitted residents, i.e., who have been admitted within the past 14 days, for possible inclusion in the sample for investigation of decline or deterioration that may have occurred before all MDS, other resident assessment information, and care planning is completed.

Have staff identify any residents for whom transfer or discharge is planned within the next 30 days.

Note residents who are interviewable or who have special factors, as listed in Task 4. When on the Initial Tour, observe and document possible quality of care and quality of life concerns in addition to those pre-selected offsite. If observed concerns involve specific residents, note the resident's name and room number on the worksheet, and the date/time when describing the observed concern. Include the details of the observation in documentation, including any effects on the residents involved.

Conduct a brief initial observation of the kitchen. (See Task 5B for further information.)

While on tour, identify the licensed and registered nursing staff who are currently on duty. At the end of the tour, compare the observed staff with the duty roster the facility is to provide. If there are discrepancies between the duty roster and the staff observed onsite, ask the person in charge to explain the discrepancies. This information will be used in Task 6 to determine if the facility is compliant with the requirements for licensed and registered nursing staff at 42 CFR 483.30(a)(2), F353 and 42 CFR 483.30(b)(1), F354.

During the tour focus on the following:

- Quality of Life

  1. Resident grooming and dress, including appropriate footwear;
  2. Staff–resident interaction related to residents' dignity; privacy and care needs, including staff availability and responsiveness to residents' requests for assistance;

3. The way staff talk to residents, the nature and manner of interactions, and whether residents are spoken to when care is given; and
4. Scheduled activities taking place and appropriateness to the residents.

• Emotional and behavioral conduct of the residents and the reactions and interventions by the staff:

1. Resident behaviors such as crying out, disrobing, agitation, rocking, pacing; and
2. The manner in which these behaviors are being addressed by staff, including nature and manner of staff interactions, response time, staff availability, and staff means of dealing with residents who are experiencing catastrophic reactions. (See "Abuse Prohibition Investigative Protocol" in Task 5G for a definition of catastrophic reaction.)

• Care issues, how care is provided, and prevalence of special care needs:

1. Skin conditions, e.g., excessive dryness, wetness;
2. Skin tears, bruising, or evidence of fractures that warrant investigation;
3. Dehydration risk factors including availability of water for most residents, and other indicators or factors, e.g., the amount and color of urine in tubing and collection bags, dependence on staff, the presence of strong urinary odors, and resident complaints of dry mouth and lips;
4. Clinical signs such as edema, emaciation, and contractures;
5. Functional risk factors such as poor positioning and use of physical restraints;
6. Side effects of antipsychotic drug use such as tardive dyskinesia, e.g., lip, tongue or other involuntary abnormal movements;
7. Presence or prevalence (numbers) of infections including antibiotic resistant strains of bacteria [e.g., Methicillin Resistant Staphylococcus Aureus (MRSA), Vancomycin Resistant Enterococcus (VRE), Clostridium Difficile (C-Diff)] or other infections [urinary tract infections, draining wounds, eye infections, skin rashes (especially if spreading, undiagnosed, and/or not responding to treatment), respiratory infections, gastroenteritis including diarrhea, etc.]
8. Pressure sores, old scars from pressure sores or evidence of surgical repair of pressure sores;
9. Amputation;
10. Significant weight loss;
11. Feeding tubes and/or improper positioning while feeding is infusing; and
12. Ventilators, oxygen, or intravenous therapies.

• Impact of the facility environment and safety issues:

1. Infection control practices, e.g., handwashing, glove use, and isolation procedures;
2. Functional and clean equipment, including kitchen equipment;
3. Presentation and maintenance of a homelike and clean environment; and
4. Availability, use, and maintenance of assistive devices.

NOTE: If the initial tour is being conducted during a mealtime, include an initial brief observation of the dining areas. Note if there are any concerns with meal service, quality of life, positioning, sufficient space, etc.

Task 4 – Sample Selection

A. General Objective

The objective of this task is to select a case-mix stratified sample (see Special Factors to Consider in Sample Selection below for further information) of facility residents based on QIs and other offsite and onsite sources of information in order to assess compliance with the resident-centered long-term care requirements.

B. General Procedures

- The Phase 1 sample is pre-selected during Task 1, "Offsite Survey Preparation," based on QM/QIs and other areas of concern. The pre-selected sample is reviewed during the sample selection meeting and residents are retained for the sample unless they are discharged, or the survey team has another reason to substitute, e.g., to select interviewable residents. Each team member is assigned a certain number of residents, completing all facets of review that have been selected including any quality of life assessment protocols selected for these residents.
- The Phase 2 sample is selected onsite, part way through the survey when surveyors have collected enough information to determine the focus of the remainder of the survey. The Phase 2 sample residents are selected to represent new concerns and/or to continue further investigation of Phase 1 concerns when Phase 1 reviews proved inconclusive or when necessary to determine scope of a problem. It is statutorily required that the sample in each facility be case-mix stratified in order to capture both interviewable and non-interviewable residents as well as residents from both heavy and light care categories.

NOTE: If the team is conducting sample selection during mealtime, delay or interrupt this task to conduct brief observations of the dining areas. Note if there are any concerns with meal service, quality of life, positioning, sufficient space, etc.

C. Definitions

- **Interviewable Resident** — This is a resident who has sufficient memory and comprehension to be able to answer coherently the majority of questions contained in the Resident Interview. These residents can make day-to-day decisions in a fairly consistent and organized manner.
- **Comprehensive Review** — For Task 5C, "Resident Review," this includes observations, interviews, and record reviews for all care areas for the sampled residents, as applicable.
- **Focused Review** — For Task 5C, "Resident Review," this includes the following:

    ✧ For Phase 1: Observations, interviews, and record reviews concerning all highlighted areas of concern and all unhighlighted areas pertinent to the resident; and

◇ For Phase 2: Observations, interviews, and record review for all highlighted areas of concern pertinent to the resident.

- **Closed Record Review** — For Task 5C, "Resident Review," this includes a record review of residents' care issues and transfer and discharge.
- **Roster/Sample Matrix** — This worksheet (Exhibit 265, Form CMS-802) is used by the survey team during Offsite Survey Preparation, and at the Phase 1 and Phase 2 Sample Selection meetings to note areas of concern for the survey, and to select residents for the sample. There are separate sets of instructions for the use of this form by the survey team and the facility. (See these instructions at Exhibits 266 and 267.)

D. Protocol

1. Phase 1 – Sample Selection

The Phase 1 sample is pre-selected during Task 1, Offsite Survey Preparation, based on the facility's QM/QIs of concern. (See Task 1 for further information.) Final Phase 1 sample selection occurs after the tour is completed and the facility has provided the completed Roster/Sample Matrix (Form CMS-802, Exhibit 265), or provided this information in some other format, e.g., computer-generated list. However, do not delay Phase 1 sample selection if the facility's Roster/Sample Matrix has not arrived. The team will complete the sample selection for Phase 1 by performing the following tasks:

NOTE: For facilities with a population of "short-stay" residents, the team may not have been able to pre-select concerns or potential sampled residents. In that instance, Phase 1 sample selection will occur during this task.

- First determine if any pre-selected concerns should be dropped due to the QM/QI data not representing the conditions of current residents. For example, there was a pre-selected QM/QI concern with residents with tube feedings, but the tour has verified there are no residents in the facility who are receiving tube feedings. Note new concerns and determine if some pre-selected residents can be evaluated for the new concerns as well as those originally selected.
- Review the Roster/Sample Matrix provided by the facility and compare it to the findings from the tour to determine if there is a reason to substitute another resident for any of the residents from the Offsite sample. A pre-selected resident who is no longer in the facility can be considered for the closed record review. The team may substitute other residents for those pre-selected, if necessary. They can select either from the QM/QI reports, the tour, or the facility's Roster/Sample Matrix.

If any resident is substituted for a pre-selected resident, record a short explanation on the Offsite Roster/Sample Matrix next to that person's name, e.g., "discharged."

- Check "Phase 1" on the copy of the Roster/Sample Matrix that will be used to denote the resident sample for Phase 1 of the survey.

✧ Highlight the column for each identified concern for Phase 1.

✧ Use Table 1 in this section and the number of the total resident census to determine the number of comprehensive and focused reviews; number of closed records; number of resident and family interviews; and the minimum number of residents who have conditions of weight loss, hydration risk and/or pressure sores, i.e., the WHP group. The number in the WHP column represents the minimum total of residents who must be selected for the Phase 1 sample to represent any or all of these conditions. For example, in a facility with 96 residents, out of 12 residents selected for the Phase 1 sample, a minimum of 6 will be those who have any of the conditions mentioned above, if any of these 3 QM/QIs were selected as concerns.

✧ Use the unnumbered blocks to the right of Resident Name to fill in the total number of residents in each sub-sample for the entire survey as listed in Table 1. For example, in a facility with a census of 100, the total number of individual interviews is 5. Enter that number in the small block below that title.

✧ All residents selected for comprehensive reviews are selected by the team during the Phase 1 sample selection. Residents selected for focused reviews, closed record reviews, individual and family interviews may be selected during Phase 1 or Phase 2 sample selection.

✧ Each resident the team selects is entered on the worksheet. Note the following about each resident:

  • Resident number and room number;
  • Surveyor assigned to complete the resident review and any quality of life assessment protocols (Resident Interview or Family Interview) that are selected for the resident;
  • Check any columns that pertain to this resident, whether or not they are highlighted as concerns for Phase 1. Each resident will be reviewed for each checked area, not just those that are highlighted; and
  • If there is anything about this resident that the team decides to investigate that is not one of the numbered columns on the worksheet, use a blank column at the far right to write the item that will be assessed and check that column for that resident. For example, if the team wants to assess ventilator use for a particular resident, write "ventilator" in one of the blank columns and make a check mark in that column for that resident.

2. Phase 2 – Sample Selection

Part way through the survey, after the team has obtained enough information to decide what concerns need further investigation, the team meets to determine the areas of concern, if any, for Phase 2 of the survey and to select the remaining sample. It is not necessary to complete all the reviews of all residents in Phase 1 before this meeting. Determine which Phase 1 concerns are ruled out as these do not need to be carried over into Phase 2 sample selection.

  • Select concerns for Phase 2 based on the following:

    ✧ Initial concerns noted during Offsite Survey Preparation or the Initial Tour that have not yet been reviewed;

♦ Currently un-reviewed concerns that are related to those under investigation, e.g., adding residents who have had falls based on results of the Phase 1 discovery of a problem with use of psychoactive drugs; and

♦ Current concerns for which the information gathered is inconclusive.

- Select residents for the Phase 2 sample based on the following:

  ♦ The statute requires selection of a "case mix stratified" sample (but not for each phase of the sample selection, just for the total sample). This stratification is defined by CMS as including residents who are interviewable and non-interviewable, and as including residents who require heavy and light care. It is important that at least one resident in the sample represent each of these categories. The requirements of the sample selection procedures make it necessary for survey teams to select interviewable and non-interviewable residents in order to complete the Task 5D, Quality of Life Assessment Interviews, so those categories of case-mix stratification will be automatically filled by complying with the sample selection procedures. At the beginning of the Phase 2 sample selection meeting, the team should review the Phase 1 sample to determine if at least one heavy care and one light care resident has been selected to fulfill this portion of the case-mix stratification requirement. If not, it is a priority to ensure that if either heavy or light care residents are missing from the Phase 1 sample, that at least one is selected from the missing category in Phase 2.

  ♦ Select residents who represent one or more of the areas of concern the team has selected for Phase 2 of the survey.

  ♦ If no residents have been selected for the Phase 1 sample for hydration, and if any residents are seen during Phase 1 of the survey who appear to have risk factors for dehydration, e.g., such as residents who are dependent on staff for activities of daily living, are immobile, receive tube feedings, or have dementias in which the resident no longer recognizes thirst, select at least one of these residents at risk and review the care area of dehydration.

- During Phase 2 sample selection, a clean copy of the Sample/Matrix worksheet is used as follows:

  ♦ Check "Phase 2" on the copy of the Roster/Sample Matrix that will be used to denote the resident sample for Phase 2 of the survey;

  ♦ Highlight the column for each identified concern for Phase 2;

  ♦ Each resident the team selects is entered on the worksheet. Note the following about each resident:

    - Resident number and room number;
    - Surveyor assigned to complete the resident review and any quality of life assessment protocols (Resident Interview, or Family Interview) that are selected for the resident;
    - Checkmarks are made only in the highlighted columns and these residents will be reviewed for these concerns, and any other concerns that are discovered during this review;

- Be sure that residents are selected to complete the required number of resident interviews, family interviews, and closed record reviews.

- If there are no outstanding areas of concern and the team has already selected interviewable, non-interviewable, heavy care, and light care residents, then select remaining residents to represent any of the following, in no particular order:

  ◈ An area of concern on the worksheet that has not been highlighted, but which the team has determined should be assessed;
  ◈ Living units that are unrepresented; and
  ◈ Special factors below that have not been reviewed.

NOTE: When selecting the sample in a facility in which there are no outstanding areas of concern, each resident will be reviewed for at least one area on the Roster/Sample Matrix that has not yet been reviewed.

3. Special Factors to Consider in Sample Selection

Residents **must** be selected for both the Phase 1 and Phase 2 samples as representatives of concerns to be investigated and to fulfill the case mix stratified sample requirement. If during sample selection, many more residents are identified than can be selected to represent the concerns of interest, consider the factors below in determining which residents to select:

- New admissions, especially if admitted during the previous 14 days. Even though the Resident Assessment Instrument (RAI) is not required to be completed for these residents, the facility must plan care from the first day of each resident's admission;
- Residents most at risk of neglect and abuse, i.e., residents who have dementia; no or infrequent visitors; psychosocial, interactive, and/or behavioral dysfunction; or residents who are bedfast and totally dependent on care;
- Residents in rooms in which variances have been granted for room size or number of beds in room;
- Residents receiving hospice services;
- Residents with end-stage renal disease;
- Residents under the age of 55;
- Residents with mental illness or mental retardation; and
- Residents who communicate with non-oral communication devices, sign language, or who speak a language other than the dominate language of the facility.

4. Other Phase 2 Tasks

- If there are any concerns about residents' funds, check that the amount of the surety bond is at least equal to the amount of residents' funds the facility is managing as of the most recent quarter.
- If concerns have been identified in the area of infection control, review policies and procedures including a focus on what preventative infection control practices the facility has in

place. For example, does the facility administer the influenza vaccine yearly to its residents, and administer pneumococcal vaccine to new residents as appropriate (does facility evaluate whether new residents have received the pneumococcal vaccine within the last 5 years)?

- Complete Task 5F Quality Assessment Assurance Review.
- If the group interview has not yet occurred, discuss what special concerns to ask of the group.
- If the facility has or has requested a nurse staffing waiver, review the requirements at 42 CFR 483.30.
- Review the Resident Census and Condition of Residents (Form CMS-672) that the facility has completed. Note any new areas of concern and determine if there appears to be large discrepancies between what is recorded by the facility and what the team has observed. For example, the team has noted 13 residents with pressure sores and the facility has listed 3. If there are large discrepancies, ask the facility to verify their totals. Answer questions F146 – F148 on the Resident Census.
- If the team has identified quality of care problems during Phase 1 of the survey, use the investigative protocol at Task 5C: Nursing Services, Sufficient Staffing to gather information and (at Task 6) to determine compliance with the following requirement: 42 CFR 483.30(a), F353 Nursing Services, Sufficient Staff. If problems with staffing have been discovered early in Phase 1, this protocol can begin in Phase 1.

5. Substituting Residents

If the team has found it necessary during the survey to remove a resident from the sample, e.g., a resident refused to complete the interview, replace this resident with another who best fulfills the reasons the first person was selected. For example, the resident who was removed had been selected because he/she was in restraints and had a pressure sore. Attempt to select another resident who meets both of these criteria. In Phase 1, the substituted resident should be selected from the pre-selected list of residents which was determined offsite, if possible, or from other information gained during the survey. Make the substitution as early in the survey as feasible. Note on the Roster/Sample Matrix that the new resident was substituted for resident #___, and briefly give the reason the first resident was dropped.

6. Supplementary Sample

If sampled residents are found not to provide enough information to make deficiency determinations concerning specific requirements under review, or to determine if there is "substandard quality of care" (see Task 6 for further information), supplement the sample with residents who represent the areas of concern under investigation. Focus review for these residents only on the concern under investigation and any other concerns that are discovered during this review. Add the names of these residents to the Phase 2 Sample Matrix worksheet, checking the relevant categories. Use the Resident Review Worksheet to complete these investigations.

Table 1 – Survey Procedures for Long-term Care Facilities – Resident Sample Selection

Survey Procedures for Long-term Care Facilities
Resident Sample Selection

Resident Census	Phase 1/ Phase 2	Comprehensive Reviews *	Focused Reviews *	Closed Rec. Reviews *	Res./Family Interviews	W, H, P Group **
1 – 4	All / 0	2	2	0	1 / 1	All
5 – 10	3 / 2	2	2	1	1 / 1	2
11 – 20	5 / 3	2	5	1	2 / 2	3
21 – 40	6 / 4	2	7	1	3 / 2	3
41 – 44	7 / 4	2	8	1	3 / 2	4
45 – 48	7 / 5	2	9	1	3 / 2	4
49 – 52	8 / 5	3	9	1	4 / 2	4
53 – 56	8 / 6	3	9	2	4 / 2	4
57 – 75	9 / 6	4	9	2	4 / 2	5
76 / 80	10 / 6	4	9	3	4 / 2	5
81 – 85	10 / 7	4	10	3	4 / 2	5
86 – 90	11 / 7	4	11	3	4 / 2	6
91 – 95	11 / 8	4	12	3	4 / 2	6
96 – 100	12 / 8	5	12	3	5 / 2	6
101 – 105	13 / 8	5	13	3	5 / 2	7
106 – 110	13 / 9	5	14	3	5 / 2	7
111 – 115	14 / 9	5	15	3	5 / 2	7
116 – 160	14 / 10	5	16	3	5 / 2	7
161 – 166	15 / 10	5	17	3	5 / 2	8
167 – 173	16 / 10	5	18	3	5 / 2	8
174 – 180	16 / 11	5	19	3	5 / 2	8
181 – 186	17 / 11	5	20	3	5 / 2	9
187 – 193	17 / 12	5	21	3	5 / 2	9
194 – 299	18 / 12	5	22	3	5 / 2	9
300 – 400	18 / 12	5	22	3	6 / 3	9
401 –	18 / 12	5	22	3	7 / 3	9

* Comprehensive reviews plus focused reviews plus closed record reviews added together equals the total sample size (Phase 1 plus Phase 2).

** For any survey in which there are identified concerns in the areas of (W) unintended weight loss, (H) hydration, and/or (P) pressure sores, this is the minimum total of residents who must be selected for the Phase 1 sample to represent any or all of these conditions.

Task 5 – Information Gathering

Task 5 provides an organized, systematic, and consistent method of gathering information necessary to make decisions concerning whether the facility has met the requirements reviewed during the Standard Survey.

Task 5 includes the following sub-tasks:

5A   General Observations of the Facility: Assessment of the environment of the facility affecting the resident's life, health, and safety;

5B   Kitchen/Food Service Observations: Assessment of the facility's food storage, preparation, and service;

5C   Resident Review: An integrated, holistic assessment of the sampled residents which includes the assessment of: drug therapies, the quality of life of the resident as affected by his/her room environment and daily interactions with staff, and assessment of those pertinent care concerns identified for each sampled resident by the survey team. Closed record reviews and dining observations are integrated into the resident review;

5D   Quality of Life Assessment: Assessment of residents' quality of life through individual interviews, a group interview, family interviews, and observations of residents who are non-interviewable;

5E   Medication Pass Observation: Application of Medication Error Detection Methodology;

5F   Quality Assessment and Assurance Review: An assessment of the facility's Quality Assessment and Assurance program to determine if the facility identifies and addresses specific care and quality issues and implements a program to resolve those issues; and

5G   Abuse Prohibition Review: A determination of whether the facility has developed and operationalized policies and procedures designed to protect residents from abuse, neglect, involuntary seclusion, and misappropriation of their property. This includes policies and procedures for hiring practices, training and ongoing supervision for employees and volunteers who provide services, and the reporting and investigation of allegations and occurrences that may indicate abuse.

Use survey worksheets and Guidance to Surveyors, also known as the Interpretive Guidelines, for each of the sub-tasks and requirements reviewed in Task 5. While these sub-tasks are discrete information gathering activities, there are a number of things to take into consideration during Task 5.

A. General Procedures

As appropriate, use the interpretations, definitions, probes, and procedures provided in the Guidance to Surveyors to guide the investigation and to help determine whether, based on the investigation and findings, the facility has met the requirements.

Worksheet documentation should be resident-centered, as appropriate. For example, if the lack of a reading light near the resident's bedroom chair is being documented, also note that this resident has said he/she prefers to read in his/her chair, and that the light over the chair is inadequate.

Relate to the requirements and provide clear evidence, as appropriate, of the facility's failure to meet a requirement. As information is collected, keep in mind that the information written on the worksheet will be used by the team to determine if there are any deficiencies, and, if so, the degree of severity and scope. Make documentation specific enough so that these decisions can be made. Include information about how the faulty facility practice affected residents, the number of residents affected, and the number of residents at risk. This documentation will be used both to make deficiency determinations and to categorize deficiencies for severity and scope. The Guidance to Surveyors assists in gathering information in order to determine whether the facility has met the requirements. For example, the facility has care plan objectives which are measurable. If the resident does not meet her/his goals, does the documentation reflect how the lack of implementation of the care plan and/or lack of quarterly assessments prevents the resident from reaching her/his goals?

In conducting the survey, use the worksheets in conjunction with the survey procedures and Guidance to Surveyors. When investigating a concern, note the tag number listed on the worksheet for that requirement and use the Guidance to Surveyors for that tag to direct the investigation.

Devote as much time as possible during the survey to performing observations and conducting formal and informal interviews. Limit record reviews to obtaining specific information, i.e., look at what is needed, not the whole record.

The information gathering tasks are interrelated. Information acquired while doing observations and interviews will direct the record review. Likewise, information obtained while doing the record review may help direct what observations or interviews are needed. Acquire the information that is necessary to make deficiency decisions in Task 6 using the survey worksheets and corresponding Guidance to Surveyors for each of the sub-tasks in Task 5.

Regardless of the task, be alert at all times to the surrounding care environment and activities. For example, while conducting the dining observations of sampled residents and the medication pass observation, observe the environment and residents, e.g., care being given, staff interactions with residents, and infection control practices.

The team should meet on a daily basis to share information, e.g., findings to date, areas of concern, any changes needed in the focus of the survey. These meetings include discussions of concerns observed, possible requirements to which those problems relate, and strategies for gathering additional information to determine whether the facility is meeting the requirements.

Throughout the survey, discuss observations, as appropriate, with team members, facility staff, residents, family members, and the ombudsman. Maintain an open and ongoing dialogue with the facility throughout the survey process. This gives the facility the opportunity to provide additional information in considering any alternative explanations before making deficiency decisions. This, however, does not mean that every negative observation is reported on a daily basis, e.g., at a nightly conference. Moreover, if the negative observation relates to a routine that needs to be monitored over time to determine whether a deficiency exists, wait until a trend has been established before notifying the facility of the problem. If it has been verified through observation and record review that a resident's condition has declined, start the investigation to determine if this decline was avoidable or unavoidable by asking a knowledgeable facility staff member, such as the nurse or other professional staff member charged with responsibility for the resident's care, to provide documentation in the resident's chart that provides the reasons for why they believe this decline occurred. Use this information to guide the investigation, but use professional judgment and team approach to determine if a deficient practice has occurred.

In conducting the tasks of the Standard Survey, situations may be identified to indicate that the facility may not be meeting a requirement not routinely reviewed in the Standard Survey.

Investigate this further. For example, residents at the council meeting say that they have not had a visit from a physician (or extender) for several months. This would lead to an investigation of facility compliance with the requirements for frequency of physician visits.

Verify information and observations in terms of credibility and reliability. If the credibility or reliability of information is doubted, validate that information or gather additional information before using it to make a compliance decision.

B. Observations

The objectives of the observational portion of information gathering are to gather resident-specific information for the residents included in the sample, and also, to be alert to the provision of care, staff-resident interactions, and quality of life for all residents.

C. Informal and Formal Interviews

The objectives of interviews are to:

- Collect information;
- Verify and validate information obtained from other survey procedures; and
- Provide the opportunity for all interested parties to provide what they believe is pertinent information.

Interview residents, staff, family, ombudsman, family council representatives, and other appropriate persons. Informal interviews are conducted throughout the duration of the information gathering tasks of the survey. Formal structured interviews are also done as part of the Quality of Life Assessment protocols. Use the information obtained from interviews to assist in deciding what additional observations and record review information is necessary. Avoid asking leading questions, but use the Guidance to Surveyors for specific requirements to focus questions and determine the significance of the answers.

In general, the individual who provides information during an interview will not be identified as providing that information. However, it is possible that their identity may be revealed if a deficiency is cited based in whole or part on their information, and that deficiency citation is appealed.

If residents appear reticent in providing information or express concern about retaliation:

- Verify that residents have information on whom to contact in the event they become the objects of retaliation by the facility; and
- With the resident's permission, notify the ombudsman of the resident's concerns.

D. Record Review

The objectives of the record review are to:

- Acquire information to direct initial and/or additional observations and interviews;
- Provide a picture of the current status of the resident as assessed by the facility; and
- Evaluate assessments, plans of care, and outcomes of care interventions for residents included in the sample. Record review of RAI information, care planning, implementation of the care plan, and evaluation of care is one facet of the resident review which determines if there has been a decline, improvement, or maintenance in identified focus areas.

NOTE: Do not spend excessive time gathering and recording information from the record. Use the record review to obtain information necessary to validate and/or clarify information obtained through observation and interviews. Ask facility staff to assist in finding any information that has not been found or that requires validation.

Sub-Task 5A – General Observations of the Facility

A. General Objective

The general objective of this task is to observe physical features in the facility's environment that affect residents' quality of life, health, and safety. Use the General Observations of the Facility worksheet (Form CMS-803, Exhibit 91) to complete this task.

B. General Procedures

During the Initial Tour, each surveyor should note and document any concerns in resident rooms and the general environment. Any concerns should be investigated and followed up either through the resident review for sampled residents or during the General Observation task. During the remainder of the survey, one surveyor is assigned to complete the General Observation of the Facility worksheet. This surveyor assures that all items on this worksheet are completed. All surveyors should share any additional concerns regarding the environment with the surveyor assigned to complete the worksheet. Begin observations as soon as possible after entering the facility, normally after introductions at the entrance conference.

During Task 5A, review the condition of the environment, e.g., cleanliness, sanitation, presence or absence of pests, accident hazards, functioning of equipment, and the proper and safe storage of drugs, biologicals, housekeeping compounds and equipment. (See Form CMS-803 worksheet for specific areas to review.)

C. Making Observations

The focus in Task 5A is on quality of life and environmental health and safety indicators in areas of the facility that would be visited or used by residents. However, some non-resident areas should also be reviewed due to their potential negative effect on residents, e.g., utility rooms.

Document thoroughly at the time of observations. If additional documentation space is needed, use the Surveyor Notes Worksheet Form CMS-807.

Plan to observe the facility's environment at different times during the survey, e.g., first and second shift, common areas when in use by residents.

Share any concerns with the team coordinator and other team members to determine the possible need to gather additional information.

Sub-Task 5B – Kitchen/Food Service Observation

A. General Objective

The general objective of the Kitchen/Food Service Observation is to determine if the facility is storing, preparing, distributing, and serving food according to 42 CFR 483.35(h)(2) to prevent foodborne illness.

B. General Procedures

One surveyor is assigned to conduct the Kitchen/Food service observation.

NOTE: The surveyor assigned to complete this task should begin the task with a brief visit to the kitchen as part of the initial tour, in order to observe the sanitation practices and cleanliness of the kitchen. Observe whether potentially hazardous foods have been left on counter tops or steam table and/or if being prepared, the manner in which foods are being thawed; the cleanliness; sanitary practices; and appearance of kitchen staff, e.g., appropriate attire, hair restraints.

Use the Kitchen/Food Service Observation worksheet to direct observations of food storage, food preparation, and food service/sanitation. (See Kitchen/Food Service Observation worksheet (Form CMS-804, Exhibit 92) for specific areas to review.)

In addition to completion of the Form CMS-804, also evaluate:

* The availability of food in relation to the number of residents; and
* Whether food being prepared is consistent with the written, planned menu.

NOTE: During team meetings, if surveyors, during the Dining Observation portion of the Resident Review, identified any concerns, such as the provision of meals that are not consistent in quality (such as color and texture of vegetables or meats, the preparation and presentation of mechanically altered foods); complaints regarding taste or texture of food and foods with an "off" or bad odor; or residents being at nutritional risk, including high prevalence of residents with unintended weight loss; then the surveyor assigned to Task 5B should review the following as appropriate.

Direct observations to the tray line and kitchen to determine:

- If recipes are available and consistent with the menu and followed by employees;
- If appropriate equipment is available and used to prepare and serve foods;
- If the food is being held for more than 30 minutes prior to food service, e.g., in the steam table, oven, refrigerator rather than freezer for frozen foods, etc.; and
- If cooked leftovers used during food preparation were stored and used within the appropriate time frames, and reheated to at least 165 degrees F.

Sub-Task 5C – Resident Review

A. General Objectives

The general objectives of the Resident Review are to determine:

- How resident outcomes and the resident's quality of life are related to the provision of care by the facility;
- If the care provided by the facility has enabled residents to reach or maintain their highest practicable physical, mental, and psychosocial well-being;
- If residents are assisted to have the best quality of life that is possible. The review will include aspects of the environment, staff interactions, and provision of services that affect sampled residents in their daily lives;
- If the facility has properly assessed its residents through the completion of the Resident Assessment Instrument (RAI), including accurate coding and transmitting of the Minimum Data Set (MDS) and has properly assessed care needs, conducted proper care planning, implemented the plan and evaluated care provided to the residents; and
- If there are additional areas of concern that need to be investigated in Phase II of the survey.

B. General Procedures

The team coordinator assigns specific residents in the sample to surveyors.

One surveyor should conduct the entire Resident Review for an assigned resident. If the resident has been chosen for a Quality of Life Assessment protocol (Task 5D), this same surveyor should also complete that protocol. If a surveyor has not passed the Surveyor Minimum Qualifications Test (SMQT) or if the complexity of a resident's care requires expertise of more than one discipline, surveyors should work jointly to complete the review. A surveyor must success-fully complete the SMQT to survey independently.

To facilitate the Resident Review, ask the charge nurse for schedules of the following, as appropriate:

1. Meals;
2. Medications;
3. Activities;
4. Tube feedings and special treatments;
5. Specialized rehabilitation therapies; and
6. Physician visits or visits of other health professionals such as dentists, podiatrists, or nurse practitioners.

For all sampled residents except closed records, parts A, B, and C (Resident Room Review, Daily Life Review, and Assessment of Drug Therapies) on the Resident Review Worksheet (Exhibit 93) are completed. The difference between the two reviews is that the focus of the part D Care Review is more extensive for Comprehensive Reviews. Determine, as appropriate, if there has been a decline, maintenance, or improvement of the resident in the identified focused care areas and/or Activities of Daily Living (ADL) functioning. If there has been a lack of improvement or a decline, determine if the decline or lack of improvement was avoidable or unavoidable.

C. Comprehensive Care Review

A Comprehensive Review includes observations, interviews, and a record review. After observing and talking with the resident, the surveyor conducts a comprehensive review which includes the following:

• A check of specific items on the MDS for accurate coding of the resident's condition. The specific items to be checked will be based on QM/QIs identified for the resident on the Resident Level Summary. At least 2 of the QM/QIs identified for the resident must be matched against the QM/QI definitions (see Exhibit 270) and against evidence other than the MDS to verify that the resident's condition is accurately recorded in the MDS. What is being verified is that the resident's condition was accurately assessed at the time the MDS was completed;
• An overall review of the facility's completion of the RAI process including their:

   ✧ Use of the Resident Assessment Protocols (RAPs);
   ✧ Evaluation of assessment information not covered by the RAPs;
   ✧ Identification of risks and causes of resident conditions;
   ✧ Completion of the RAP Summary;
   ✧ Development of a care plan that meets the identified needs of the resident;

• A review of the implementation of the care plan and resident response;
• A review of the relationship of the resident's drug regimen to the resident's condition (see the description of procedures for completing part C below);

- A thorough review of any of the following conditions that apply to the resident: weight loss, dehydration, pressure sores. This review is completed using the investigative protocols found below as a guide. (**NOTE**: All the residents selected for comprehensive reviews should have one or more of these concerns checked on the QM/QI reports [unless there are no residents with these concerns in the facility]); and
- An evaluation of the resident's dining experience (see Dining Observation Protocol below).

D. Focused Care Review Phase 1

This focused review includes observations, interviews, and a record review. This review focuses on care areas that were checked for the resident on the Resident Level Summary and any additional care items checked by the team as pertinent to the resident, e.g., all areas that are checked on the Roster/Sample Matrix by the team for the resident are reviewed, whether or not they have been highlighted as concerns for the survey. The dining observation is done for a resident if the resident has any checkmarks related to dining or the investigating team member has any concerns about the resident related to dining, such as weight loss.

The Phase 1 focused care review includes all care areas the team has checked for the resident: a review of the MDS, the facility's use of the RAPs, care planning, implementation of the care plan, and the resident's response to the care provided.

E. Focused Care Review Phase 2

This focused review includes observations, interviews, and a record review which concentrates only on those areas of concern for which the team requires additional information. For example, if the team needs additional information concerning facility compliance with the requirements for tube feeding, review only those RAI areas related to tube feeding; make observations of nutritional status, complications, and techniques of tube feeding, and interview residents, family, and staff concerning related areas.

F. Closed Record Review

This includes a record review of the resident's care issues and transfer and discharge requirements. It may be possible to select some or all of the closed records from the preselected list of residents for the Phase 1 sample, if any of these preselected residents were noted onsite to be discharged or deceased.

Assess quality of care and quality of life requirements that relate to the identified care areas for the sampled resident. While assessing these, note and investigate concerns with any other requirements.

G. Conducting the Resident Review

The Resident Review consists of 4 main sections: Resident Room Review, Daily Life Review, Assessment of Drug Therapies, and Care Review. See Resident Review Worksheet and instructions (Form CMS-805, Exhibit 93) for specific areas to review.

1. **Section A** – The Resident Room Review assesses aspects of accommodation of needs, environmental quality, and quality of life in the resident's room. Through observations and interviews, evaluate how the resident's environment affects his/her quality of life.

2. **Section B** – The Daily Life Review is a review of the resident's daily quality of life, especially in the areas of staff responsiveness to resident grooming and other needs, staff interactions, choices, and activities. Through ongoing observations and interviews, evaluate the resident's daily life routines and interactions with staff.

3. **Section C** – The Assessment of Drug Therapies is a review of the medications the resident is receiving to evaluate whether the effectiveness of the therapeutic regimen, including all drugs that may play a significant role in the resident's everyday life, is being monitored and assessed.

General Procedures

Conduct an assessment of drug therapies for residents selected for comprehensive and focused review. In addition, if the team has identified a concern that relates to the medication regimen, include a review of medication regimen in closed record reviews.

- Record the information on the Resident Review Worksheet, Form CMS-805. Review and record, as pertinent, all non-prescription and prescription medications taken by the resident during the past 7 days.
- Evaluate for the presence of any unnecessary drugs. (Review of the unnecessary drug requirements includes drugs and protocols or circumstances described in all sections of 42 CFR 483.25(l) and as pertinent, 42 CFR 483.60(c)(2).) The surveyor is to review the medication regimen for the following:

  ♦ Indications/reason for use;
  ♦ Effectiveness of therapeutic goal;
  ♦ Dose;
  ♦ Presence of monitoring, including drug regimen review and response to identified irregularities;
  ♦ Presence of duplicative therapy; and
  ♦ Presence of possible Adverse Drug Reactions (ADR) or side effects. In addition, review for the presence of any medications with "High Potential for Severe ADRs" or "High Potential for Less Severe ADRs" as identified in the Guidance to Surveyors. If any of these medications are identified, use the "Investigative Protocol: Adverse Drug Reactions" below.

NOTE: An ADR is a secondary effect of a drug that is usually undesirable and different from the therapeutic and helpful effects of the drug. The term "side effect" is often used interchangeably with ADR. Technically, however, side effects are but one of five ADR categories, the others being hypersensitivity, idiosyncratic response, toxic reactions, and adverse drug interactions. Formal definitions stress an ADR is any response to a drug that is noxious and unintended and occurs in doses used for prophylaxis, diagnosis, or therapy.

- Correlate the review of the drugs with the resident's clinical condition and any extenuating circumstances, such as recent admission, a change in the resident's environment, and hospitalization, etc.
- Evaluate how the drugs the resident receives affect his/her quality of care and quality of life through the following methods:

  ✧ A review of the clinical record, i.e., any section that has useful information pertaining to the resident;
  ✧ Observations of the resident; and
  ✧ Interviews with the resident or interested parties.

- Allow the facility the opportunity to provide their rationale for use of drugs which are prescribed contrary to CMS guidelines.
- If problems or concerns with drug therapy are noted, review the results of the pharmacist's drug regimen review, and the response from the attending physician/director of nurses. The Medical Director may have provided additional information regarding the specific issues identified during the resident's medication review.

Use the following investigative protocol for the review of apparent adverse drug reaction.

Investigative Protocol – Adverse Drug Reactions (ADR)

Objectives:

- To determine if the resident may be experiencing any Adverse Drug Reactions (ADRs) as a result of receiving one or more of the medications identified with high potential for severe ADRs or high potential for less severe ADRs.
- To determine whether the facility's drug regimen review process identified and reported any potential irregularities associated with the use of medications listed as having a high potential for ADRs, and whether there was any response to this notification.

Task 5C: Use:

Use this protocol if the resident meets the following criteria:

- Is over 65 years old;
- Has been in the facility over 7 days (or appears to be having a noticeable ADR within the first 7 days); and
- Is receiving any of the medications which has a high potential for severe ADRs or a high potential for less severe ADRs at 42 CFR 483.25(l) and 42 CFR 483.60(c)(2) in the guidance to surveyors, respectively.

NOTE: An Adverse Drug Reaction (ADR) is a secondary effect of a drug that is usually undesirable and different from the therapeutic and helpful effects of the drug. The term "side effect" is often used interchangeably with ADR. Technically, however, side effects are but one of five ADR categories, the others being hypersensitivity, idiosyncratic response, toxic reactions, and adverse drug interactions. An ADR is any response to a drug that is noxious and unintended and occurs in doses for prophylaxis, diagnosis or therapy.

Procedures:

These procedures are not intended to instruct surveyors to determine if a resident outcome is an actual ADR (except in obvious circumstances), but are guidelines intended to guide surveyors to find the pertinent facts that will assist them in determining compliance. In addition, the list of drugs and adverse reactions in the guidelines are not all inclusive and other medication sources may be reviewed for evaluation of the drug regimen.

1. **Screening** — If the criteria for use of the protocol are met, use the following (additional resources may be used, e.g., information provided by the facility, journals, etc.) to identify whether the resident may be experiencing a potential ADR.

   - **Review of Drugs with High Potential for Severe ADRs** — For this review, refer to the drugs and the Adverse Drug Reactions found in the surveyor guidance at 42 CFR 483.25(l), Section H, Unnecessary Drugs.

     ✧ Determine if there is evidence in the record explaining why the benefit of this medication outweighs the risk of a potential ADR, that is, the facility notes indicate the reasons that the medication is the one of choice for a particular resident.
     ✧ Determine if the resident is experiencing decline or other negative outcome as a result of the apparent ADR.

   - **Review of Drugs with High Potential for Less-Severe ADRs** — For this review, refer to the list of drugs in the surveyor guidance at F429, Drug Regimen Review.

     ✧ Determine if there is evidence in the record explaining why the benefit of this medication outweighs the risk of a potential ADR, that is, the facility notes indicate the reasons that the medication is the one of choice for a particular resident.

2. **Analyze** — Base evidence that an apparent ADR occurred or is occurring on two sources of information (clinical record review, interview with the resident or interested party, and observation, or one source for closed records).
3. **Review Facility Response** — If the resident is experiencing any potential ADR, determine whether the facility has identified and addressed/acknowledged the potential ADR.
4. **Additional Considerations** — When conducting the review, consider the following:

   - The use of any medication that appears in the Guidance to Surveyors at 42 CFR 483.25(l) and 42 CFR 483.60(c)(2) could be an appropriate therapy if valid documentation supporting its use is provided;

- The prescribing of medication should always take into consideration its risks and benefits, e.g., the benefits of a pain medication versus the risk of worsened constipation in a person already prone to constipation;
- The side effects of many medications are similar or the same as for other medications or disease processes; and
- In some cases, the benefits of a particular medication may not be self-evident and additional pertinent information, either written or verbal, should be requested from the facility.
- This protocol does not supercede current regulation. The surveyor has the option to cite at F329 (Unnecessary Drugs) or F429 (Drug Regimen Review) based on the situation.

Task 6 – Determination of Compliance

- Compliance with 42 CFR 483.25(l)(1)(i-vi), of F329: Unnecessary Drugs.

  ◇ For this resident, the medication is not an unnecessary drug if the facility identified the risks; determined that the benefit of this drug outweighs the risk or development of a potential ADR, that is, the facility indicates the reasons that the drug is the one of **choice** for a particular resident; and the facility continually assessed the use of the drug and determined that this continued to be a valid therapeutic intervention for the resident. If not, the medication is an unnecessary drug—Cite F329.

- Compliance with 42 CFR 483.60(c)(2), F429, Drug Regimen Review:

  ◇ For this resident, the drug regimen review is in compliance if the facility identified the risks, assessed, and determined if the benefit of this drug outweighs the risk of a potential ADR, that is, the facility notes indicate the reasons the drug is the one of choice for a particular resident. If the facility has not completed the above review and assessment, but the pharmacist has identified and reported the apparent irregularity to the attending physician/director of nursing as part of the drug regimen review process, the drug regimen review is in compliance. If not—Cite F429.

4. **Section D** — The care review is an assessment of those quality of care areas (see 42 CFR 483.25) that are pertinent to the sampled resident. The survey team, through use of the Roster/Sample Matrix, determines what care areas will be reviewed for each sampled resident. Additional areas for evaluation may be identified during the review.

   There are a designated number of comprehensive, focused, and closed record care reviews completed, depending on the size of the sample.

H. Care Observations and Interviews

Make resident observations and conduct interviews which include those factors or care areas as determined by the Roster/Sample Matrix. For example, if the resident was chosen because he/

she is receiving tube feedings, observe the care and the outcomes of the interventions, facility monitoring and assessment, and nutritional needs/adequacy related to tube feeding.

Complete the following tasks:

- Observe the resident and caregivers during care and treatments, at meals, and various times of the day, including early morning and evening, over the entire survey period. Observe residents in both informal and structured settings, e.g., receiving specialized rehabilitation services, participating in formal and informal activities. Also, observe staff-resident interactions;
- Gather resident-specific information, including information on the resident's functional ability, potential for increasing ability, and any complications concerning special care needs;
- Evaluate implementation of the care plan. Determine if the care plan is consistently implemented by all personnel at all times of the day, and if the care plan is working for the resident. If the care plan is not working, look for evidence that the facility has identified this and acted on it even if the care plan has not formally been revised;
- Determine if there is a significant difference between the facility's assessment of the resident and observations; and
- Evaluate the adequacy of care provided to the resident using the Guidance to Surveyors.

Do not continue to follow residents once enough information has been accrued to determine whether the resident has received care in accordance with the regulatory requirements.

If there are indicators to suggest the presence of a quality of care problem that is not readily observable, e.g., a leg ulcer covered with a dressing, or a sacral pressure sore, ask facility staff to assist in making observations by removing, for example, a dressing or bedclothes.

Resident care observations should be made by those persons who have the clinical knowledge and skills to evaluate compliance.

When observing residents, respect their right to privacy, including the privacy of their bodies. If the resident's genital or rectal area or female breast area must be observed in order to document and confirm suspicions of a care problem, a member of the nursing staff must be present at this observation, and the resident must give clear consent.

If the resident is unable to give consent, e.g., is unresponsive, incompetent, and a legal surrogate (family member who can act on the resident's behalf or legal representative as provided by State law) is present, ask this individual to give consent.

An observation of a resident's rectal or genital area (and for females, the breast area) may be made without a resident's or legal surrogate's consent, under the following conditions:

1. It is determined that there is a strong possibility that the resident is receiving less than adequate care which can only be confirmed by direct observation;
2. The resident is unable to give clear consent; and
3. A legal surrogate is not present in the facility.

Only a surveyor who is a licensed nurse, a physician's assistant, or a physician may make an observation of a resident's genitals, rectal area, or, for females, the breast area.

I. Record Review

Conduct a record review to provide a picture of the current status of the resident as assessed by the facility; information on changes in the resident's status over the last 12 months for those areas identified for review; and information on planned care, resident goals, and expected outcomes.

Use the record review to help determine whether the assessments accurately reflect the resident's status and are internally consistent. An example of inconsistency may be that the facility assessed the resident's ADLs as being independently performed yet had indicated that the resident requires task segmentation for performing ADLs.

For sampled residents selected for either a comprehensive or focused review, conduct a review of the RAI information including:

- The face sheet of the MDS for background information including customary routines and demographic information to provide an understanding of the resident prior to admission. This assists in assessing the quality of life of the resident.
- The latest MDS to determine which RAPs were triggered. For a sampled resident receiving a comprehensive review, note all triggered areas. Also, review the facility's assessment of the resident's level of functioning and note particularly drug therapy and cognitive, behavior, and ADL function. For a resident receiving a focused review in Phase I of the survey, review both the areas of concern specific to the resident and the other care areas that have been identified with the Roster/Sample Matrix. For Phase 2 residents, review only those areas that have been identified by the team as areas of concern.

If the RAI is less than 9 months old, review and compare with the previous RAI and the most recent quarterly review. If the RAI is 9 months or older, compare the current RAI with the most recent quarterly review. Review the following:

- The RAP summary sheet to see where the assessment documentation is located for any RAP triggered;
- The information summarizing the assessments (RAPs) and decision to proceed or not to proceed to care planning. Determine if the assessments indicate that the facility used the RAPs and considered the nature of the problem, the causal and risk factors, the need for referrals, complications, and decisions for care planning. If this is a reassessment, review whether the facility determined if the care plan required revision or was effective in moving the resident toward his/her goals;
- The care plan to identify whether the facility used the RAI to make sound care planning decisions. Determine whether the facility identified resident strengths, needs, and problems which needed to be addressed to assist the resident to maintain or improve his/her current functional status. Determine whether the facility identified resident-centered, mea-

surable goals and specific interventions to achieve those goals. With observations, interviews, and record review, determine if the facility implemented the interventions defined; and

- Determine whether the facility documentation and resident status as observed indicate the decision to proceed or not to proceed to care planning was appropriate. This information will assist in determining whether a resident's decline or failure to improve was avoidable or unavoidable.
- It is not necessary to review the entire resident record. Review only those sections that are necessary to verify and clarify the information necessary to make compliance decisions. These sections may include, for example, laboratory reports, progress notes, and drug regimen review reports.
- In any care area in which it is determined that there has been a lack of improvement, a decline, or failure to reach highest practicable well-being, assess if the change for the resident was avoidable or unavoidable. Note both the faulty facility practice and its effect on resident(s). Determine if a reassessment based on significant change should have been conducted, and if the absence of reassessment contributed to the resident's decline or lack of improvement.
- Verify the information needed has been obtained to determine if the facility fulfilled its obligation to provide care that allowed the resident to attain or maintain the highest practicable physical, mental, and psychosocial well-being.

NOTE: When conducting either a focused or comprehensive review, if there are areas of concern which fall outside the care areas identified, investigate these, as necessary.

The following are special investigative protocols which should be used in Task 5C to gather information and in Task 6, to determine facility compliance in the care areas of pressure sore/ulcer(s), hydration, unintended weight loss, sufficient nursing staffing, and dining and food services.

NOTE: "Although the RAI assessments discussed in the following [investigative protocols] must occur at specific times, by Federal regulation, a facility's obligation to meet each resident's needs through ongoing assessment is not neatly confined to these mandated time frames. Likewise, completion of the RAI in the prescribed time frame does not necessarily fulfill a facility's obligation to perform a comprehensive assessment. Facility's are responsible for assessing areas that are relevant to individual residents regardless of whether these areas are included in the RAI." ("CMS Long-Term Care Facility Resident Assessment Instrument User's Manual," Version 2.0.)

Investigative Protocol

Hydration

Objectives:

- To determine if the facility identified risk factors which lead to dehydration and developed an appropriate preventative care plan; and

- To determine if the facility provided the resident with sufficient fluid intake to maintain proper hydration and health.

Task 5C: Use:

Use this protocol for the following situations:

- A sampled resident who flagged for the sentinel event of dehydration (QM/QI 7.3);
- A sampled resident who has one or more of the following QM/QI conditions:

  ⬦ 5.4 – Prevalence of fecal impaction;
  ⬦ 6.1 – Residents with a urinary tract infection;
  ⬦ 7.1 – Residents who lose too much weight;
  ⬦ 7.2 – Prevalence of tube feeding;
  ⬦ 9.1 – Residents whose need for help with daily activities has increased; and
  ⬦ Any of the three pressure ulcer QM/QIs: 12.1, 12.2, or 13.3.

- A sampled resident who was discovered to have any of the following risk factors: vomiting/diarrhea resulting in fluid loss; elevated temperatures and/or infectious processes; dependence on staff for the provision of fluid intake; use of medications including diuretics, laxatives, and cardiovascular agents; renal disease; dysphagia; a history of refusing fluids; limited fluid intake; or lacking the sensation of thirst.

Procedures:

- Observations/interviews conducted as part of this procedure should be recorded on the Forms CMS-805 and/or the Form CMS-807.
- Determine if the resident was assessed to identify risk factors that can lead to dehydration, such as those listed above and also whether there were abnormal laboratory test values which may be an indicator of dehydration.

NOTE: A general guideline for determining baseline daily fluid needs is to multiply the resident's body weight in kilograms (kg) × 30ml (2.2 lbs = 1 kg), except for residents with renal or cardiac distress, or other restrictions based on physician orders. An excess of fluids can be detrimental for these residents.

- Determine if an interdisciplinary care plan was developed utilizing the clinical conditions and risk factors identified, taking into account the amount of fluid that the resident requires. If the resident is receiving enteral nutritional support, determine if the tube feeding orders include a sufficient amount of free water, and whether the water and feeding are being administered in accordance with physician orders?
- Observe the care delivery to determine if the interventions identified in the care plan have been implemented as described.

  ⬦ What is the resident's response to the interventions? Do staff provide the necessary fluids as described in the plan? Do the fluids provided contribute to dehydration, e.g., caffeinated beverages, alcohol? Was the correct type of fluid provided with a resident with dysphagia?

✧ Is the resident able to reach, pour, and drink fluids without assistance and is the resident consuming sufficient fluids? If not, are staff providing the fluids according to the care plan?

✧ Is the resident's room temperature (heating mechanism) contributing to dehydration? If so, how is the facility addressing this issue?

✧ If the resident refuses water, are alternative fluids offered that are tolerable to the resident?

✧ Are the resident's beverage preferences identified and honored at meals?

✧ Do staff encourage the resident to drink? Are they aware of the resident's fluid needs? Are staff providing fluids during and between meals?

✧ Determine how the facility monitors to assure that the resident maintains fluid parameters as planned. If the facility is monitoring the intake and output of the resident, review the record to determine if the fluid goals or calculated fluid needs were met consistently.

• Review all related information and documentation to look for evidence of identified causes of the condition or problem. This inquiry should include interviews with appropriate facility staff and health care practitioners, who by level of training and knowledge of the resident, should know of, or be able to provide information about the causes of a resident's condition or problem.

NOTE: If a resident is at an end of life stage and has an advance directive, according to State law (or a decision has been made by the resident's surrogate or representative, in accordance with State law) or the resident has reached an end of life stage in which minimal amounts of fluids are being consumed or intake has ceased, and all appropriate efforts have been made to encourage and provide intake, then dehydration may be an expected outcome and does not constitute noncompliance with the requirement for hydration. Conduct observations to verify that palliative interventions, as described in the plan of care, are being implemented and revised as necessary, to meet the needs/ choices of the resident in order to maintain the resident's comfort and quality of life. If the facility has failed to provide the palliative care, cite noncompliance with 42 CFR 483.25, F309, Quality of Care.

• Determine if the care plan is evaluated and revised based on the response, outcomes, and needs of the resident.

Task 6: Determination of Compliance:

• Compliance with 42 CFR 483.25(j), F327, Hydration:

✧ For this resident, the facility is compliant with this requirement to maintain proper hydration if they properly assessed, care planned, implemented the care plan, evaluated the resident outcome, and revised the care plan as needed. If not, cite at F327.

- Compliance with 42 CFR 483.20(b)(1) & (2), F272, Comprehensive Assessments:

  ✧ For this resident in the area of hydration, the facility is compliant with this requirement if they assessed factors that put the resident at risk for dehydration, whether chronic or acute. If not, cite at F272.

- Compliance with 42 CFR 483.20(k)(1), F279, Comprehensive Care Plans:

  ✧ For this resident in the area of hydration, the facility is compliant with this requirement if they developed a care plan that includes measurable objectives and timetables to meet the resident's needs as identified in the resident's assessment. If not, cite at F279.

- Compliance with 42 CFR 483.20(k)(3)(ii), F 282, Provision of care in accordance with the care plan:

  ✧ For this resident in the area of hydration, the facility is compliant with this requirement if qualified persons implemented the resident's care plan. If not, cite at F282.

Investigative Protocol

Unintended Weight Loss

Objectives:

- To determine if the identified weight loss is avoidable or unavoidable; and
- To determine the adequacy of the facility's response to the weight loss.

Task 5C: Use:

Utilize this protocol for a sampled resident with unintended weight loss.

Procedures:

- Observations/interviews conducted as part of this procedure should be recorded on the Form CMS-805 if they pertain to a specific sampled resident and on the Form CMS-807 if they relate to general observations of the dining service/dining room.
- Determine if the resident was assessed for conditions that may have put the resident at risk for unintended weight loss such as the following:

  ✧ Cancer; renal disease; diabetes; depression; chronic obstructive pulmonary disease; Parkinson's disease; Alzheimer's disease; malnutrition; infection; dehydration; constipation; diarrhea; Body Mass Index (BMI) below 19; dysphagia; chewing and swallowing problems; edentulous; ill-fitting dentures; mouth pain; taste/sensory changes; bedfast; totally dependent for eating; pressure ulcer; abnormal laboratory values (review in accordance with the facility's laboratory norms) associated with malnutrition (serum albumin, plasma transferrin, magnesium, hct/hgb, BUN/creatinine ratio, potassium, cholesterol); and use of medications such as diuretics, laxatives, and cardiovascular agents.

NOTE: Amputation of a body part will contribute to a significant decrease in previously targeted weight range. Once the new weight goals are established the resident should be assessed within the parameters of the unintended weight loss investigative protocol.

NOTE: Body Mass Index (BMI) estimates total body mass and is highly correlated with the amount of body fat. It provides important information about body composition, making it a useful indicator of nutritional status. BMI is easy to calculate because only information about height and weight are needed.

$$BMI = weight\ (Kg)/height\ (M^2)\ or$$

$$BMI = weight\ (lbs.)/height\ (inches^2) \times 703$$

- Determine if the facility has assessed the resident's nutritive and fluid requirements, dining assistance needs (such as assistive devices), food cultural/religious preferences, food allergies, and frequency of meals.
- Review all related information and documentation to look for evidence of identified causes of the condition or problem. This inquiry should include interviews with appropriate facility staff and health care practitioners, who by level of training and knowledge of the resident should know of, or be able to provide information about the causes of a resident's condition or problem.
- Determine if the care plan was developed utilizing the clinical conditions and risk factors identified in the assessment for unintended weight loss. Were the care plan interventions, such as oral supplements, enteral feeding, alternative eating schedule, liberalized diet, nutrient supplements, adaptive utensils, assistance, and/or increased time to eat developed to provide an aggressive program of consistent intervention by all appropriate staff?
- Determine if the care plan was evaluated and revised based on the response, outcomes, and needs of the resident.

NOTE: If a resident is at an end of life stage and has an advance directive according to State law (or a decision has been made by the resident's surrogate or representative in accordance with State law) or the resident has reached an end of life stage in which minimal amounts of nutrients are being consumed or intake has ceased, and all appropriate efforts have been made to encourage and provide intake, then the weight loss may be an expected outcome and may not constitute noncompliance with the requirement for maintaining nutritional parameters. Conduct observations to verify that palliative interventions, as described in the plan of care, are being implemented and revised as necessary, to meet the needs/choices of the resident in order to maintain the resident's comfort and quality of life. If the facility has failed to provide the palliative care, cite noncompliance with 42 CFR 483.25, F309, Quality of Care.

• Observe the delivery of care as described in the care plan, e.g., staff providing assistance and/or encouragement during dining; serving food as planned with attention to portion sizes, preferences, nutritional supplements, and/or between-meal snacks, to determine if the interventions identified in the care plan have been implemented. Use the Dining and Food Service Investigative Protocol to make this determination.

Task 6: Determination of Compliance:

• Compliance with 42 CFR 483.25(I), F325, Nutrition

 ✧ For this resident, the unintended weight loss is unavoidable if the facility properly assessed, care planned, implemented the care plan, evaluated the resident outcome, and revised the care plan as needed. If not, the weight loss is avoidable; cite at F325.

• Compliance with 42 CFR 483.25, F309, Quality of Care:

 ✧ For the resident who is in an end-of-life stage and palliative interventions, as described in the plan of care, are being implemented and revised as necessary, to meet the needs/choices of the resident in order to maintain the resident's comfort and quality of life, then for this resident, in the area of palliative care, the facility is compliant with this requirement. If not, cite F309.

• Compliance with 42 CFR 483.20(b)(1) and (2), F272, Comprehensive Assessments:

 ✧ For this resident in the area of unintended weight loss, the facility is compliant with this requirement if they assessed the factors that put the resident at risk for weight loss. If not, cite at F272.

• Compliance with 42 CFR 483.20(k)(1), F279, Comprehensive Care Plans:

 ✧ For this resident in the area of unintended weight loss, the facility is compliant with this requirement if they developed a care plan that includes measurable objectives and timetables to meet the resident's needs as identified in the resident's assessment. If not, cite at F279.

• Compliance with 42 CFR 483.20(k)(3)(ii), F 282, Provision of care in accordance with the care plan:

 ✧ For this resident in the area of unintended weight loss, the facility is compliant with this requirement if qualified persons implemented the resident's care plan. If not, cite at F282.

Investigative Protocol

Dining and Food Service

Objectives:

- To determine if each resident is provided with nourishing, palatable, attractive meals that meet the resident's daily nutritional and special dietary needs;
- To determine if each resident is provided services to maintain or improve eating skills; and
- To determine if the dining experience enhances the resident's quality of life and is supportive of the resident's needs, including food service and staff support during dining.

Task 5C: Use

This protocol will be used for:

- All sampled residents identified with malnutrition, unintended weight loss, mechanically altered diet, pressure sores/ulcers, and hydration concerns; and
- Food complaints received from residents, families, and others.

General Considerations:

- Use this protocol at two meals during the survey, preferably the noon and evening meals.
- Record information on the Form CMS-805 if it pertains to a specific sampled resident, or on the Form CMS-807 if it relates to the general observations of the dining service/dining room.

    ✧ Discretely observe all residents, including sampled residents, during meals keeping questions to a minimum to prevent disruption in the meal service.

- For each sampled resident being observed, identify any special needs and the interventions planned to meet their needs. Using the facility's menu, record in writing what is planned in writing to be served to the resident at the meal observed.
- Conduct observations of food preparation and quality of meals.

Procedures:

1. During the meal service, observe the dining room and/or resident's room for the following:

    - Comfortable sound levels;
    - Adequate illumination, furnishings, ventilation; absence of odors; and sufficient space;
    - Tables adjusted to accommodate wheelchairs, etc.; and
    - Appropriate hygiene provided prior to meals.

2. Observe whether each resident is properly prepared for meals. For example:

    - Resident's eyeglasses, dentures, and/or hearing aids are in place;
    - Proper positioning in chair, wheelchair, gerichair, etc., at an appropriate distance from the table (tray table and bed at appropriate height and position); and
    - Assistive devices/utensils identified in care plans provided and used as planned.

3. Observe the food service for:

    - Appropriateness of dishes and flatware for each resident. Single use disposable dining ware is not used except in an emergency and, other appropriate dining activities. Except those with fluid restriction, each resident has an appropriate place setting with water and napkin;
    - Whether meals are attractive, palatable, served at appropriate temperatures, and are delivered to residents in a timely fashion.

        ◇ Did the meals arrive 30 minutes or more past the scheduled meal time?
        ◇ If a substitute was needed, did it arrive more than 15 minutes after the request for a substitute?

    - Are diet cards, portion sizes, preferences, and condiment requests being honored?

4. Determine whether residents are being promptly assisted to eat or provided necessary assistance/cueing in a timely manner after their meal is served.

    - Note whether residents at the same table, or in resident room's, are being served and assisted concurrently.

5. Determine if the meals served were palatable, attractive, nutritious, and met the needs of the resident. Note the following:

    - Whether the resident voiced concerns regarding the taste, temperature, quality, quantity, and appearance of the meal served;
    - Whether mechanically altered diets, such as pureed, were prepared and served as separate entree items (except when combined food, e.g., stews, casseroles, etc.);
    - Whether attempts to determine the reason(s) for the refusal and a substitute of equal nutritive value was provided, if the resident refused/rejected food served; and
    - Whether food placement, colors, and textures were in keeping with the resident's needs or deficits, e.g., residents with vision or swallowing deficits.

Sample Tray Procedure

If residents complain about the palatability/temperature of food served, the survey team coordinator may request a test meal to obtain quantitative data to assess the complaints. Send the meal to the unit that is the greatest distance from the kitchen or to the affected unit or dining room. Check food temperature and palatability of the test meal at about the time the last resident on the unit is served and begins eating.

6. Observe for institutional medication pass practices that interfere with the quality of the residents' dining experience. This does not prohibit the administration of medications during meal service for medications that are necessary to be given at a meal, nor does this prohibit a medication to be given during a meal upon request of a resident who is accustomed to taking the medication with the meal, as long as it has been determined that this practice does not interfere with the effectiveness of the medication.

- Has the facility attempted to provide medications at times and in a manner to support the dining experience of the resident, such as:

  ✧ Pain medications being given prior to meals so that meals could be eaten in comfort;
  ✧ Foods served are not routinely or unnecessarily used as a vehicle to administer medications (mixing the medications with potatoes or other entrees).

7. Determine if the sampled resident consumed adequate amounts of food as planned.

- Determine if the facility is monitoring the foods/fluids consumed. Procedures used by the facility may be used to determine percentage of food consumed, if available; otherwise, determine the percentage of food consumed using the following point system:

  ✧ Each food item served except for water, coffee, tea, or condiments equals one point. Example: Breakfast: juice, cereal, milk, bread and butter, coffee (no points) equals four points. If the resident consumes all four items in the amount served, the resident consumes 100% of breakfast. If the resident consumes two of the four food items served, then 50% of the breakfast would have been consumed. If three-quarters of a food item is consumed, give one point; for one-half consumed, give .5 points; for one-fourth or less, give no points. Total the points consumed × 100 and divide by the number of points given for that meal to give the percentage of meal consumed. Use these measurements when determining the amount of liquids consumed: Liquid measurements: 8 oz. cup = 240 cc, 6 oz. cup = 180 cc, 4 oz. cup = 120 cc, 1 oz. cup = 30 cc.
  ✧ Compare these findings with the facility's documentation to determine if the facility has accurately recorded the intake. Ask the staff if these findings are consistent with the resident's usual intake; and
  ✧ Note whether plates are being returned to the kitchen with 75% or more of food not eaten.

8. If concerns are noted with meal service, preparation, quality of meals, etc., interview the person(s) responsible for dietary services to determine how the staff are assigned and monitored to assure meals are prepared according to the menu, that the meals are

delivered to residents in a timely fashion, and at proper temperature, both in the dining rooms/areas and in resident rooms.

NOTE: If concerns are identified in providing monitoring by supervisory staff during dining or concerns with assistance for residents to eat, evaluate nursing staffing in accord with 42 CFR 483.30(a), F353, and quality of care at 42 CFR 483.25(a)(2) and (3).

Task 6: Determination of Compliance:

- Compliance with 42 CFR 483.35(d)(1)(2), F364, Food

    ◇ The facility is compliant with this requirement when each resident receives food prepared by methods that conserve nutritive value and are palatable, attractive, and at the proper temperatures. If not, cite F364.

- Compliance with 42 CFR 483.35(b), F362, Dietary services, sufficient staff

    ◇ The facility is compliant with this requirement if they have sufficient staff to prepare and serve palatable and attractive, nutritionally adequate meals at proper temperatures. If not, cite F362.

NOTE: If serving food is a function of the nursing service rather than dietary, refer to 42 CFR 483.30(a), F353.

- Compliance with 42 CFR 483.15(h)(1), F252, Environment

    ◇ The facility is compliant with this requirement if they provide a homelike environment during the dining services that enhances the resident's quality of life. If not, cite F252.

- Compliance with 42 CFR 483.70(g)(1)(2)(3)(4), F464, Dining and Resident Activities

    ◇ The facility is compliant with this requirement if they provide adequate lighting, ventilation, furnishings, and space during the dining services. If not, cite F464.

Investigative Protocol

Nursing Services, Sufficient Staffing

Objectives:

- To determine if the facility has sufficient nursing staff available to meet the residents' needs.

- To determine if the facility has licensed registered nurses and licensed nursing staff available to provide and monitor the delivery of resident care.

Task 5C: Use:

NOTE: This protocol is not required during the standard survey, unless it is triggered in the event of care concerns/problems which may be associated with sufficiency of nursing staff. It is required to be completed for an extended survey.

This protocol is to be used when:

- Quality of care problems have been identified, e.g., residents not receiving the care and services to prevent pressure sore/ulcer(s), unintended weight loss and dehydration, and to prevent declines in their condition as described in their comprehensive plans of care, such as bathing, dressing, grooming, transferring, ambulation, toileting, and eating; and
- Complaints have been received from residents, families, or other resident representatives concerning services, e.g., care not being provided, call lights not being answered in a timely fashion, and residents not being assisted to eat.

Procedures:

- Determine if the registered/licensed nursing staff are available to:

  - ◇ Supervise and monitor the delivery of care by nursing assistants according to residents' care plans;
  - ◇ Assess resident condition changes;
  - ◇ Monitor dining activities to identify concerns or changes in residents' needs;
  - ◇ Respond to nursing assistants' requests for assistance;
  - ◇ Correct inappropriate or unsafe nursing assistants' techniques; and
  - ◇ Identify training needs for the nursing assistants.

- If problems were identified with care plans/services not provided as needed by the resident, focus the discussion with supervisory staff on the situations which led to using the protocol: how do they assure that there are adequate staff to meet the needs of the residents; how do they assure that staff are knowledgeable about the needs of the residents and are capable of delivering the care as planned; how do they assure that staff are appropriately deployed to meet the needs of the residents; how do they provide orientation for new or temporary staff regarding the resident needs and the interventions to meet those needs; and how do they assure that staff are advised of changes in the care plan?
- Determine if nursing assistants and other nursing staff are knowledgeable regarding the residents' care needs, e.g., the provision of fluids and foods for residents who are unable to provide these services for themselves; the provision of turning, positioning, and skin care for those residents identified at risk for pressure sore/ulcers; and the provision of incontinence care as needed;

- If necessary, review nursing assistant assignments in relation to the care and/or services the resident requires to meet his/her needs;
- In interviews with residents, families, and/or other resident representatives, inquire about the staff's response to requests for assistance, and the timeliness of call lights being answered; and
- Determine if the problems are facility-wide, cover all shifts or if they are limited to certain units or shifts, or days of the week. This can be based on information already gathered by the team with additional interviews of residents, families, and staff, as necessary.

Task 6: Determination of Compliance:

NOTE: Meeting the State-mandated staffing ratio, if any, does not preclude a deficiency of insufficient staff if the facility is not providing needed care and services to residents.

- Compliance with 42 CFR 483.30(a), F353, Sufficient Staff:

  ◇ The facility is compliant with this requirement if the facility has provided a sufficient number of licensed nurses and other nursing personnel to meet the needs of the residents on a 24-hour basis. If not, cite F353.

J. Closed Record Reviews

Closed records are included in the total resident sample. If possible, select closed records of residents who have been identified through the use of offsite information concerning a particular care issue. If there is a care area that is an identified concern, try to obtain the closed records of residents who had the same care needs before death, discharge, or transfer. Document information on the Form CMS-805, Sections C and D, as appropriate.

Look for information to determine compliance with quality of care and other requirements such as:

- Assessment and care of infections;
- Pressure sores;
- Significant weight loss;
- Restraints;
- Multiple falls or injuries;
- Discharge planning; and
- Transfer and discharge requirements.

Unless there is a reason to review the entire record, focus the review on the appropriateness of care and treatment surrounding the resident's discharge or transfer, and the events leading up to that discharge or transfer. For example, if the survey team has identified a concern with inadequate identification and care of residents with infections, and several residents have recently been hospitalized with serious infections, the review would be a focused review on the care and assessment these residents received before they were hospitalized. In addition:

- Look for documentation related to transfer, discharge, and bed-hold, including facility's discharge planning, notices, and reasons for facility-initiated moves, e.g., proper planning and transferring subsequent to a change in payor or care needs; and
- Determine if within 30 days of the death of a resident, the facility conveyed the deceased resident's personal funds and a final accounting to the individual or probate jurisdiction administering the individual's estate as provided by State law (see 42 CFR 483.10(c)(6), F160).

K. Review of a Resident Receiving Hospice Care

When a facility resident has also elected the Medicare hospice benefit, the hospice and the nursing home must communicate, establish, and agree upon a coordinated plan of care for both providers which reflects the hospice philosophy, and is based on an assessment of the individual's needs and unique living situation in the facility. The plan of care must include directives for managing pain and other uncomfortable symptoms and be revised and updated as necessary to reflect the individual's current status.

The hospice must designate a registered nurse from the hospice to coordinate the implementation of the plan of care.

This coordinated plan of care must identify the care and services which the SNF/NF and hospice will provide in order to be responsive to the unique needs of the patient/resident and his/her expressed desire for hospice care.

The SNF/NF and the hospice are responsible for performing each of their respective functions that have been agreed upon and included in the plan of care. The hospice retains overall professional management responsibility for directing the implementation of the plan of care related to the terminal illness.

For residents receiving Hospice benefit care, evaluate if:

- The plan of care reflects the participation of the hospice, the facility, and the patient to the extent possible;
- The plan of care includes directives for managing pain and other uncomfortable symptoms and is revised and updated as necessary to reflect the individual's current status;
- Drugs and medical supplies are provided as needed for the palliation and management of the terminal illness and related conditions;
- The hospice and the facility communicate with each other when any changes are indicated to the plan of care;
- The hospice and the facility are aware of the other's responsibilities in implementing the plan of care;
- The facility's services are consistent with the plan of care developed in coordination with the hospice (the hospice patient residing in a SNF/NF should not experience any lack of SNF/NF services or personal care because of his/her status as a hospice patient); and

- The SNF/NF offers the same services to its residents who have elected the hospice benefit as it furnishes to its residents who have not elected the hospice benefit. The patient/resident has the right to refuse any services.

NOTE: If there are concerns about the resident in relation to care provided by the hospice agency, refer the issue to the State Agency responsible for surveying hospices.

L. Review of a Resident Receiving Dialysis Services

When dialysis is provided in the facility by an outside entity, or the resident leaves the facility to obtain dialysis, the nursing home must have an agreement or arrangement with the entity in accordance with 42 CFR 483.75 (h). This agreement/arrangement should include all aspects of how the resident's care is to be managed, including:

- Medical and non-medical emergencies;
- Development and implementation of the resident's care plan;
- Interchange of information useful/necessary for the care of the resident; and
- Responsibility for waste handling, sterilization, and disinfection of equipment.

If there is a sampled resident who is receiving dialysis care, evaluate the following, in addition to the standard Resident Review protocol:

- Whether medication is given at times for maximum effect;
- Whether staff know how to manage emergencies and complications, including equipment failure and alarm systems (if any), bleeding/hemorrhaging, and infection/bacteremia/septic shock;
- Whether facility staff are aware of the care of shunts/fistulas, infection control, waste handling, nature and management of end stage renal disease (including nutritional needs, emotional and social well-being, and aspects to monitor); and
- Whether the treatment for this (these) resident(s), affects the quality of life, rights or quality of care for other residents, e.g., restricting access to their own space, risk of infections.

Sub-Task 5D – Quality of Life Assessment

A. Introduction

The assessment of the quality of life and rights of residents incorporates review of selected tags within the following requirements:

- 42 CFR 483.10, Resident Rights;
- 42 CFR 483.12, Admission, Transfer, and Discharge Rights;
- 42 CFR 483.13, Resident Behavior and Facility Practices;
- 42 CFR 483.15, Quality of Life; and
- 42 CFR 483.70, Physical Environment.

Since quality of life and quality of care are closely interrelated concepts, the survey process holistically integrates the quality of life assessment into the following tasks or sub-tasks:

- Task 5A, General Observations of the Facility (see Task 5A for further description);
- Task 5C, Resident Review, Sections A and B (see Task 5C for further description); and
- Task 5D, Quality of Life Assessment.

B. General Objectives

The general objectives of the quality of life assessment are:

- To determine if the facility protects and promotes the rights of residents;
- To assess the impact of the facility's environment, facility schedules and policies, and staff interactions with residents on the quality of residents' lives;
- To determine if the facility is assisting residents to achieve and maintain their highest practicable well-being; and
- To determine if the facility provides equal access to quality care for all residents, regardless of payment source.

C. Quality of Life Protocols

Task 5D includes the following sub-tasks: interviews of interviewable residents, a meeting with the resident group or council, family interviews of residents who are not interviewable, and observations of these same non-interviewable residents. These are each described below.

1. Resident Interview

These interviews are conducted with a subsample of interviewable residents from the resident sample. Refer to Table 1 in Task 4 to determine how many residents to interview. For example, in a facility with a census of 100, Table 1 directs the team to select 5 residents to interview.

It is helpful to divide the interview into two or more short segments. Seeing the resident more than once helps to establish rapport and also gives the resident a chance to think over the questions and provide more information later. Surveyors are encouraged to have several short conversations with interviewable residents during the course of the survey.

Locate a private place for the interview, and arrange interview times at the resident's convenience. Resident interviews should be conducted privately unless the resident expresses a preference to have a family member, staff member, or the ombudsman present.

Prior to the interview, complete Question 11 by writing any concerns that have been discovered about this resident or about the facility that you would like to discuss with the resident. Issues that are already covered in the other questions of the interview need not be listed.

For example, during Offsite Survey Preparation, the team has noted that the facility has had repeated deficiencies for pest control of roaches. On the Initial Tour, it may have been noticed the resident and her roommate were speaking angrily to each other. During the survey, the team has discovered disagreeable smells in this resident's unit, low levels of lighting in the dining room and some residents who go into others' rooms and rummage through drawers. Also add items discovered in the Resident Review about any of this resident's special needs and preferences that the facility should be taking into account. For example, a preference for a shower instead of a bath, or a need to have extra strong lighting because of a vision deficit. Add all these items to Question 11.

At the beginning of the first interview segment, use the probes on the first page of the interview to guide the explanation to the resident of the purpose of the interview. Discuss with the resident that some of his/her answers may be written down, and ask if that is all right. Then take a few minutes to establish rapport by letting the resident direct the conversation. For residents who are uncommunicative at first, use cues from their surroundings or from what is known about this resident to begin the conversation. Try to seek some commonality that will allow the resident to develop some ease in talking. For example, remark on family pictures and other personal items seen in the resident's room, or bring up a past occupation or hobby or a current activity preference of the resident that is of mutual interest. Share a little about yourself, as appropriate.

Use the resident interview protocol to guide the conversation with the resident, but bring up topics in an order that is sensible to the conversation. Probe for further information if the answer the resident is giving is incomplete or unclear. After the interview, follow-up on the concerns the resident has raised. Include in the documentation both the facility practice in question and its effect on the resident. Share these concerns with team members so that they can pursue them during the remainder of the survey. (See the tag numbers in parentheses after particular questions for interpretive guidance on following up on resident comments.)

NOTE: There are some problems that a resident will express that are not within the scope of the long-term care requirements. For example, a resident is complaining during an interview that he/she is displeased that he/she does not have a private room. This facility does not have private rooms, nor do the requirements mandate private rooms. If there is no issue related to one of the requirements, further investigation is not needed.

2. Group Interview

This interview is conducted with members of the resident council if one exists, or with an informal group of residents if there is no council. Staff members and residents' family members are not to be present at this interview unless the group specifically requests a certain person's presence. The group need not be restricted to officers of the resident council. The survey team members should feel free to invite other residents they encounter who are able to converse and provide information. The resident council should also be encouraged to invite other residents at their discretion. It is preferable to keep the group size manageable, e.g., usually no more than 12, to facilitate communication. Residents who are not able to participate should not be included in this interview.

Prior to the meeting, review council minutes if they were provided by the council. Determine if there are any particular concerns you would like to discuss. Write in Question 13 these concerns and any other special concerns the team has learned about this facility during Offsite Survey Preparation, the Initial Tour, or during other observations and interviews. Concerns that are already covered in other questions of the interview need not be written.

During the meeting, it may be helpful to have one surveyor conduct the interview while another takes notes. At the beginning of the meeting, use the probes on the first page of the protocol to guide introductions and describing the purpose of the interview. Spend a few minutes establishing rapport with the group by letting them direct the conversation. If residents have nothing to say at this time, use a general question such as, "Tell me what life is like in this facility," or "What makes a good day for you here?" Then continue with the protocol questions, probing for more information where necessary and presenting questions in an order that is sensible to the conversation. Get residents to talk in terms of actual situations or examples, using open-ended probes such as: "Can you tell me more about that? Can you give me an example?" or "How does that work here?"

After the meeting, follow-up on any concerns the residents have raised that are within the scope of the long-term care requirements. Share these concerns with the team to focus their investigations.

3. Interview with Family Member or Friend of Non-Interviewable Resident

The family interview is the first part of a two part protocol. The purpose of this interview is to obtain information about the prior and current preferences of a subsample of non-interviewable residents to help assess whether the facility is individualizing daily life activities, care, and services to the highest practicable level. The information gained through the interview will be used to complete Part D. below, the Observation of Non-Interviewable Resident. Follow-up on any concerns raised by the family member about the resident's treatment by the facility.

Use Table 1 in Task 4, to determine how many residents will receive the family interview and resident observation. For example, in a facility with a census of 100, 2 residents are selected.

Prior to the interview, review the relevant sections of the Minimum Data Set about past activities and preferences, and the resident's social history and activities assessment, if any. Begin completing this worksheet with information from the chart, and then use the interview to fill in missing information.

Information about a resident's past lifestyle and preferences may be more or less relevant, depending on the resident's condition and on the length of time spent in the nursing home. However, even after years of institutionalization, some features of a resident's prior life may still be relevant, even if the resident is now debilitated and uncommunicative. Collect information about how the resident's current cognitive status and physical condition have changed his/her past preferences.

Family members do not always know the prior history of a nursing home resident. Therefore, Question 1 of this interview serves to obtain information about the family member's knowledge of the resident. If the family member's answers to Question 1 show that he/she has little or no knowledge of the resident's past history, this interview may be discontinued. If discontinued, end the interview with a general question such as, "What would you like to tell me about this facility and how your relative is treated?" This resident can still remain as part of the survey sample. Select another non-interviewable resident from the sample for a family interview and observation of non-interviewable resident protocol.

If the family member has partial knowledge, the interview may be partially completed with whatever information is obtained in answer to the protocol questions.

Be aware that family members may have strong emotions about their relative's decline and institutionalization. Allow them to express their feelings, but gently direct them back to the questions of the protocol.

The interview may be conducted in person with a family member who was met on tour or by telephone, if necessary.

The second part of this protocol is the Observation of Non-Interviewable Resident. The purpose of this protocol is to obtain information through direct observation about the quality of life of the non-interviewable residents who have received family interviews.

Combine the information gained during the interview with what has been learned about the resident during the Resident Review to write any special items to observe in item 1. What special needs and preferences does this resident have that the nursing home should be taking into account? For example, a resident is ambulatory with Alzheimer's Disease. Her prior life included meeting the school bus at 3 p.m. every day to pick up her children. Now she attempts to leave the facility around that time. What is the facility doing to accommodate this agenda of the resident? Another resident enjoyed being outdoors, and the family member stated she believes this resident would still like the opportunity to go outdoors. Is the facility responding to this preference? Another resident preferred tea to coffee. Is this preference taken into account? A resident preferred to be addressed as Mrs. Hernandez. How do staff address this resident? A resident liked to ski, but can no longer do so due to her condition. However, she may like to see a movie on skiing, have a skiing picture in her room, or go outside in the snow. Has the facility noted this preference? A resident always watched a certain soap opera every day. The family member says that even though she is now confused, this show may still attract her interest. Is this show being made available to the resident?

Use this protocol to complete approximately 1 hour of observations per resident, divided into short segments in at least three settings, at different times of the day. This need not be dedicated time — surveyors can complete other tasks while conducting this observation. Part of the time should be spent in a location in which what is happening as staff interact with the resident in his/her room can be observed. The remainder of the time should be divided among other locations frequented by the resident, including the dining room, activities rooms, other common areas, and therapy rooms. Some observations of this resident may have already been completed prior to the interview, as part of the Resident Review. Continue making observations until all probes on the worksheet are covered, including the special items noted for observation. When making observations of the resident in particular settings, e.g., an activity or physical therapy, observations need not be for the entire duration of the activity or therapy session.

Use the probes in this protocol to guide observations. Note the areas of concern on the Resident Review Worksheet. For each concern, be specific in noting time, location, and exact observations. Record what is seen and heard, rather than a judgment of the situation. Instead of writing that the resident's dignity was violated by some interaction, simply record the interaction.

NOTE: During the individual, group and family interviews, ask questions regarding their awareness of to whom and how to report allegations, incidents and/or complaints. Share this information with the surveyor assigned to complete Task 5G.

Follow-up on areas of concern observed. For example, at lunch it was observed that the resident was given only one food item at a time. The resident was reaching out for other food and his/her drink. Determine through staff interview and chart review if this method of feeding this resident has a therapeutic purpose or if it is an unnecessary restriction on his/her freedom to select the food he/she wishes to eat.

Share observations with the team to assist them in their investigations of quality of life of other residents.

D. Follow-Up on Concerns Raised Through Interviews

Whenever information is obtained about areas of concern through resident interviews, attempt to investigate these areas through whatever means are appropriate. These might include interviews with other residents, staff, and families, and reviews of written facility information such as policies and procedures, and the admission rights information given to residents.

Sometimes these other sources will provide no other corroborating information. If that is the case, the team will determine during decision-making if the requirement is met or not met through the information obtained in resident interviews.

E. Confidentiality

If residents or family members have stated during interviews that they do not want certain information they have shared in confidence to be shared with the facility, respect their wishes. However, the issue can still be investigated. During the survey, discuss the issue with the team and make the topic the subject of other interviews and observations. For example, a resident has said that certain staff "make fun" of him/her, but he/she asks you to keep that in confidence. The resident's comment may not be referred to in the statement of deficiencies. However, discuss this with the team and decide how best to pursue the matter while respecting the resident's wishes. Team members may want to address this topic with other residents, family members, or the resident group. When aware of which staff are involved, attempt to observe these staff interacting with residents.

If other residents have complained about the same problem, their comments may be referred to generally as a group. For example, "Three out of five residents interviewed reported that . . . " Use judgment to determine if the statement would compromise the resident's confidentiality.

Sub-Task 5E – Medication Pass

A. General Objective

The general objective of the medication pass is to observe the actual preparation and administration of medications in order to assess compliance with 42 CFR 483.25(m).

B. General Procedures

Record observations on the Medication Pass Worksheet (Form CMS-677, Exhibit 88). The column marked "Record" is for the purpose of recording the physician's actual order. Do this only if the physician's order differs from the observation of the administration of the drug. When observing the medication pass, do the following:

- See Guidance to Surveyors for specific information on conducting the medication pass.
- Be as neutral and unobtrusive as possible during the medication pass observation.
- Initially observe a minimum of 20-25 opportunities for errors (opportunities are both the drugs being administered and the doses ordered but not administered). Strive to observe as many individuals administering medications as possible. This provides a better overall picture of the accuracy of the facility's entire drug distribution system. Ideally, the medication observation could include residents representative of the care needs in the sample, or the actual sampled residents. This would provide additional information on these residents, and provide a more complete picture of the care they actually receive. For example, if blood sugars are a problem, insulin administration may be observed. If eye infections are a problem, antibiotic eye drops may be observed, if residents are in pain, as needed pain medications may be observed, etc. Observe different routes of administration, i.e., eye drops, injections, NG administration, inhalation. If no errors are found after reconciliation of the pass with the medical records, this task is complete. If one or more errors are found, observe another 20–25 opportunities for errors.
- Calculate the facility's medication error rate. If it is determined that the facility's significant and non-significant error rate is 5 percent or more, or that one significant error has occurred, a medication error deficiency exists.

Sub-Task 5F – Quality Assessment and Assurance Review

A. General Objectives

The quality assessment and assurance review protocol is designed to determine if:

1. A Quality Assessment and Assurance Committee (QA) exists and meets in accordance with the regulatory requirements of 42 CFR 483.75(o); and

2. The committee has a method, on a routine basis, to identify, respond to, and evaluate its response to issues which require quality assessment and assurance activity.

Facility compliance with 42 CFR 483.75(o) is not dependent upon identification of quality deficiencies identified by the survey team, but rather by survey team identification of an effective QA committee that is constituted and meets according to the regulatory requirements, and identifies and resolves quality deficiencies pertinent to the quality of care and quality of life of facility residents.

B. General Procedures

1. The review of requirements at 42 CFR 483.75(o) will be conducted only after the Phase 2 sampling meeting.
2. The review is postponed until this time to ensure that facility quality deficiencies are not identified by the survey team through the use of records of the facility's quality assessment and assurance activities.
3. The protocol has 2 parts:
    a. Part 1 applies to all facilities; and
    b. Part 2 is initiated and builds upon Part 1, when the survey team has identified actual or probable quality deficiencies during the first phase of the survey.

C. Protocol

1. **Part 1 – All Facilities**

    Through interview with administrative staff and Quality Assessment and Assurance Committee members, determine if:

    - The facility has a Quality Assessment and Assurance Committee;
    - The committee consists of, at a minimum, the Director of Nursing, a physician designated by the facility, and 3 members of the facility staff;
    - The committee meets at least quarterly;
    - The committee has a formal method to identify issues in the facility which require quality assessment and assurance activities; and
    - The committee has a formal method to respond to identified quality deficiencies and evaluate the effectiveness of that response.

Part 1 should not include a review of committee minutes that address actual quality deficiencies. A written description of the Committee's process or protocol for identifying quality deficiencies, coupled with interviews indicating that this process is actually followed, is satisfactory documentation for Part 1.

2. **Part 2 – Facilities with Identified Actual or Probable Quality Deficiencies**

    The survey team conducts this investigation through interviews with Committee members and, as necessary, directs care staff to determine if the facility:

- Has identified quality deficiencies;
- Has developed and implemented a plan to address those quality deficiencies; and
- Has evaluated, or has a plan to evaluate, the effectiveness of the planned implementation.

The surveyors' goal in this part of the survey is to determine whether the facility has an effective method of identifying quality deficiencies and dealing with them.

This may be done by asking the facility to describe a sample of the quality deficiencies they have identified and dealt with. Surveyors should be guided by the following principles in this part of the survey:

- The surveyors' goal during this part of the survey is to ascertain whether the facility has a QA committee which addresses quality concerns and that staff know how to access that process;
- Surveyors may ask QA committee members and/or direct care staff how the QA committee functions, what the quality assurance and assessment process in the facility is, whether direct care staff know how to access the QA process and committee, and whether the QA committee is responsive to QA concerns submitted to it;
- Committee records and/or minutes, including those identifying details of the specific quality deficiencies which have been dealt with or are currently being dealt with should not be reviewed;
- Surveyors may also ask the facility, e.g., the QA committee, to describe a sample of the types of quality deficiencies the facility has identified and how it addressed them. These need not be practices that the survey team has identified as concerns. Such a sample should consist only of quality deficiencies which the facility believes it has resolved through its quality assurance process, i.e., past corrected problems;
- Determine compliance in this phase by interviewing direct care staff to determine if they are familiar with the specific plan(s) for care described by the QA committee and have implemented them. It is not necessary that direct care staff know that the care they are providing is the result of a quality assurance plan, however, they should be implementing the plan as developed as a routine part of their resident care. Also, if the plan described by the QA committee is not being followed, determine whether there is a justifiable reason, e.g., the facility replaced the process described by the QA committee with a different process based on updated protocols, medical knowledge, etc.;

  ✧ For guidance on citations of past noncompliance, see Chapter 7 of the State Operations Manual.

Sub-Task 5G – Abuse Prohibition Review

A. General Objective

To determine if the facility has developed and operationalized policies and procedures that prohibit abuse, neglect, involuntary seclusion, and misappropriation of property for all residents.

The review includes components of the facility's policies and procedures as contained in the Guidance to Surveyors at 42 CFR 483.13(c), F226. (See Guidance to Surveyors for further information.)

These include policies and procedures for the following:

- Screening of potential hirees;
- Training of employees (both for new employees, and ongoing training for all employees);
- Prevention policies and procedures;
- Identification of possible incidents or allegations which need investigation;
- Investigation of incidents and allegations;
- Protection of residents during investigations; and
- Reporting of incidents, investigations, and facility response to the results of their investigations.

B. General Procedures:

- Utilize the Abuse Prohibition Investigative Protocol to complete this task.

Investigative Protocol

Abuse Prohibition

Objective:

To determine if the facility has developed and operationalized policies and procedures that prohibit abuse, neglect, involuntary seclusion, and misappropriation of property for all residents.

Use:

Use this protocol on every standard survey.

Task 5G Procedures:

- Obtain and review the facility's abuse prohibition policies and procedures to determine that they include the key components, i.e. screening, training, prevention, identification, investigation, protection, and reporting/response. (See Guidance to Surveyors at F226.) It is not necessary for these items to be collected in one document or manual.
- Interview the individual(s) identified by the facility as responsible for coordinating the policies and procedures to evaluate how each component of the policies and procedures is operationalized, if not obvious from the policies. How do you monitor the staff providing and/or supervising the delivery of resident care and services to assure that care service is provided as needed to assure that neglect of care does not occur? How do you determine which injuries of unknown origin should be investigated as alleged occurrences of abuse?

How are you ensuring that residents, families, and staff feel free to communicate concerns without fear of reprisal?

- Request written evidence of how the facility has handled alleged violations. Select 2–3 alleged violations (if the facility has this many) since the previous standard survey or the previous time this review has been done by the State.

  ✧ Determine if the facility implemented adequate procedures:

  - For reporting and investigating;
  - For protection of the resident during the investigation;
  - For the provision of corrective action;

  NOTE: The reporting requirements at 483.13(c) specify both a report of the alleged violation and a report of the results of the investigation to the State survey agency.

  ✧ Determine if the facility reevaluated and revised applicable procedures as necessary.

- Interview several residents and families regarding their awareness of to whom and how to report allegations, incidents, and/or complaints. This information can be obtained through the resident, group, and family interviews at Task 5D.
- Interview at least five direct care staff, representing all three shifts, including activity staff and nursing assistants, to determine the following:

  ✧ If staff are trained in and are knowledgeable about how to appropriately intervene in situations involving residents who have aggressive or catastrophic reactions.

  NOTE: Catastrophic reactions are extraordinary reactions of residents to ordinary stimuli, such as the attempt to provide care. One definition in current literature is: " . . . catastrophic reactions [are] defined as reactions or mood changes of the resident in response to what may seem to be minimal stimuli (e.g., bathing, dressing, having to go to the bathroom, a question asked of the person) that can be characterized by weeping, blushing, anger, agitation, or stubbornness. "Catastrophic reactions and other behaviors of Alzheimer residents: Special unit compared to traditional units." Elizabeth A Swanson, Meridean L. Maas, and Cathleen Buckwalter. Archives of Psychiatric Nursing. Vol. VII No. 5 (October, 1993). Pp. 292-299.

  ✧ If staff are knowledgeable regarding what, when, and to whom to report according to the facility policies.

- Interview at least three front line supervisors of staff who interact with residents (Nursing, Dietary, Housekeeping, Activities, Social Services). Determine how they monitor the provision of care/services, the staff/resident interactions, deployment of staff to meet the residents' needs, and the potential for staff burnout which could lead to resident abuse.

- Obtain a list of all employees hired within the previous 4 months, and select five from this list. Ask the facility to provide written evidence that the facility conducted pre-screening based on the regulatory requirements at 42 CFR 483.13(c).

Task 6 Determination of Compliance:

Take account of all the information gained during this review as well as all other information gained during the survey. When a deficiency exists, determine if F225 or F226 provides the best regulatory support for the deficiency.

- 483.13(c), F226, Staff Treatment of Residents:

    ◇ The facility is compliant with this requirement if they have developed and implemented written policies and procedures that prohibit mistreatment, neglect, and abuse of residents and misappropriation of resident property. If not, cite at F226.

- 483.13(c)(1)(2)(3) and (4), F225, Staff Treatment of Residents:

    ◇ The facility is compliant with this requirement if they took appropriate actions in the areas of screening, reporting, protecting, investigating, and taking appropriate corrective actions. If not, cite at F225.

Task 6 – Information Analysis for Deficiency Determination

A. General Objectives

The objectives of information analysis for deficiency determination are:

- To review and analyze all information collected and to determine whether or not the facility has failed to meet one or more of the regulatory requirements; and
- To determine whether to conduct an extended survey.

B. Overview

The worksheets and procedures are designed to assist the surveyor in gathering, investigating, organizing, and analyzing information about the quality of services provided by the facility in order to determine whether the facility has failed to meet long term care requirements.

The information gathering portions of the survey have focused on the resident and the delivery of services by the facility using observation, interview, and record review as sources of information. The information analysis and decision-making portion of the survey focuses on making determinations about whether the facility meets requirements.

Information analysis and decision making builds on discussions of the daily team meetings, which should include discussions of observed problems, areas of concern, and possible failure to meet requirements.

Decisions about deficiencies are to be team decisions with each member of the team, including specialty surveyors (see Section I.C.), having input into the decisions. The team coordinator or designee should document the deficiency decisions and the substance of the evidence on the Form CMS-807.

For initial surveys, a determination must be made regarding whether the facility meets every long-term care requirement.

C. Decision-making Process

Each member of the team should review his/her worksheets to identify concerns and specific evidence relating to requirements that the facility has potentially failed to meet. In order to identify the facility's deficient practices and to enable collating and evaluating the evidence, worksheets should reflect the source of the evidence and should summarize the concerns on relevant data tags.

- Begin the decision-making task by taking into account the daily discussions, the findings documented on the worksheets, discussions with the facility, observations over the course of the survey, and the discussions regarding definitions of deficiencies in the following section. At a minimum, focus on the regulatory groupings 42 CFR 483.10, Resident Rights; 42 CFR 483.13, Resident Behavior and Facility Practices; 42 CFR 483.15, Quality of Life; 42 CFR 483.20, Resident Assessment; and 42 CFR 483.25, Quality of Care. Gather information from all worksheets pertinent to the particular requirements being reviewed (e.g., documentation from all worksheets concerning resident rights). In general, what is the facility's performance in meeting these requirements? Does the facility protect and promote resident rights? Discuss results of the information gathering phase in the context of facility conformance with these resident-centered requirements and the examples of resident-facility interactions that cause you to believe there may be deficiencies.
- Prioritize the review of worksheets so that the first information the team discusses relates to those requirements that the facility has potentially failed to meet. For example, what documentation on the Quality of Life Assessment worksheet supports the belief that the facility does not protect and promote resident rights? What information on other worksheets supports or does not support the team's assessment of Resident Rights? Evaluate the specifics of the regulatory language and the specific data collected (e.g., observation, resident, family, and staff interview information) with respect to the facility's performance in each requirement. Review the worksheets on an individual tag-by-tag basis. If data indicate that the facility has not met a specific requirement (see Task 6, Section D), document that deficiency.
- In order to ensure that no requirements are missed, proceed through the requirements sequentially as they appear in the interpretive guidelines, preferably section by section. Findings/evidence within each section should be shared by each team member during this discussion. Consider all aspects of the requirements within the tag/section being discussed and evaluate how the information gathered relates to the specifics of the regulatory language and to the facility's performance in each requirement. The team should come to consensus on each requirement for which problems have been raised by any member. If

no problems are identified for a particular tag number during the information gathering process, then no deficiency exists for that tag number.

- The team coordinator, or a designee, collates all information and records the substance of the decision-making discussion on the Form CMS-807. (See Exhibit 95.)
- Determine if there is substandard quality of care.
- If substandard quality of care exists, conduct an extended survey.

D. Deficiency Criteria

To determine if a deficiency exists, use the following definitions and guidance:

- A "deficiency" is defined as a facility's failure to meet a participation requirement specified in the Social Security Act or in Part 483, Subpart B (i.e., 42 CFR 483.5 – 42 CFR 483.75).
- To help determine if a deficiency exists, look at the language of the requirement. Some requirements need to be met for each resident. Any violation of these requirements, even for one resident, is a deficiency.
- Other requirements focus on facility systems.

For some requirements, especially those in the regulatory grouping of Quality of Life (42 CFR 483.15), the team will evaluate the sum of the staff actions and/or decisions for an individual resident to determine if the requirement is met for that individual. Quality of Life requirements are best evaluated comprehensively, rather than in terms of a single incident. However, a single incident which is considered severe enough may result in a deficiency.

Certain facility systems requirements must be met in an absolute sense, e.g., a facility must have a RN on duty 7 days a week unless it has received a waiver. Other facility system requirements are best evaluated comprehensively, rather than in terms of a single incident. In evaluating these requirements the team will examine both the individual parts of the system, e.g., the adequacy of the infection control protocol, the adequacy of facility policy on hand washing, as well as the actual implementation of that system.

E. Evidence Evaluation

The survey team must evaluate the evidence documented during the survey to determine if a deficiency exists due to a failure to meet a requirement and if there are any negative resident outcomes due to the failure. Failure to meet requirements related to quality of care, resident rights, and quality of life generally fall into two categories:

1. Potential or Actual Physical, Mental, or Psychosocial Injury or Deterioration to a Resident Including Violation of Residents' Rights

    Some situations which illustrate this level of harm could be:

    a. Development of, or worsening of, a pressure sore;

    b. Loss of dignity due to lying in a urine-saturated bed for a prolonged period; and

c. Social isolation caused by staff failure to assist the resident in participating in scheduled activities.

This category of negative outcome may be identified when an identified facility practice is so divergent from accepted principles of practice that harm has occurred or a future negative outcome or harm is probable. An example would be nurse aides in a facility who often fail to wash their hands between caring for residents. In this example, there is a strong potential for harm although there has been no evidence of a high facility infection rate, or of infections spreading from one resident to another. Should a resident contract an infection or become colonized with a highly contagious bacteria, there is a high potential for a major outbreak of nosocomial infection.

2. Lack of (or the Potential for Lack of) Reaching the Highest Practicable Level of Physical, Mental, or Psychosocial Well-Being

No deterioration occurred, but the facility failed to provide necessary care for resident improvement. For example:

a. The facility identified the resident's desire to reach a higher level of ability, e.g., improvement in ambulation, and care was planned accordingly. However, the facility failed to implement, or failed to consistently implement the plan of care, and the resident failed to improve, i.e., did not reach his/her highest practicable well-being;

b. The facility identified a need in the comprehensive assessment, e.g., the resident was withdrawn/depressed, but the facility did not develop a care plan or prioritize this need of the resident, planning to address it at a later time. The resident received no care or treatment to address the need and did not improve, i.e., remained withdrawn/depressed. Therefore, the resident was not given the opportunity to reach his/her highest practicable well-being;

c. The facility failed to identify the resident's need/problem/ability to improve, e.g., the ability to eat independently if given assistive devices, and, therefore, did not plan care appropriately. As a result, the resident failed to reach his/her highest practicable well-being, i.e., eat independently.

d. A facility's written procedures or oral explanations do not provide information about which residents are supposed to be fully informed, e.g., the resident is provided treatment which they may have wished to refuse.

If the resident is the primary source of information, the team should conduct further information-gathering and analysis. This may include additional interviews with family and staff or record reviews to supplement or corroborate the resident's report. If additional sources of information are not available, determine if the interviewees are reliable sources of information and if the information received is accurate. If so, citation of a deficiency may be based on resident information alone.

In cases where residents are unable to speak for themselves, the survey team should assess how most people would react to the situation in question. For example, a female resident who is unable to express herself is wheeled down the hall in a wheelchair on the way to her shower with only a towel partially covering her body. The team will decide if this incident is inappropriate because the resident is unable to express herself. Quality of Life and Residents' Rights requirements are most often evaluated using this type of analysis.

F. Determination of Substandard Quality of Care

The team must determine if substandard quality of care exists. Substandard quality of care is defined as one or more deficiencies related to participation requirements under 42 CFR 483.13, Resident Behavior and Facility Practices; 42 CFR 483.15, Quality of Life; or 42 CFR 483.25, Quality of Care which, constitute either immediate jeopardy to resident health or safety, pattern or widespread deficiencies at severity level 3, or widespread deficiencies at severity level 2. (See Section IV., Deficiency Categorization.)

G. Special Circumstances

Substandard quality of care and immediate jeopardy determinations trigger additional survey tasks and must be determined during the information gathering tasks of the survey and/or during information analysis and decision-making.

Immediate jeopardy is defined as a situation in which the facility's failure to meet one or more requirements of participation has caused, or is likely to cause, serious injury, harm, impairment, or death to a resident. At any time during the survey, if one or more team members identifies possible immediate jeopardy, the team should meet immediately to confer. The guiding principles to determine immediate jeopardy and serious threat make it clear that the threat can be related to mental, as well as physical well-being, and that the situation in question need not be a widespread problem. If the team concurs, the team coordinator must consult immediately with his/her supervisor. If the supervisor concurs that the situation constitutes immediate jeopardy, the team coordinator informs the facility Administrator or designee that the immediate jeopardy termination procedures are being invoked. The team coordinator should explain the nature of the immediate jeopardy to the Administrator or designee. The survey team should complete the entire survey. See Appendix Q for guidance regarding determination of immediate jeopardy, and §3010 for procedures to follow if the immediate jeopardy termination procedures are invoked.

When surveyors suspect substandard quality of care (SQC), they expand the standard (or abbreviated) survey sample as necessary to determine scope (Refer to Task 4, Supplementary Sample for further information). If there is no deficiency(ies) classified as substandard quality of care and there is a deficiency under the regulatory Groupings of 42 CFR 483.13, 42 CFR 483.15, and/or 42 CFR 483.25, that are classified as an isolated incident of severity level 3, or, as a pattern of severity level 2, then determine if there is sufficient evidence to make the decision that there is **not** substandard quality of care.

If the evidence is not adequate and the number of observations only allowed for isolated scope when there is a severity level 3, or pattern for scope when there is a severity level 2, then expand the sample to include additional reviews of that requirement. For example, if residents in the facility are receiving care for a colostomy, and for the one resident with a colostomy in the sample, it is determined that care provided caused actual harm to the resident, there would be a deficiency of isolated actual harm, but there would not be sufficient evidence to determine that there was substandard quality of care. Thus, the sample would need to be expanded before determining that substandard quality of care did or did not exist. On the other hand, if the number of individuals with a colostomy in the facility was the same (6), and 4 residents with colostomies were included in the sample and only one had deficient care, there would be no need to expand the sample. If the team verifies the existence of SQC, the Administrator should be informed that the facility is in SQC and an extended (or partial extended) survey will be conducted. If expanding the sample determines that SQC does not exist, no extended or partial extended survey will be conducted.

Task 7 – Exit Conference

A. General Objective

The general objective of the exit conference is to inform the facility of the survey team's observations and preliminary findings.

B. Conduct of Exit Conference

Conduct the exit conference with facility personnel. Invite the ombudsman and an officer of the organized residents group, if one exists, to the exit conference. Also, invite one or two residents to attend. The team may provide an abbreviated exit conference specifically for residents after completion of the normal facility exit conference. If two exit conferences are held, notify the ombudsman and invite the ombudsman to attend either or both conferences.

Do not discuss survey results in a manner that reveals the identity of an individual resident. Provide information in a manner that is understandable to those present, e.g., say the deficiency "relates to development of pressure sores," not "Tag F314."

Describe the team's preliminary deficiency findings to the facility and let them know they will receive a report of the survey which will contain any deficiencies that have been cited (Form CMS-2567). If requested, provide the facility with a list of residents included in the standard survey sample. Do not give the team's Roster/Sample Matrixes to the facility, because they contain confidential information.

If an extended survey is required and the survey team cannot complete all or part of the extended survey prior to the exit conference, inform the Administrator that the deficiencies, as discussed in the conference, may be amended upon completion of the extended survey. (See §2724 for additional information concerning exit conferences.)

During the exit conference, provide the facility with the opportunity to discuss and supply additional information that they believe is pertinent to the identified findings. Because of the ongoing dialogue between surveyors and facility staff during the survey, there should be few instances where the facility is not aware of surveyor concerns or has not had an opportunity to present additional information prior to the exit conference.

II.B – The Traditional Survey

I.B.2. – The Traditional Extended and/or Partial Extended Survey

Conduct an extended survey subsequent to a standard survey and conduct a partial extended survey subsequent to an abbreviated survey when you have determined that there is a substandard quality of care in:

- 42 CFR 483.13, Resident behavior and facility practices;
- 42 CFR 483.15, Quality of life; and/or
- 42 CFR 483.25, Quality of care.

When conducting the extended/partial extended survey, at a minimum, fully review and verify compliance with each tag number within 42 CFR 483.30, Nursing Services; 42 CFR 483.40, Physician Services; and 42 CFR 483.75, Administration. Focus on the facility's policies and procedures that may have produced the substandard quality of care. As appropriate, include a review of staffing, inservice training, and the infection control program. An extended/partial extended survey explores the extent to which structure and process factors such as written policies and procedures, staff qualifications and functional responsibilities, and specific agreements and contracts of the facility may have contributed to the outcomes. If the extended/partial extended survey was triggered by a deficiency in quality of care, conduct a detailed review of the accuracy of resident assessment. During the partial extended survey, consider expanding the scope of the review to include a more comprehensive evaluation of the requirements at 42 CFR 483.13, 42 CFR 483.15, and/or 42 CFR 483.25 in which substandard quality of care was found.

Document the observations from the extended or partial extended survey on the Form CMS-805, (see Exhibit 93) or the Form CMS-807 (see Exhibit 95).

Review of the Accuracy of Resident Assessments During an Extended/Partial Extended Survey

The objective of this review is to determine if resident assessments are accurate.

If an extended/partial extended survey is conducted based on substandard quality of care in Quality of Care (42 CFR 483.25), review the accuracy of resident assessments by:

- Reviewing a sample of comprehensive resident assessments completed no more than 30 days prior to conducting the survey;
- Comparing observations of the resident with the facility's assessment;

- Conducting the number of assessment reviews needed to make a decision concerning the accuracy of the facility's resident assessments; and
- Determining if observations of the resident, and interviews with resident/staff/family, "match" the facility's assessment (or specific portions of the assessment) of the resident. If observations and interviews do not "match," investigate further.

Record the indepth review of the accuracy of resident assessments on page 3 of the Form CMS-805. (See Exhibit 93.)

Timing for Conducting the Extended Survey and Partial Extended Survey

Conduct the extended or partial extended survey:

- Prior to the exit conference, in which case the facility will be provided with information from the standard, abbreviated standard, partial extended, or extended surveys; or,
- Not later than 2 weeks after the standard/abbreviated survey is completed, if the team is unable to conduct the extended survey or partial extended survey concurrent with the standard survey or the abbreviated survey. Advise the facility's Administrator that there will be an extended or partial extended survey conducted and that an exit conference will be held at the completion of the survey.

II.B. – The Traditional Survey

II.B.3 – The Traditional Post Survey Revisit (Follow-up)

In accordance with §7317, the State agency conducts a revisit, as applicable, to confirm that the facility is in compliance and has the ability to remain in compliance. The purpose of the post-survey revisit (follow-up) is to re-evaluate the specific care and services that were cited as noncompliant during the original standard, abbreviated standard, extended, or partial extended survey(s). Ascertain the status of corrective actions being taken on all requirements not in substantial compliance. Section 7304 contains the 5 elements a facility must address in developing an acceptable plan of correction. One of these elements is what continuous quality improvement system(s) a facility has in place to monitor its performance in identifying the deficient practice/care and assuring that it does not recur.

Because this survey process focuses on the care of the resident, revisits are generally necessary to ascertain whether the deficient practices have been corrected. The nature of the noncompliance dictates the scope of the revisit. For example, do not perform another drug pass if no drug distribution related deficiencies were cited on the initial survey. Do interviews and closed record reviews, as appropriate. Prior to the revisit, review appropriate documents, including the plan of correction, to focus the revisit review.

Conduct as many survey tasks as needed to determine compliance status. However, the team is not prohibited from gathering information related to any requirement during a post-survey revisit.

When selecting the resident sample for the revisit survey, determine the sample size using 60% of the sample size for a standard survey as described in Table 1, Resident Sample Selection. (Phase 1 sample size is 60%.) The follow-up survey does not require a 2 Phase sample selection.

Focus on selecting residents who are most likely to have those conditions/needs/problems cited in the original survey. If possible, include some residents identified as receiving substandard quality of care during the prior survey. If, after completing the revisit activities, you determine that the cited incidence(s) of noncompliance was not corrected, initiate enforcement action, as appropriate. (See §7400 for specific guidance concerning initiation of enforcement action.)

Use appropriate CMS forms during this survey. However, if the need for documentation is minimal, use the Surveyor Notes Worksheet (Form CMS-807). (See Exhibit 95 to record the results of the revisit.)

II.B. – The Traditional Survey

II.B.4 – The Traditional Abbreviated Standard Survey

A. Complaint Investigations

(See also Chapter 5)

B. Substantial Changes in a Facility's Organization and Management

If a facility notifies the survey agency of a change in organization or management, review the change to ensure compliance with the regulations. Request copies of the appropriate documents, e.g., written policies and procedures, personnel qualifications and agreements. If changes in a facility's organization and management are significant and raise questions of its continued compliance, determine, through a survey, whether certain changes have caused a decline in quality of care furnished by a SNF or NF.

III. Writing the Statement of Deficiencies

A. General Objective

The general objective of this section is to write the statement of deficiencies in terms specific enough to allow a reasonably knowledgeable person to understand the aspect(s) of the requirement(s) that is (are) not met. Indicate the data prefix tag and regulatory citation, followed by a summary of the evidence and supporting observations using resident identifiers. This documentation must be written in language specific enough to use to identify levels of severity and scope at the completion of the survey. If information was identified during confidential resident interviews, do not include a resident identifier when recording the source of the evidence. List the data tags in the order specified in the Code of Federal Regulations.

When a facility is in substantial compliance, but has deficiencies which are isolated with no actual harm and potential for only minimal harm, the deficiencies are recorded on the "Notice of Isolated Deficiencies" instead of on the Form CMS-2567. A plan of correction is not required but a facility is expected to correct all deficiencies.

The statement of deficiencies should:

- Specifically reflect the content of each requirement that is not met;
- Clearly identify the specific deficient entity practices and the objective evidence concerning these practices;
- Identify the extent of the deficient practice, including systemic practices, where appropriate; and
- Identify the source(s) of the evidence, e.g., interview, observation, or record review.

Following deficiency categorization (Section IV), enter on Form CMS-2567L the letter corresponding to the box of the scope and severity grid (Chapter 7, §7400.E.) for at least any deficiency which constitutes substandard quality of care and any deficiency which drives the choice of a required remedy category. Enter these letters in ID prefix tag column immediately below the tag number of the Form CMS-2567L.

IV. Deficiency Categorization

A. General Objective

After the survey team determines that a deficiency(ies) exists, assess the effect on resident outcome (severity level) and determine the number of residents potentially or actually affected (scope level). Use the results of this assessment to determine whether or not the facility is in substantial compliance or is noncompliant. When a facility is noncompliant, consider how the deficient practice is classified according to severity and scope levels in selecting an appropriate remedy. (See §7400 for discussion of remedies.)

Scope and severity determinations are also applicable to deficiencies at §483.70(a), Life Safety from Fire.

B. Guidance on Severity Levels

There are four severity levels. Level 1, no actual harm with potential for minimal harm; Level 2, no actual harm with potential for more than minimal harm that is not immediate jeopardy; Level 3, actual harm that is not immediate jeopardy; Level 4, immediate jeopardy to resident health or safety. These four levels are defined accordingly:

1. Level 1 is a deficiency that has the potential for causing no more than a minor negative impact on the resident(s).
2. Level 2 is noncompliance that results in no more than minimal physical, mental, and/or psychosocial discomfort to the resident and/or has the potential (not yet realized) to

compromise the resident's ability to maintain and/or reach his/her **highest** practicable physical, mental, and/or psychosocial well-being as defined by an accurate and comprehensive resident assessment, plan of care, and provision of services.

3. Level 3 is noncompliance that results in a negative outcome that has compromised the resident's ability to maintain and/or reach his/her highest practicable physical, mental, and psychosocial well-being as defined by an accurate and comprehensive resident assessment, plan of care, and provision of services. This does not include a deficient practice that only could or has caused limited consequence to the resident.

4. Level 4 is immediate jeopardy, a situation in which immediate corrective action is necessary because the facility's noncompliance with one or more requirements of participation has caused, or is likely to cause, serious injury, harm, impairment, or death to a resident receiving care in a facility. (See Appendix Q.)

C. Guidance on Scope Levels

Scope has three levels: isolated, pattern, and widespread. The scope levels are defined accordingly:

1. Scope is isolated when one or a very limited number of residents are affected and/or one or a very limited number of staff are involved, and/or the situation has occurred only occasionally or in a very limited number of locations.

2. Scope is a pattern when more than a very limited number of residents are affected, and/or more than a very limited number of staff are involved, and/or the situation has occurred in several locations, and/or the same resident(s) have been affected by repeated occurrences of the same deficient practice. The effect of the deficient practice is not found to be pervasive throughout the facility.

3. Scope is widespread when the problems causing the deficiencies are pervasive in the facility and/or represent systemic failure that affected or has the potential to affect a large portion or all of the facility's residents. Widespread scope refers to the entire facility population, not a subset of residents or one unit of a facility. In addition, widespread scope may be identified if a systemic failure in the facility (e.g., failure to maintain food at safe temperatures) would be likely to affect a large number of residents and is, therefore, pervasive in the facility.

D. General Procedures

After the team makes a decision to cite a deficiency(ies), evaluate the deficient practice's impact on the resident(s) and the prevalence of the deficient practice. Review deficiency statements, worksheets, and results of team discussions for evidence on which to base these determinations. The team may base evidence of the impact or prevalence for residents of the deficient practices on record reviews, interviews, and/or observations. Whatever the source, the evidence must be credible.

After determining the severity level of a deficient practice, determine scope. When determining scope, evaluate the cause of the deficiency. If the facility lacks a system/policy (or has an inadequate system) to meet the requirements and this failure has the potential to affect a large number of residents in the facility, then the deficient practice is likely to be widespread. If an adequate system/policy is in place but is being inadequately implemented in certain instances, or if there is an inadequate system with the potential to impact only a subset of the facility's population, then the deficient practice is likely to be pattern. If the deficiency affects or has the potential to affect one or a very limited number of residents, then the scope is isolated.

If the evidence gathered during the survey for a particular requirement includes examples of various severity or scope levels, surveyors should generally classify the deficiency at the highest level of severity, even if most of the evidence corresponds to a lower severity level. For example, if there is a deficiency in which one resident suffered a severity 3 while there were widespread findings of the same deficiency at severity 2, then the deficiency would be generally classified as severity 3, isolated.

V. Confidentiality and Respect for Resident Privacy

Conduct the survey in a manner that allows for the greatest degree of confidentiality for residents, particularly regarding the information gathered during the in-depth interviews. Use the resident identifier (e.g., a code number the survey team has assigned to each resident in the sample) on the Form CMS-2567 in place of the resident's name, which should never be used on the Form CMS-2567.

When communicating to the facility about substandard quality of care, fully identify the resident(s) by name if the situation was identified through observation or record review. Improperly applied restraints, medication error, cold food, gloves not worn for a sterile procedure, and diet inconsistent with order are examples of practices that can be identified to the facility by resident name. Information about injuries due to broken equipment, prolonged use of restraints, and opened mail is more likely to be obtained through resident and family interviews. Do not identify residents or family members providing this information without their permission.

Notes and worksheets contain pre-decisional information and are, therefore, not required to be disclosed to the facility at the time of the survey. However, once the Form CMS-2567 has been written, portions of the worksheets explaining the findings reported on the Form CMS-2567 may become subject to release under the Freedom of Information Act (FOIA). Information on the worksheets that was not subsequently used as a basis for writing a deficiency remains pre-decisional and is exempt from disclosure. That information would have to be deleted, according to FOIA guidelines, before the worksheets could be released.

The requirements of the FOIA apply only to those documents held by the Federal government. They do not apply to State or local governments. Therefore, surveyor worksheets held by the State are subject to State disclosure laws only.

VI. Information Transfer

In conjunction with conducting surveys, the State should provide information to the facility about care and regulatory topics that would be useful to the facility for understanding and applying best practices in the care and treatment of long-term care residents.

This information exchange is not a consultation with the facility, but is a means of disseminating information that may be of assistance to the facility in meeting long-term care requirements. States are not liable, nor are they to be held accountable if training which occurs during information transfer does not "correct" problems at the facility.

Performance of the function is at the discretion of the State and can be performed at various times, including during the standard survey, during follow-up or complaint surveys, during other conferences or workshops or at another time mutually agreeable to the survey agency and the facility. The time allotted for this information transfer should not usually exceed one hour. In no instance should the information transfer delay the survey process.

The Centers for Medicare & Medicaid Services, in cooperation with State survey agencies and consumer and provider groups, will develop and provide packages of training materials suitable for use in this activity.

VII. Additional Procedures for Medicare Participating Long-term Care Facilities

Medicare-participating long-term care facilities are obligated to inform Medicare beneficiaries about specific rights related to billing, and to submit bills to the Medicare intermediary when requested by the beneficiary. In a Medicare-participating long-term care facility, verify compliance with these requirements. Listed below are the requirements and the survey process to follow:

- If a Medicare SNF provider believes, on admission, or during a resident's stay, that Medicare will not pay for skilled nursing or specialized rehabilitative services, the facility must inform the resident or his/her legal representative in writing why these specific services may not be covered. The facility must use the mandatory denial notice found in §358 of the Skilled Nursing Facility Manual, and keep a copy of this uniform denial notice on file. Failure to give notice using the uniform facility denial notice or to submit the bill, if requested by a resident, may constitute a violation of the facility's provider agreement to submit information to the intermediary. (See 42 CFR 489.21(b).)
- The facility is also required to inform each Medicare resident of his/her right to request that the facility submit the bill to the Medicare payor (demand bill). If the resident requests that the bill be submitted to the intermediary or carrier for a Medicare decision, then evidence that the submission has occurred should also appear in the resident's record. The facility must not charge the resident while the demand bill is under review by the Medicare payor.
- During the entrance conference, obtain a list of Medicare residents who requested demand bills in the past 6 months. From this list, randomly select one resident's file to determine if the bill was properly submitted to the intermediary. In addition, draw a sample of all residents in the facility.

The number sampled for this procedure must be equal to the sample size selected for quality of life resident interviews. Use the sample selection table, Table 1, to obtain the correct sample size. Check to determine that the denial letters included appropriate notice information and that bills were submitted upon request. Review billing records for the last 6 months for each resident selected. During resident interviews use the following probes:

- [Individual] Do you know what things or services you pay for out of your own pocket? Who handles the payment for these items?
- [Individual] How do you find out how much these services or things cost?
- [Individual] Tell me how you find out what you have to pay for here?
- [Individual] When you receive a bill to pay for services out-of-pocket, does the facility explain why it believes Medicare will not pay for the services? Does the facility let you know that, if you disagree, you can have a bill submitted to Medicare?
- [Individual] Have you received a bill which you asked to have submitted to Medicare or your insurance company? How has the facility helped you or discouraged you from submitting the bill?
- [Group] Have there been any changes in the charges since you've been here? How do you find out about these changes?
- [Group] How does the facility give you information about your Medicare or Medicaid benefits?
- [Group] Did you or your family receive an explanation of any charges or monthly bills?

If residents are not clear about the scope of services they are entitled to, or the additional services provided by the facility and the cost of these services, or their right to have bills submitted to Medicare, and/or problems are identified during the review of resident records, either in the uniform notice or the bill submittal process, interview administrative staff to determine how the facility informs residents about their Medicare and Medicaid benefits, the non-covered services the facility provides, and the facility's charges for these services. Review additional resident records to assure the facility is using the uniform facility denial notice.

If the facility is in violation of the provider agreement with respect to resident billing requirements, cite tag F492, 42 CFR 483.75(b), Compliance with Federal, State and local laws and professional standards. If the facility is in violation of notice requirements, cite tag F156.

When reviewing facility plans of correction, if a deficiency is noted with respect to billing procedures, it may be appropriate to expect submission of past claims.

Background

1000 – Medicare and Medicaid – Background

(Rev. 1, 05-21-04)

The Social Security Act (the Act) mandates the establishment of minimum health and safety and Clinical Laboratory Improvement Amendments (CLIA) standards that must be met by providers and suppliers participating in the Medicare and Medicaid programs. The Secretary of the Department of Health and Human Services (DHHS) has designated CMS to administer the standards compliance aspects of these programs.

1000A – Medicare Provisions

(Rev. 1, 05-21-04)

Medicare is a Federal insurance program providing a wide range of benefits for specific periods of time through providers and suppliers participating in the program. Providers, in Medicare terminology, include patient care institutions such as hospitals, critical access hospitals (CAHs), hospices, nursing homes, and home health agencies (HHAs). Suppliers are agencies for diagnosis and therapy rather than sustained patient care, such as laboratories, clinics, and ambulatory surgery centers (ASCs). The Act designates those providers and suppliers that are subject to Federal health care quality standards. Benefits are payable for most people over age 65, Social Security beneficiaries under age 65 entitled to disability benefits, and individuals needing renal dialysis or renal transplantation. The Federal Government makes payment for services through designated fiscal intermediaries (FIs) and carriers to the providers and suppliers. Section 1802 of the Act provides that any individual entitled to Medicare may obtain health services from any institution, agency, or person qualified to participate in Medicare if that institution, agency, or person undertakes to provide that individual such services.

1000B – Medicaid Provisions

(Rev. 1, 05-21-04)

Medicaid is a State program that provides medical services to clients of the State public assistance program and, at the State's option, other needy individuals, as well as augments hospital and nursing facility (NF) services that are mandated under Medicaid. States may decide on the amount, duration, and scope of additional services, except that care in institutions primarily for the care and treatment of mental disease may not be included for persons over age 21 and under age 65. When services are furnished through institutions that must be certified for Medicare, the institutional standards must be met for Medicaid as well. In general, the only types of institutions participating solely in Medicaid are NFs, Psychiatric Residential Treatment Facilities (PRTF), and Intermediate Care Facilities for the Mentally Retarded (ICFs/MR). Medicaid requires NFs to meet virtually the same requirements that SNFs participating in Medicare must meet. ICFs/MR must comply with special Medicaid standards. Section 1902 (a)(23) of the Act provides Medicaid recipients a free choice of providers if the provider undertakes to provide the recipients with medical services. However, such freedom may be restricted under §1932(a) of the Act if the State determines that an individual must receive his or her medical assistance from a managed care organization.

1008C – Compliance with Title VI of the Civil Rights Act of 1964

(Rev. 1, 05-21-04)

Providers are direct recipients of Federal funds and are thus subject to title VI of the Civil Rights Act of 1964. The U.S. Office for Civil Rights (OCR) has the authority to determine whether Medicare providers comply with this non-discrimination statute, and the conditions of participation (CoPs) make OCR approval a requirement for Medicare approval by CMS. Before OCR will issue its approval, it also determines compliance with §504 of the Rehabilitation Act of 1973, as amended by the Rehabilitation Act Amendments of 1974, which includes a cross reference to the Uniformed Federal Accessibility Standards concerning architectural barriers to the handicapped. The OCR must also determine compliance with the Age Discrimination Act of 1975, and with title IX of the Education Amendments of 1972. See 45 CRF Part 84; see also Exhibit 2 of this manual.

Regarding Medicaid-only providers, the States themselves are considered the direct recipients of the Federal funds and may be considered to have a direct obligation to assure OCR of **their** compliance by assuring that funds go to providers who are in compliance. As with Medicare, determinations of civil rights compliance of providers are under the authority of OCR and are preconditions to approving the provider's participation in the Medicaid program.

Hospices

2080 – Hospice – Citations and Description

(Rev. 1, 05-21-04)

2080A – Citations

(Rev. 1, 05-21-04)

Section 1861(u) of the Act created hospices as a provider category. Section 1861(dd) of the Act defines hospice care and the hospice program. 42 CFR 418 sets forth the CoPs. 42 CFR Part 418.100 is an additional Condition applicable only to hospices that provide short-term inpatient care and respite care directly, rather than under arrangements with other participating providers. Section 1866(a)(1)(Q) of the Act requires hospices, among other providers, to file an agreement with the Secretary to comply with the requirements found in §1866 of the Act regarding advance directives.

The CMS has a Web site for hospice at http://www.cms.hhs.gov/providers/hospiceps. This site contains recent policy memos, hospice provisions enacted by the Balanced Budget Act (BBA) of 1997, State Operations Manual, §§2080-2087 and Appendix M, Hospice Survey Procedures and Interpretive Guidelines.

Definition

A hospice is a public agency or private organization or a subdivision of either that is primarily engaged in providing care to terminally ill individuals, meets the conditions of participation for hospices, and has a valid Medicare provider agreement. The law governing the provision of Medicare hospice services is found at §1861(dd) of the Act. The law further clarifies that "terminally ill individuals" are individuals having a "medical prognosis that their life expectancy is 6 months or less if the illness runs its normal course. Although the law does not explicitly define its expectations for "primarily engaged," CMS has interpreted it to mean exactly what it says, that a hospice provider must be primarily engaged in providing hospice care and services (§1861(dd)(2)(A)(i)). "Primarily" does not mean "exclusively." This requirement does not preclude provision of non-hospice services to terminally ill individuals who have not been accepted into the hospice program or services to individuals, who are not terminally ill, so long as the primary activity of the hospice is the provision of hospice services to terminally ill individuals and the hospice meets all requirements for participation in Medicare.

Hospice Benefit Periods

An individual may elect to receive Medicare coverage for an unlimited number of election periods of hospice care. The periods consist of two 90-day periods, and an unlimited number of 60-day periods.

Eligibility Requirements

In order to be eligible to elect hospice care under Medicare, an individual must be entitled to Part A of Medicare and be certified as being terminally ill. An individual is considered to be terminally ill if the individual has a medical prognosis that his or her life expectancy is 6 months or less if the illness runs its normal course.

The hospice must obtain the certification that an individual is terminally ill in accordance with the following procedures.

For the first 90 calendar-day period of hospice coverage, the hospice must obtain, no later than two calendar days after hospice care is initiated (that is, by the end of the third calendar day), certification of the terminal illness by the medical director of the hospice or the physician member of the hospice interdisciplinary group and the individual's attending physician (if the individual has an attending physician). If the written certification is not obtained within two calendar days following the initiation of hospice care, a verbal certification must be made within two calendar days following the initiation of hospice care, with a written certification obtained before billing for hospice care. If these requirements are not met, no payment is made for the days prior to the certification. Instead, payment begins with the day of certification, i.e., the date verbal certification is obtained. These certifications may be completed up to two weeks before hospice care is elected. The attending physician is a doctor of medicine or osteopathy and is identified by the individual, at the time he or she elects to receive hospice care, as having the most significant role in the determination and delivery of the individual's medical care.

For the subsequent periods, the hospice must obtain, no later than two calendar days after the first day of each period, a verbal certification statement from the medical director of the hospice or the physician member of the hospice's interdisciplinary group. A written certification from the medical director of the hospice or the physician member of the interdisciplinary group must be on file in the beneficiary's record prior to the submission of a claim to the intermediary. The certification must include: (1) the statement that the individual's medical prognosis is that his or her life expectancy is 6 months or less if the terminal illness runs its normal course and (2) the signature(s) of the physician(s). The provider must retain a copy of the certification statement in the patient's clinical record.

2080B – Description

(Rev. 1, 05-21-04)

Hospice care is an approach to caring for terminally ill individuals that stresses palliative care (relief of pain and uncomfortable symptoms), as opposed to curative care. In addition to meeting the patient's medical needs, hospice care addresses the physical, psychosocial, and spiritual needs of the patient, as well as the psychosocial needs of the patient's family/caregiver. The emphasis of the hospice program is on keeping the hospice patient at home with family and friends as long as possible.

Although some hospices are located as a part of a hospital, SNF, and HHA, hospices must meet specific CoPs and be separately certified and approved for Medicare participation. (See Exhibit 129 for "Hospice Survey and Deficiencies Report," Form CMS-643 and Exhibit 72 for "Hospice Request for Certification in the Medicare Program," Form CMS-417.)

Services and Items Provided

Substantially all core services must be provided directly by hospice employees on a routine basis. The following are hospice core services and must be provided directly by hospice employees:

- Nursing care (on a 24-hour basis) provided by or under the supervision of an RN functioning within a medically approved plan of care;
- Medical social services under the direction of a physician; and
- Counseling (including dietary and bereavement counseling) with respect to care of the terminally ill individual and adjustment to death.

A hospice may use contracted staff for core services only under extraordinary circumstances (i.e., to supplement hospice employees in order to meet patients' needs during periods of peak patient load). If contracting is used, the hospice must continue to maintain professional, financial, and administrative responsibility for the services in accordance with 42 CFR 418.56.

Substantially all hospice core services must be routinely provided directly by hospice employees and cannot be delegated or otherwise furnished under arrangement. For example, nursing services are core services and as such are subject to the core services requirements contained in 42 CFR 418.80. Just because a service is highly specialized, such as managing a peripherally inserted central catheter (PICC) line or other highly specialized nursing services, does not relieve the hospice of this requirement. It is expected that the hospice employ sufficient RNs who have the educational preparation and attainment of clinical competence to manage the ongoing needs of the hospice patients. For hospices that are unable to hire a sufficient number of nurses directly due to the nursing shortage, CMS has instituted a temporary measure.[1]

2082 – Election of Hospice Benefit by Resident of SNF, NF, ICF/MR, or Non-Certified Facility

(Rev. 1, 05-21-04)

There is no indication in the statute that the term "home" is to be limited for a Hospice patient. A patient's home is where he or she resides. A Hospice may furnish routine or continuous home care to a Medicare beneficiary who resides in a SNF, NF, ICF/MR, or any residence or facility not certified by Medicare or Medicaid. The facility is considered to be the beneficiary's place of residence (the same as a house or apartment), and the patient/resident may elect the Hospice benefit if he/she also meets the Hospice eligibility criteria. The hospice then assumes full responsibility for professional management of the individual's hospice care in accordance with the hospice CoPs and makes any arrangements necessary for inpatient care in a participating Medicare or Medicaid facility.

When a Nursing Facility Resident elects the Hospice Benefit, the Hospice and Nursing Facility should have a written agreement outlining key elements in the relationship before the hospice provides care (42 CFR 418.56). Issues in the agreement should include the following:

- Services to be provided by the Hospice;
- Services to be provided by the Facility;
- Manner and frequency in which the services are coordinated, supervised, documented, and evaluated;
- Identification of the role(s) of the Hospice and the Nursing Facility in the admission process, patient/family assessment, and interdisciplinary group care conferences;
- Qualifications of the personnel providing services;
- Orientation/ongoing education to Hospice staff by Nursing Facility;
- Orientation/ongoing education to Nursing Facility staff by Hospice;
- Applicable state/Federal health & safety regulations and standards of practice;
- Process by which the Hospice & Nursing Facility staff address service issues and complaints;

- Methods and frequency of communication between Hospice and Nursing Facility staff;
- Financing of medications, supplies, and durable medical equipment related to the terminal illness;
- Payment to the Nursing Facility for a Medicaid patient's "room & board" services;
- Resident eligibility, desire, and election of hospice;
- Resident rights and confidentiality;
- Professional management responsibility of the hospice; and
- Liability and insurance.

In entering into the relationship, each provider retains responsibility for the quality and appropriateness of the care it provides. Both providers must comply with applicable conditions/requirements for participation in Medicare/Medicaid.

In addition, the hospice and nursing facility negotiate an agreement on how they will coordinate their services. These issues include, but are not limited to, the following areas:

- Hospice staff access to and communication with nursing facility staff;
- Development of coordinated plan of care;
- Documentation in both respective entities' clinical records or other means to ensure continuity of communication and easy access to ongoing information;
- Role of any hospice vendor in delivering supplies or medications;
- Ordering, renewal, delivery, and administration of medications;
- Role of the attending physician and process for obtaining and implementing physician orders;
- Communicating resident change of condition; and
- Change in level of care and transfer from facility.

The hospice and nursing facility review this agreement as appropriate for needed changes and/ or improvement in the working relationship between the two entities and/or the care and services provided to residents electing the hospice benefit.

2082A – Compliance with SNF/NF Requirements

(Rev. 1, 05-21-04)

The SNF/NF Requirements are applicable to all of the residents in a SNF/NF facility. Neither the statute nor the regulations setting out SNF/NF requirements exempt hospice patients in a SNF/NF from those regulations. Sections 1819(c)(4) and 1919(c)(4) provide that a SNF or NF must "establish and maintain identical policies and practices" regarding transfer, discharge, and the provision of covered services under Medicare or Medicaid "for all individuals regardless of source of payment."

Sections 1819 and 1919 of the Act set forth requirements for SNFs and NFs to ensure that these facilities provide quality care and services to their residents. Even though the SNF/NF is the hospice patient's residence for purposes of the hospice benefit, the SNF/NF must still comply with all SNF/NF requirements for participation in Medicare or Medicaid.

Responsibility of the Facility

When a Hospice patient resides in a Nursing Facility, the facility staff is the patient/resident's primary caregiver. As the primary caregiver, facility staff provides services in a safe and comfortable environment to meet the needs of the patient/resident. SNF/NF services offered to a patient/resident should be the same whether or not he/she has elected hospice. The patient/ resident has the right to refuse any service.

It is the nursing facility's responsibility to assure that the care outlined in the care plan is performed by qualified staff and consistent with acceptable professional standards of practice. Those services include:

- Performing personal care services;
- Assisting with activities of daily living;
- Administering medication;
- Socializing activities;
- Maintaining the cleanliness of a patient's/resident's room; and
- Supervising and assisting in the use of durable medical equipment and prescribed therapies.

The responsibilities of the Nursing Facility also include:

- Notifying the hospice when the resident experiences a change in condition. The nursing facility must continue to meet the requirements for notifying the attending physician and family of significant change in condition. As part of a coordinated plan of care, procedures will be identified and addressed.
- Facilitating orientation of new staff by the hospice.
- Assessing the patient/resident according to the requirements for participation in Medicare/ Medicaid. In completing the assessment, the Nursing Facility may consult with the Hospice. The Medicare/Medicaid regulations for completion and submission of RAI/MDS data do not change when the patient/resident elects the Hospice Benefit.

Responsibility of the Hospice

The Hospice provides services in accordance with the Medicare Hospice Regulations (42 CFR 418) based upon the needs of the patient/resident. Services are provided at the same level as those provided a patient residing in his/her home. These include:

- Ongoing assessment, care planning, monitoring, coordination and provision of care by the Hospice IDG;
- Assessment, coordination, and provision of any needed General Inpatient or Continuous Care;
- Professional management of the patient's care with input from nursing facility staff;
- Coordination by the hospice RN of the implementation of the plan of care for resident;

- Provision, in a timely manner, of all supplies, medications, and durable medical equipment that are needed for the palliation and management of the terminal illness and related conditions;
- Financial responsibility for all medical supplies, appliances, medications and biologicals related to the terminal illness;
- Determining the appropriate level of care to be given to the patient/resident (routine homecare, inpatient, or continuous care) and making arrangements for any necessary transfers from the nursing facility in consultation with the nursing facility staff.

When the patient/resident elects the Medicare Hospice Benefit, hospice assumes responsibility for the professional management of the patient's/resident's care. Professional management involves the assessment, planning, monitoring, directing, and evaluation of the patient's/resident's care across all settings. All hospice services including nursing services, physician services, medical social services, and counseling must be routinely provided by the hospice and cannot be delegated to the facility unless circumstance requires nursing facility intervention to meet the immediate needs of the patient/resident. Nursing facility staff should notify the hospice of these unplanned interventions.

Coordinated Care Plan

The Facility/Hospice are jointly responsible for developing a coordinated plan of care based upon their assessments and needs of the patient/resident. Input from the patient/resident and their family/significant other is incorporated into the plan. The plan of care must be consistent with the hospice philosophy of care. This coordinated plan of care must identify the care and services, which the SNF/NF and hospice will provide in order to be responsive to the unique needs of the patient/resident and his/her expressed desire for hospice care. The plan of care must include directives for managing pain and other uncomfortable symptoms and be revised and updated as necessary to reflect the individual's current status. The plan of care must be written in accordance with 42 CFR Part 418.58 and include the individual's current medical, physical, psychosocial, family, and spiritual needs. The hospice must designate an RN from the hospice to coordinate the implementation of the plan of care. (See 42 CFR 418.68(d).) The coordinated plan of care identifies the discipline and provider to be held responsible/accountable for each intervention. For example, the hospice aide visits on Tuesday and Thursday to bathe the resident. The nursing facility aide bathes the resident on Monday, Wednesday, and Friday. If there is an unanticipated need to change the schedule, notification must be given to the other provider and resident to assure that the resident's needs continue to be met.

The hospice and the SNF/NF must communicate with each other when any changes are indicated to the plan of care, and each provider must be aware of the other's responsibilities in implementing the plan of care. The hospice must approve any changes to the plan of care proposed by the SNF/NF staff prior to implementation. Evidence of this coordinated plan of care must be present in the clinical records of both providers. All aspects of the plan of care should reflect the hospice philosophy.

The providers may develop one common care plan to be utilized by both providers, or two care plans following the documentation policies for each provider. The hospice and nursing facility may continue to utilize their individual processes/forms for care planning. Regardless of the number, when compared, care plans should reflect the identification of:

- A common problem list;
- Palliative interventions;
- Palliative outcomes;
- Responsible discipline; and
- Responsible provider.

The care plans are to be implemented, evaluated, and updated to meet the identified needs of the patient/resident as changes occur.

Procedures are in place to ensure that the patient receives timely medication and treatments for optimal palliation. The hospice provides education to the nursing facility on the hospice resident's pain management regime.

The hospice works with the nursing facility to monitor the effectiveness of treatments related to pain and symptom control. The hospice and nursing facility coordinate care to assure that the patient does not experience a delay in receiving needed drugs and treatment.

The hospice and nursing facility determine a process by which information from the hospice interdisciplinary team and the nursing facility team will be exchanged when developing and evaluating outcomes of care and updating the plan of care to assure that the resident receives the necessary care and services. The teams actively seek input from the resident/family on desired goals.

Documentation

Both respective provider's should agree on documentation issues to ensure continuity of communication and easy access to ongoing information. For example, the providers can agree that the nursing facility clinical record will contain a copy of the hospice election form, physician certification of terminal illness, assessments from core team members, current documentation of visits, and plan of care. In addition, the providers need to ensure that hospice documents are accessible to staff caring for the patient/resident. Both providers may document physician orders. Orders are to be signed in accordance with state regulations. Implementation of the plan of care changes resulting from physician orders received by the nursing facility must have **prior** hospice approval.

Provider Survey

If the surveyor of either provider identifies a potential compliance issue related to hospice patients, the respective surveying agency responsible for oversight of the other provider shall be notified.

2186 – Health Facility-Based HHAs

(Rev. 1, 05-21-04)

An HHA based to a hospital, SNF, hospice, or rehabilitation facility is expected to be an integral but subordinate part of the institution. Administrative and fiscal controls may be exercised over the HHA. However, the HHA's policies, personnel files, and clinical records must be separate and identifiable. Time records must be maintained for all personnel who provide home health services and must be identifiable as home health regardless of whether they are part-time or full-time. The HHA's concurrent use of personnel employed by a hospital, SNF, hospice, or rehabilitation facility is acceptable provided the HHA's operating hours are definite and not arbitrarily subject to the operation of the other institution, and provided the other institution's operation does not interfere with the HHA's maintaining compliance with the CoPs.

An HHA's services must be supervised by an employee of the HHA. If members of the institution's governing body serve the HHA as the group of professional personnel, minutes must reflect meetings of this group. Clinical records may be maintained in the record room or department. However, the clinical records must contain information pertinent only to the delivery of home health services, and should be readily available for either claims review or review by the SA.

In surveying the health facility-based HHA, the SA considers the institution's ability to share its administrative structure and personnel in fulfilling the needs and requirements of the HHA on a continuing basis. The CoPs for HHAs must be applied and met independently.

Life Safety Code (LSC)

2470 – LSC – Citations and Applicability

(Rev. 1, 05-21-04)

(Also see Chapter 7, §7410)

2470A – Background

(Rev. 1, 05-21-04)

The LSC is a set of fire protection requirements designed to provide a reasonable degree of safety from fire. It covers construction, protection, and operational features designed to provide safety from fire, smoke, and panic. The LSC, which is revised periodically, is a publication of National Fire Protection Association (NFPA), which was founded in 1896 to promote the science and improve the methods of fire protection.

The basic requirement for facilities participating in the Medicare and Medicaid programs is compliance with the 2000 edition of the LSC. Facilities with waivers of the health occupancy provisions of the LSC or with an acceptable PoC are considered "in compliance."

2480B – Meeting Intent of LSC

(Rev. 1, 05-21-04)

The requirements of the LSC are directed to a series of factors or areas. These may be classified as follows:

1. **Fire Load** – All materials which might contribute to the fuel aspect of a fire within the building and requirements pertaining to construction, interior finish, draperies, furnishings, and building service equipment;

2. **Fire Containment** – Those elements which tend to restrict the spread of flame, smoke, or fire gases throughout the building, such as corridor wall construction, subdivision of floor areas, and protection for vertical openings;

3. **Fire Extinguishment** – Elements which help to put out the fire as quickly as possible. They include alarm systems, portable extinguishers, sprinkler systems, and special requirements for protection of hazardous areas;

4. **Evacuation** – Those elements which facilitate the removal of occupants from the scene of the fire. They include details of the emergency plan and exiting capability from the building;

5. **Operating Features** – The administrative and operational features such as housekeeping techniques, smoking regulations, and the fire emergency plan which, if not properly implemented, could result in hazardous fire situations;

The following additional considerations should also be evaluated by the fire authority since they may have an important bearing on the safety of patients in facilities which request a waiver:

1. Staffing considerations such as staff-patient ratios, staffing patterns, and scope of staff training to handle fire emergencies;

2. Availability and adequacy of compartment and horizontal exits, such as areas to hold patients during a fire emergency;

3. Location and number of ambulatory and nonambulatory patients;

4. Availability, extent, and type of automatic fire detection and fire extinguishment systems provided in the facility;

5. Means for notifying the fire department in case of fire; and

6. Effectiveness of fire department (e.g. types of equipment available, number of personnel normally responding to a fire call, distance to the nearest fire station, and normal response time of the fire department).

The total fire safety of a building is dependent upon the combined effect of the factors mentioned above. Each building is a unique problem from a fire safety point of view and should be evaluated by the fire authority on its own merits. Not all requirements are of equal importance in all situations.

If it can be established that a particular deficiency does not materially affect the overall level of safety, it is reasonable to hold that the fire safety characteristics of the facility have not been compromised and that the intent of the LSC has been met.

2762B – Definitions of Terms Used on Form CMS-1539

(Rev. 1, 05-21-04)

1 – Facility

For Form CMS-1539 purposes, facility means the provider entity or the business establishment of a provider or supplier that is subject to certification and approval in order for the provider or supplier's services to be approved for payment. If a provider operates separate provider institutions or a supplier operates separate businesses, they are regarded as separate facilities for Form CMS-1539 purposes. A LTC facility with a SNF and a NF distinct part is one facility, even though the distinct parts are separately certified for Medicare and Medicaid. Although an agency, such as an HHA with subunits, is one facility, the subunits must be separately certified. "One enterprise; one facility; one certification" is NOT always the rule. Rather, the way CMS assigns provider identification numbers determines how many certifications the SA prepares for any given institution. (See §2764.)

2 – Certified Beds

The Medicare/Medicaid program does not actually "certify" beds. This term means counted beds in the certified provider or supplier facility or in the certified component. A count of facility beds may differ depending on whether the count is used for licensure, eligibility for Medicare payment formulas, eligibility for waivers, or other purposes. For Form CMS-1539, all the following are **excluded** from "certified beds": pediatric visitors, newborn nursery cribs, maternity labor and delivery beds, intensive therapy beds which a patient occupies for only a short time (such as in radiation therapy units), and temporary extra beds. The following are **included**: designated bed locations (even though an actual bed is not in evidence) and beds which a patient occupies for an extensive period of time in special care units such as cancer treatment units as well as all routine inpatient beds.

3 – Dually-Participating

Simultaneous participation of an institution, in the Medicare and Medicaid programs.

4 – Distinct Part

The term "distinct part" refers to a portion of an institution or institutional complex (e.g., a nursing home or a hospital) that is certified to provide SNF and/or NF services. A distinct part must be physically distinguishable from the larger institution and fiscally separate for cost reporting purposes. An institution or institutional complex can only be certified with one distinct part SNF and/or one distinct part NF. Multiple certifications within the same institution or institutional complex are strictly prohibited. The distinct part must consist of all beds within the designated area. The distinct part can be a wing, separate building, a floor, a hallway, or one side of a corridor. The beds in the certified distinct part area must be physically separate from (that is, not commingled with) the beds of the institution or institutional complex in which it is located. However, the distinct part need not be confined to a single location within the institution or institutional complex's physical plant. It may, for example, consist of several floors or wards in a single building or floors or wards that are located throughout several different buildings within the institutional complex. In each case, however, all residents of the distinct part would have to be located in units that are physically separate from those units housing other patients of the institution or institutional complex. Where an institution or institutional complex owns and operates a distinct part SNF and/or NF, that distinct part SNF and/or NF is a single distinct part even if it is operated at various locations throughout the institution or institutional complex. The aggregate of the SNF and/or NF locations represents a single distinct part subprovider, not multiple subproviders, and must be assigned a single provider number.

5 – Fully Participating

Participation of an institution in its entirety either in the Medicare or Medicaid program, or both.

Changes in Provider Status or Services

3200 – Action Based on Changes in Provider Organization, Services, or Action of Other Approving Agencies

(Rev. 1, 05-21-04)

Notification that an entity has undergone organizational changes, added or relocated units, or received an accreditation may require a change in SA scheduling.

3202 – Change in Size or Location of Participating SNF and/or NF

(Rev. 1, 05-21-04)

Under §1866 of the Social Security Act (the Act), the Secretary has the authority to enter into an agreement with an institution or an institutional complex to provide covered services to our beneficiaries. The provider agreement requires compliance with the requirements the Secretary deems necessary for participation in the Medicare or Medicaid program. See §1866(b)(2) and §1902(a)(27) of the Act. On the effective date of the provider agreement, the institution or institutional complex is deemed to have met the requirements for participation based upon a survey of the institution or institutional complex as it was configured (i.e., bed size/bed location configuration) on the date(s) of the survey. The CMS' authority to regulate bed size changes in a SNF or a NF is based on the authority to ensure compliance with the provider agreement under §1866 of the Act and to further ensure that the configuration that has been approved for the institution or institutional complex does not so drastically change from that of the original certified configuration so as to endanger resident health and safety or otherwise change in a material fashion the identity of the entity that CMS originally certified for program participation.

An institution or institutional complex may choose to participate in the Medicare and/or Medicaid programs either in its entirety (i.e., fully participating), or a portion thereof (i.e., a distinct part), **but not both.** If only a portion of an institution or institutional complex actually participates in either program it is classified as a distinct part and must meet the criteria found in §2762. For example, an institution has 4 wings that consist of 25 beds each. Three contiguous wings that contain 75 beds are dually participating (i.e., participating in Medicare and Medicaid). The fourth wing is only certified to participate in Medicare. It consists of 25 beds. Therefore, in this instance the institution is fully participating for purposes of Medicare (i.e., 100 beds) and a distinct part for purposes of Medicaid (i.e., 75 beds). The policies on bed size changes and changes in designated bed locations that are included in this section apply, regardless of whether an institution is fully participating (i.e., all beds within the institution or institutional complex are certified to participate in the Medicare and/or Medicaid program) or participating as or with a distinct part.

A SNF or NF may be:

- An entire institution for skilled nursing or rehabilitative care, such as a nursing home; or
- A distinct part of an institution such as, a hospital, personal care home, assisted living facility, board and care home, domiciliary care facility, rest home, continuing care retirement community, or nursing home.

An institution that is primarily for the care and treatment of mental diseases cannot be a SNF or NF.

3202A – Requirements for Distinct Part Certification

(Rev. 1, 05-21-04)

If the institution or institutional complex is participating as a distinct part SNF and/or NF, for a change to be approved, the requested change in bed size must conform to the requirements to be classified as a distinct part. The term "distinct part" refers to a portion of an institution or institutional complex (e.g., a nursing home or a hospital) that is certified to provide SNF and/or NF services. A distinct part must be physically distinguishable from the larger institution and fiscally separate for cost reporting purposes.

An institution or institutional complex can only be certified with one distinct part SNF and/or one distinct part NF. A hospital-based SNF is by definition a distinct part. Multiple certifications within the same institution or institutional complex are strictly prohibited.

The distinct part must consist of all beds within the designated area. The distinct part can be a wing, separate building, a floor, a hallway, or one side of a corridor. The beds in the certified distinct part area must be physically separate from (that is, not commingled with) the beds of the institution or institutional complex in which it is located. However, the distinct part need not be confined to a single location within the institution or institutional complex's physical plant. It may, for example, consist of several floors or wards in a single building or floors or wards that are located throughout several different buildings within the institutional complex. In each case, however, all residents of the distinct part would have to be located in units that are physically separate from those units housing other patients of the institution or institutional complex.

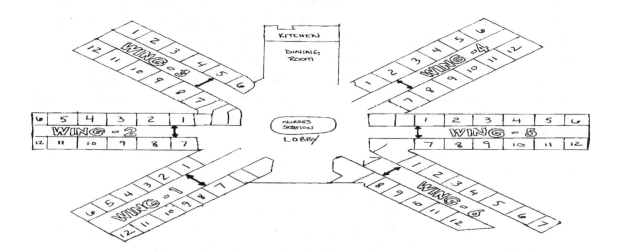

Illustration I – Floor Plan of Nursing Facility

Where an institution or institutional complex owns and operates a distinct part SNF and/or NF, that distinct part SNF and/or NF is a single distinct part even if it is operated at various locations throughout the institution or institutional complex. The aggregate of the SNF and/or NF locations represents a single distinct part subprovider, not multiple subproviders, and must be assigned a single provider number.

Illustration I, above, is an illustration of a floor plan of a nursing facility followed below by examples that meet the requirements for a distinct part, as well as examples that do not meet the requirements for a distinct part. The purpose of the Illustration is to assist the State and the RO in ensuring proper distinct part certification.

3202A1 – Meet Distinct Part Certification

(Rev. 1, 05-21-04)

An institution or institutional complex can select any **one** of the following examples discussed in the context of Illustration I above that meets the requirements for distinct part certification.

- All rooms numbered 1 through 12 in wing 1 and all rooms numbered 1 through 12 in wing 2 constitute a distinct part. This option is approvable because it constitutes all beds in each wing.
- All rooms numbered 1 through 12 in wing 5. This option is approvable because it includes all beds in the wing.
- Room numbers 1 through 6 in wing 4 constitute a distinct part. This option is approvable because it includes all beds that constitute a single side of the corridor.
- Room numbers 7 through 12 in wing 2 and all rooms 1 through 12 in wing 1 constitute a distinct part. This option is approvable because it includes all beds in wing 1 and all beds that constitute a single side of the corridor in wing 2.

4009 – Federal Surveyor Qualifications Standards

(Rev. 1, 05-21-04)

(Also see §7201)

In accordance with the "Personnel" clause of the State agreement, SA personnel must be under a merit system that meets Federal standards. Minimum standards specifically applicable to surveyors for Medicare and Medicaid Programs are as follows:

4009A – Persons Covered

(Rev. 1, 05-21-04)

The term "surveyor" means a person who investigates, evaluates, and/or makes official reports of situations and conditions in a health facility, and who determines the degree to which the facility meets specific criteria contained in regulations issued pursuant to titles XVIII and XIX of the Act.

4009B – Health Professional Qualifications

(Rev. 1, 05-21-04)

To perform the surveyor functions requires an appropriate background in the health professions or health administration, in addition to basic investigative skills. Therefore, one element in the standard is that the surveyor be qualified in one of the following professions:

- Hospital administrator;
- Industrial hygienist;
- Laboratory or medical technologist, bacteriologist, microbiologist, or chemist;
- Medical record librarian;
- Nurse;
- Nursing home administrator;
- Nutritionist;
- Pharmacist;
- Physical therapist;
- Physician;
- Qualified Mental Retardation Professional;
- Sanitarian;
- Social worker; or
- Any other professional category used within State merit systems for health professional positions, provided the State has determined the position classification skill level to be commensurate with any of the above professions.

This does not mean that the surveyor must belong to a professional organization or have prior work experience in the profession. It means that he/she must satisfy necessary requirements to be employed in one of these specialties by the State.

4009C – Education, Training, and Experience

(Rev. 1, 05-21-04)

To assure that individuals have the necessary knowledge, skills, and abilities to carry out survey functions, the following prerequisites apply:

- The amount of academic education required is that which is necessary to qualify in a profession listed in §4009B;
- Newly hired surveyors must successfully complete an orientation program approved by CMS that includes the core elements of the CMS-developed orientation program. (See Exhibit 42.) The CMS provides this program for Federal surveyors and the States provide it for theirs;
- The CMS and States assure that the health facility surveyors, laboratory surveyors, and Life Safety Code (LSC) surveyors have successfully completed, within the first 12 months of employment, the basic surveyor training course developed under CMS auspices, including all course prerequisites. LSC surveyors are required to complete a LSC basic course (there is self-paced training on a CD-ROM) as a prerequisite. No individual may serve on a survey team until he or she fulfills this requirement, except as a trainee who is accompanied onsite by a surveyor, who has successfully completed the required training and testing program;
- Before any State or Federal surveyor may serve on a survey team (except as a trainee) for an ICF/MR, End-Stage Renal Disease (ESRD) facility, HHA, or Hospice survey, he/she must have successfully completed the relevant provider-specific Basic course and any course prerequisites;
- Some State position classifications may require additional education, training, and experience as State minimums, as requirements for promotion, or entry at a higher scale of position classification; and
- SAs must have a mechanism to identify and respond to the in-service training needs of the surveyors.

5000 – Management of Complaints and Incidents

(Rev. 1, 05-21-04)

The following procedures provide direction and guidance in the management of complaints and reported incidents for nursing homes, home health agencies, end-stage renal disease facilities, hospitals, suppliers of portable x-ray services, providers of outpatient physical therapy or speech pathology services, rural health clinics, and comprehensive outpatient rehabilitation facilities.

For these providers, the management of complaints and reported incidents is supported by the national implementation of the ASPEN Complaints/Incidents Tracking System (ACTS).

Sections 5000 to 5060 supercede §§5100 to 5590, where inconsistencies may exist.

5010 – Intake Process

(Rev. 1, 05-21-04)

An allegation is an assertion of improper care or treatment against a Medicare, Medicaid, or CLIA participating program that could result in the citation of a Federal deficiency. The point of receipt of the allegation is a critical fact-finding and decision-making point. Information regarding the care, treatment, and services provided to beneficiaries can come from a variety of sources and in a number of formats. Allegations may come directly from beneficiaries themselves, beneficiaries' family members, health care providers, concerned citizens, public agencies, or in published or broadcast media reports. Report sources may be verbal or written. In some instances, the complainant may request anonymity.

The SA and RO ensure the privacy and anonymity of every complainant. Generally, the SA follows the disclosure procedures under §3308. The SA discloses the complainant's identity only to those individuals with a need to know who are acting in an official capacity to investigate the complaint.

In addition to these Federal requirements, the SA abides by any State procedures not in direct conflict with CMS instructions. The SA notifies the RO if State regulations conflict directly with any part of these complaint procedures.

5400 – Additional Provisions for the Investigation of Complaints in Nursing Homes

(Rev. 1, 05-21-04)

SOM 7700

NOTE: Sections 5000 to 5040 supersede §§5400 through 5460, where inconsistencies may exist.

The survey agency must review all complaint allegations and conduct a standard or an abbreviated standard survey to investigate complaints of violations of requirements if its review of the allegation concludes that:

- A deficiency in one or more of the requirements may have occurred;
- Only a survey can determine whether a deficiency or deficiencies exist; and
- The complaint is general or specific and may involve staff, residents, volunteers, the physical environment, or administration.

Complaint investigations follow, as appropriate, the pertinent survey tasks, and information gathered is recorded on the appropriate survey worksheets. However, if the documentation required is minimal, use the Form CMS-807 to record information during the complaint investigation. Record deficiencies on the Form CMS-2567, the "Notice of Isolated Deficiencies," or both as applicable.

The survey agency does not conduct a survey if the complaint raises issues that are outside the purview of Federal participation requirements.

The timing, scope, duration and conduct of a complaint investigation are at the discretion of the State survey agency, except when the complaint involves an allegation of immediate jeopardy to resident health and safety, which must be investigated within 2 working days of receipt. In cases where the SA makes the determination that a higher level of harm is present, the investigation is to be initiated within 10 days of its receipt. The team should conduct the necessary investigation to resolve the complaint. If the complaint concerns conditions on a certain day (e.g., on weekends), or on a certain shift (e.g., 11 p.m. – 7 a.m.), the survey agency should make an attempt to investigate it at the time relevant to the complaint. In most cases, the following tasks, or portion of tasks, should be performed in a complaint investigation:

If necessary, a specialized team may be used to investigate complaints. Team members may include, but are not limited to, an attorney, auditor, and appropriate health professionals. The specialized team is not necessarily composed of qualified surveyors. However, specialized team members provide unique talents and expertise that assist at least one qualified surveyor in identifying, gathering, and preserving documented evidence. Further information regarding the composition of the survey team is provided in Chapter 7.

5410 – Task 1: Offsite Survey Preparation

(Rev. 1, 05-21-04)

Obtain as much information as possible about the complaint before beginning to plan the investigation, including:

a. Name of complainant;
b. Nature of the complaint – describe exactly the facts of the complaint situation;
c. Information about when the complaint situation occurred, whether it was an isolated event or an ongoing situation – date, time, time between different events;
d. Place where the incident happened – care unit, resident room;
e. How it happened – sequence of events;
f. Whether a resident or a family member of a resident was involved;
g. Witnesses to complaint situation – anyone who saw incident happen;
h. Staff or other residents involved; and
i. Other persons involved – volunteers or visitors.

Review any information about the facility that would be helpful to know in planning the investigation. Contact the ombudsman to discuss the nature of the complaint and whether there have been any similar complaints reported to and substantiated by the ombudsman.

Review the related regulatory requirements or standards that pertain to the complaint. For example, if it is a complaint about abuse, review the requirements at 42 CFR 483.13.

Plan the investigation. Before going to the facility, plan what information is needed to obtain during the complaint investigation based on the information already acquired. Consider practical methods to obtain that information.

5420 – Task 2: Entrance Conference/Onsite Preparatory Activities

(Rev. 1, 05-21-04)

Onsite complaint investigations should always be unannounced. Upon entrance, advise the facility's Administrator of the general purpose of the visit. It is important to let the facility know why you are there, but protect the confidentiality of those involved in the complaint. Do not release information that will cause opportunities to be lost for pertinent observations, interviews, and record reviews required for a thorough investigation. For example, if the complaint is that food that is intended to be served hot is always served cold, do not tell the facility the exact complaint. Rather, tell them it is a situation related to dietary requirements.

5430 – Task 5: Information Gathering

(Rev. 1, 05-21-04)

The order and manner in which information is gathered will depend on the type of complaint that is being investigated. Conduct comprehensive, focused, and/or closed record reviews as appropriate for the type of complaint. It is very important to remember that the determination of whether the complaint happened is not enough. The surveyor needs to determine noncompliant facility practices related to the complaint situation and which, if any, requirements are not met by the facility.

Perform information gathering in order of priorities, i.e., obtain the most critical information first. Based on this critical information about the incident, determine what other information to obtain in the investigation.

Observations, record review, and interviews can be done in any order necessary. As information is obtained, use what has been learned to determine what needs to be clarified or verified as the investigation continues.

Observe the physical environment, situations, procedures, patterns of care, delivery of services to residents, and interactions related to the complaint. Also, if necessary, observe other residents with the same care need. After determining what occurred, i.e., what happened to the resident and the outcome, investigate what facility practice(s) or procedures affected the occurrence of the incident.

EXAMPLE

It was verified through the investigation that a resident developed a pressure sore/ulcer which progressed to a Stage IV, became infected and resulted in the resident requiring hospitalization for aggressive antibiotic therapy. Observe as appropriate: dressing changes, especially to any other residents with Stage III or IV pressure sores; infection control techniques such as hand washing, linen handling, and care of residents with infections; care given to prevent development of pressure sores (such as turning and repositioning, use of specialized bedding when appropriate, treatments done when ordered, keeping residents dry, and provision of adequate nutritional support for wound healing).

Record review: If a specific resident is involved, focus on the condition of the resident before and after the incident. If there are care issues, determine whether the appropriate assessments, care planning, implementation of care, and evaluations of the outcome of care have been done as specified by the regulatory requirements.

EXAMPLE

For a complaint of verbal and physical abuse, review the record to determine the resident's mood and demeanor before and after the alleged abuse. Determine if there are any other reasons for the change in the resident's demeanor and behavior. Determine whether an assessment has been done to determine the reason for the change in mood and behavior. Does the record document any unexplained bruises and/or complaints of pain, and whether they occurred in relation to the alleged incident?

Interviews: Interview the person who made the complaint. If the complainant is not at the facility at the time of the survey, he/she should be interviewed by telephone, if possible. Also, interview the person the complaint is about. Then, interview any other witnesses or staff involved. In order to maintain the confidentiality of witnesses, change the order of interviews if necessary. It may not always be desirable to interview the person who made the complaint first, as that may identify the person as the complainant to the facility. Interview residents with similar care needs at their convenience.

As interviews proceed, prepare outlines needed for other identified witnesses and revise outlines as new information is obtained.

5440 – Task 6: Information Analysis

(Rev. 1, 05-21-04)

Review all information collected. If there are inconsistencies, do additional data collection as needed, to resolve the inconsistencies. Determine if there is any other information still needed.

Determine whether:

- The complaint is substantiated;
- The facility failed to meet any of the regulatory requirements; and

- The facility practice or procedure that contributed to the complaint has been changed to achieve and/or maintain compliance.

5450 – Task 7: Exit Conference

(Rev. 1, 05-21-04)

Advise the Administrator of the complaint investigation findings and any present deficiencies. Do not inform him/her of confidential information unless the individual who provided the information specifically authorizes you to do so.

If a deficiency is not present now, but was present and has been corrected, notify the facility orally and in writing that the complaint was substantiated because deficiencies existed at the time that the complaint situation occurred. (See Appendix P, Task 5F, Section A and §7510 for specific information about imposing a civil money penalty (CMP) for egregious past non-compliance.)

If the complaint is unsubstantiated, i.e., the surveyor(s) cannot determine that it occurred and there is no indication of deficient practice, notify the facility of this decision.

Follow usual office procedure in notifying the resident and/or person who made the complaint of the findings.

Appendix

Survey Form Exhibits

List of Exhibits

EXHIBIT 85

DEPARTMENT OF HEALTH AND HUMAN SERVICES
CENTERS FOR MEDICARE & MEDICAID SERVICES

LONG TERM CARE FACILITY APPLICATION FOR MEDICARE AND MEDICAID

Standard Survey   **Extended Survey**

From: F1 ☐☐ ☐☐ ☐☐ To: F2 ☐☐ ☐☐ ☐☐   From: F3 ☐☐ ☐☐ ☐☐ To: F4 ☐☐ ☐☐ ☐☐
　　　MM   DD YY　　　　MM DD YY　　　　　　　MM   DD YY　　　　MM DD YY

Name of Facility		Provider Number	Fiscal Year Ending: F5 ☐☐ ☐☐ ☐☐ MM DD YY
Street Address	City	County	State	Zip Code
Telephone Number: F6	State/County Code: F7		State/Region Code: F8

A. F9 ☐☐

　　01 Skilled Nursing Facility (SNF) - Medicare Participation
　　02 Nursing Facility (NF) - Medicaid Participation
　　03 SNF/NF - Medicare/Medicaid

B. Is this facility hospital based? F10   Yes ☐   No ☐

　　If yes, indicate Hospital Provider Number: F11 ☐☐☐☐☐☐

Ownership: F12 ☐☐

For Profit	**NonProfit**	**Government**	
01 Individual	04 Church Related	07 State	10 City/County
02 Partnership	05 Nonprofit Corporation	08 County	11 Hospital District
03 Corporation	06 Other Nonprofit	09 City	12 Federal

Owned or leased by Multi-Facility Organization: F13   Yes ☐   No ☐

Name of Multi-Facility Organization: F14

Dedicated Special Care Units (show number of beds for all that apply)

F15 ☐☐☐ AIDS	F16 ☐☐☐ Alzheimer's Disease
F17 ☐☐☐ Dialysis	F18 ☐☐☐ Disabled Children/Young Adults
F19 ☐☐☐ Head Trauma	F20 ☐☐☐ Hospice
F21 ☐☐☐ Huntington's Disease	F22 ☐☐☐ Ventilator/Respiratory Care
F23 ☐☐☐ Other Specialized Rehabilitation	

Does the facility currently have an organized residents group?	F24	Yes ☐	No ☐
Does the facility currently have an organized group of family members of residents?	F25	Yes ☐	No ☐
Does the facility conduct experimental research?	F26	Yes ☐	No ☐
Is the facility part of a continuing care retirement community (CCRC)?	F27	Yes ☐	No ☐

If the facility currently has a staffing waiver, indicate the type(s) of waiver(s) by writing in the date(s) of last approval. Indicate the number of hours waived for each type of waiver granted. If the facility does not have a waiver, write NA in the blanks.

　　Waiver of seven day RN requirement.　　　　Date: F28 ☐☐ ☐☐ ☐☐   Hours waived per week: F29_____
　　Waiver of 24 hr licensed nursing requirement.　Date: F30 ☐☐ ☐☐ ☐☐   Hours waived per week: F31_____
　　　　　　　　　　　　　　　　　　　　　　　　　　MM DD YY

Does the facility currently have an approved Nurse Aide Training
　　　　and Competency Evaluation Program?　　　　　　　　　　　　F32　　Yes ☐　　　No ☐

Form CMS-671 (12/02)

EXHIBIT 85 *(continued)*

FACILITY STAFFING

	Tag Number	A Services Provided			B Full-Time Staff (hours)					C Part-Time Staff (hours)					D Contract (hours)				
		1	2	3															
Administration	F33																		
Physician Services	F34																		
Medical Director	F35																		
Other Physician	F36																		
Physician Extender	F37																		
Nursing Services	F38																		
RN Director of Nurses	F39																		
Nurses with Admin. Duties	F40																		
Registered Nurses	F41																		
Licensed Practical/ Licensed Vocational Nurses	F42																		
Certified Nurse Aides	F43																		
Nurse Aides in Training	F44																		
Medication Aides/Technicians	F45																		
Pharmacists	F46																		
Dietary Services	F47																		
Dietitian	F48																		
Food Service Workers	F49																		
Therapeutic Services	F50																		
Occupational Therapists	F51																		
Occupational Therapy Assistants	F52																		
Occupational Therapy Aides	F53																		
Physical Therapists	F54																		
Physical Therapists Assistants	F55																		
Physical Therapy Aides	F56																		
Speech/Language Pathologist	F57																		
Therapeutic Recreation Specialist	F58																		
Qualified Activities Professional	F59																		
Other Activities Staff	F60																		
Qualified Social Workers	F61																		
Other Social Services	F62																		
Dentists	F63																		
Podiatrists	F64																		
Mental Health Services	F65																		
Vocational Services	F66																		
Clinical Laboratory Services	F67																		
Diagnostic X-ray Services	F68																		
Administration & Storage of Blood	F69																		
Housekeeping Services	F70																		
Other	F71																		

Name of Person Completing Form	Time
Signature	Date

Form CMS-671 (12/02)

EXHIBIT 85 *(continued)*

GENERAL INSTRUCTIONS AND DEFINITIONS
(use with CMS-671 Long Term Care Facility Application for Medicare and Medicaid)
This form is to be completed by the Facility

For the purpose of this form "the facility" equals certified beds (i.e., Medicare and/or Medicaid certified beds).

Standard Survey - LEAVE BLANK - Survey team will complete
Extended Survey - LEAVE BLANK - Survey team will complete

INSTRUCTIONS AND DEFINITIONS

Name of Facility - Use the official name of the facility for business and mailing purposes. This includes components or units of a larger institution.

Provider Number - Leave blank on initial certifications. On all recertifications, insert the facility's assigned six-digit provider code.

Street Address - Street name and number refers to physical location, not mailing address, if two addresses differ.

City - Rural addresses should include the city of the nearest post office.

County - County refers to parish name in Louisiana and township name where appropriate in the New England States.

State - For U.S. possessions and trust territories, name is included in lieu of the State.

Zip Code - Zip Code refers to the "Zip-plus-four" code, if available, otherwise the standard Zip Code.

Telephone Number - Include the area code.

State/County Code - LEAVE BLANK - State Survey Office will complete.

State/Region Code - LEAVE BLANK - State Survey Office will complete.

Block F9 - Enter either 01 (SNF), 02 (NF), or 03 (SNF/NF).

Block F10 - If the facility is under administrative control of a hospital, check "yes," otherwise check "no."

Block F11 - The hospital provider number is the hospital's assigned six-digit Medicare provider number.

Block F12 - Identify the type of organization that controls and operates the facility. Enter the code as identified for that organization (e.g., for a for profit facility owned by an individual, enter 01 in the F12 block; a facility owned by a city government would be entered as 09 in the F12 block).

Definitions to determine ownership are:

FOR PROFIT - If operated under private commercial ownership, indicate whether owned by individual, partnership, or corporation.

NONPROFIT - If operated under voluntary or other nonprofit auspices, indicate whether church related, nonprofit corporation or other nonprofit.

GOVERNMENT - If operated by a governmental entity, indicate whether State, City, Hospital District, County, City/County, or Federal Government.

Block F13 - Check "yes" if the facility is owned or leased by a multi-facility organization, otherwise check "no." A Multi-Facility Organization is an organization that owns two or more long term care facilities. The owner may be an individual or a corporation. Leasing of facilities by corporate chains is included in this definition.

Block F14 - If applicable, enter the name of the multi-facility organization. Use the name of the corporate ownership of the multi-facility organization (e.g., if the name of the facility is Soft Breezes Home and the name of the multi-facility organization that owns Soft Breezes is XYZ Enterprises, enter XYZ Enterprises).

Block F15 – F23 - Enter the number of beds in the facility's Dedicated Special Care Units. These are units with a specific number of beds, identified and dedicated by the facility for residents with specific needs/diagnoses. They need not be certified or recognized by regulatory authorities. For example, a SNF admits a large number of residents with head injuries. They have set aside 8 beds on the north wing, staffed with specifically trained personnel. Show "8" in F19.

Block F24 - Check "yes" if the facility currently has an organized residents' group, i.e., a group(s) that meets regularly to discuss and offer suggestions about facility policies and procedures affecting residents' care, treatment, and quality of life; to support each other; to plan resident and family activities; to participate in educational activities or for any other purposes; otherwise check "no."

Block F25 - Check "yes" if the facility currently has an organized group of family members of residents, i.e., a group(s) that meets regularly to discuss and offer suggestions about facility policies and procedures affecting residents' care, treatment, and quality of life; to support each other, to plan resident and family activities; to participate in educational activities or for any other purpose; otherwise check "no."

EXHIBIT 85 *(continued)*

GENERAL INSTRUCTIONS AND DEFINITIONS

(use with CMS-671 Long Term Care Facility Application for Medicare and Medicaid)

Block F26 - Check "yes" if the facility conducts experimental research; otherwise check "no." Experimental research means using residents to develop and test clinical treatments, such as a new drug or therapy, that involves treatment and control groups. For example, a clinical trial of a new drug would be experimental research.

Block F27 - Check "yes" if the facility is part of a continuing care retirement community (CCRC); otherwise check "no." A CCRC is any facility which operates under State regulation as a continuing care retirement community.

Blocks F28 – F31 - If the facility has been granted a nurse staffing waiver by CMS or the State Agency in accordance with the provisions at 42CFR 483.30(c) or (d), enter the last approval date of the waiver(s) and report the number of hours being waived for each type of waiver approval.

Block F32 - Check "yes" if the facility has a State approved Nurse Aide Training and Competency Evaluation Program; otherwise check "no."

FACILITY STAFFING

GENERAL INSTRUCTIONS

This form requires you to identify whether certain services are provided and to specify the number of hours worked providing those services. Column A requires you to enter "yes" or "no" about whether the services are provided onsite to residents, onsite to nonresidents, and offsite to residents. Columns B-D requires you to enter the specific number of hours worked providing the service. To complete this section, base your calculations on the staff hours worked in the most recent complete pay period. If the pay period is more than 2 weeks, use the last 14 days. For example, if this survey begins on a Tuesday, staff hours are counted for the previous complete pay period.

Definition of Hours Worked - Hours are reported rounded to the nearest whole hour. Do not count hours paid for any type of leave or non-work related absence from the facility. If the service is provided, but has not been provided in the 2-week pay period, check the service in Column A, but leave B, C, or D blank. If an individual provides service in more than one capacity, separate out the hours in each service performed. For example, if a staff person has worked a total of 80 hours in the pay period but has worked as an activity aide and as a Certified Nurse Aide, separately count the hours worked as a CNA and hours worked as an activity aide to reflect but not to exceed the total hours worked within the pay period.

Completion of Form

Column A - Services Provided - Enter Y (yes), N (no) under each sub-column. For areas that are blocked out, do not provide the information.

Column A-1 - Refers to those services provided onsite to residents, either by employees or contractors.

Column A-2 - Refers to those services provided onsite to non-residents.

Column A-3 - Refers to those services provided to residents offsite/or not routinely provided onsite.

Column B - Full-time staff, C - Part-time staff, and D - Contract - Record hours worked for each field of full-time staff, part-time staff, and contract staff (do not include meal breaks of a half an hour or more). Full-time is defined as 35 or more hours worked per week. Part-time is anything less than 35 hours per week. Contract includes individuals under contract (e.g., a physical therapist) as well as organizations under contract (e.g., an agency to provide nurses). If an organization is under contract, calculate hours worked for the individuals provided. Lines blocked out (e.g., Physician services, Clinical labs) do not have hours worked recorded.

REMINDER - Use a 2-week period to calculate hours worked.

DEFINITION OF SERVICES

Administration - The administrative staff responsible for facility management such as the administrator, assistant administrator, unit managers and other staff in the individual departments, such as: Health Information Specialists (RRA/ARTI), clerical, etc., who do not perform services described below. Do not include the food service supervisor, housekeeping services supervisor, or facility engineer.

Physician Services - Any service performed by a physician at the facility, except services performed by a resident's personal physician.

Medical Director - A physician designated as responsible for implementation of resident care policies and coordination of medical care in the facility.

Other Physician - A salaried physician, other than the medical director, who supervises the care of residents when the attending physician is unavailable, and/or a physician(s) available to provide emergency services 24 hours a day.

Physician Extender - A nurse practitioner, clinical nurse specialist, or physician assistant who performs physician delegated services.

Nursing Services - Coordination, implementation, monitoring and management of resident care plans. Includes provision of personal care services, monitoring resident responsiveness to environment, range-of-motion exercises, application of sterile dressings, skin care, naso-gastric tubes, intravenous fluids, catheterization, administration of medications, etc.

EXHIBIT 85 *(continued)*

GENERAL INSTRUCTIONS AND DEFINITIONS

(use with CMS-671 Long Term Care Facility Application for Medicare and Medicaid)

Director of Nursing - Professional registered nurse(s) administratively responsible for managing and supervising nursing services within the facility. Do not additionally reflect these hours in any other category.

Nurses with Administrative Duties - Nurses (RN, LPN, LVN) who, as either a facility employee or contractor, perform the Resident Assessment Instrument function in the facility and do not perform direct care functions. Also include other nurses whose principal duties are spent conducting administrative functions. For example, the Assistant Director of Nursing is conducting educational/in-service, or other duties which are not considered to be direct care giving. Facilities with an RN waiver who do not have an RN as DON report all administrative nursing hours in this category.

Registered Nurses - Those persons licensed to practice as registered nurses in the State where the facility is located. Includes geriatric nurse practitioners and clinical nurse specialists who primarily perform nursing, not physician-delegated tasks. Do not include Registered Nurses' hours reported elsewhere.

Licensed Practical/Vocational Nurses - Those persons licensed to practice as licensed practical/vocational nurses in the State where the facility is located. Do not include those hours of LPN/LVNs reported elsewhere.

Certified Nurse Aides - Individuals who have completed a State approved training and competency evaluation program, or competency evaluation program approved by the State, or have been determined competent as provided in 483.150(a) and (3) and who are providing nursing or nursing-related services to residents. Do not include volunteers.

Nurse Aides in Training - Individuals who are in the first 4 months of employment and who are receiving training in a State approved Nurse Aide training and competency evaluation program and are providing nursing or nursing-related services for which they have been trained and are under the supervision of a licensed or registered nurse. Do not include volunteers.

Medication Aides/Technicians - Individuals, other than a licensed professional, who fulfill the State requirement for approval to administer medications to residents.

Pharmacists - The licensed pharmacist(s) who a facility is required to use for various purposes, including providing consultation on pharmacy services, establishing a system of records of controlled drugs, overseeing records and reconciling controlled drugs, and/or performing a monthly drug regimen review for each resident.

Dietary Services - All activities related to the provision of a nourishing, palatable, well-balanced diet that meets the daily nutritional and special dietary needs of each resident.

Dietitian - A person(s), employed full, part-time or on a consultant basis, who is either registered by the Commission of Dietetic Registration of the American Dietetic Association, or is qualified to be a dietitian on the basis of experience in identification of dietary needs, planning and implementation of dietary programs.

Food Service Workers - Persons (excluding the dietitian) who carry out the functions of the dietary service (e.g., prepare and cook food, serve food, wash dishes). Includes the food services supervisor.

Therapeutic Services - Services, other than medical and nursing, provided by professionals or their assistants, to enhance the residents' functional abilities and/or quality of life.

Occupational Therapists - Persons licensed/registered as occupational therapists according to State law in the State in which the facility is located. Include OTs who spend less than 50 percent of their time as activities therapists.

Occupational Therapy Assistants - Person(s) who, in accord with State law, have licenses/certification and specialized training to assist a licensed/certified/registered Occupational Therapist (OT) to carry out the OT's comprehensive plan of care, without the direct supervision of the therapist. Include OT Assistants who spend less than 50 percent of their time as Activities Therapists.

Occupational Therapy Aides - Person(s) who have specialized training to assist an OT to carry out the OT's comprehensive plan of care under the direct supervision of the therapist, in accord with State law.

Physical Therapists - Persons licensed/registered as physical therapists, according to State law where the facility is located.

Physical Therapy Assistants - Person(s) who, in accord with State law, have licenses/certification and specialized training to assist a licensed/certified/registered Physical Therapist (PT) to carry out the PT's comprehensive plan of care, without the direct supervision of the PT.

Physical Therapy Aides - Person(s) who have specialized training to assist a PT to carry out the PT's comprehensive plan of care under the direct supervision of the therapist, in accord with State law.

Speech-Language Pathologists - Persons licensed/registered, according to State law where the facility is located, to provide speech therapy and related services (e.g., teaching a resident to swallow).

3

EXHIBIT 85 *(continued)*

GENERAL INSTRUCTIONS AND DEFINITIONS
(use with CMS-671 Long Term Care Facility Application for Medicare and Medicaid)

Therapeutic Recreation Specialist - Person(s) who, in accordance with State law, are licensed/registered and are eligible for certification as a therapeutic recreation specialist by a recognized accrediting body.

Qualified Activities Professional - Person(s) who meet the definition of activities professional at 483.15(f)(2)(i)(A) and (B) or 483.15(f)(2)(ii) or (iii) or (iv) and who are providing an on-going program of activities designed to meet residents' interests and physical, mental or psychosocial needs. Do not include hours reported as Therapeutic Recreation Specialist, Occupational Therapist, OT Assistant, or other categories listed above.

Other Activities Staff - Persons providing an on-going program of activities designed to meet residents' needs and interests. Do not include volunteers or hours reported elsewhere.

Qualified Social Worker(s) - Person licensed to practice social work in the State where the facility is located, or if licensure is not required, persons with a bachelor's degree in social work, a bachelor's degree in a human services field including but not limited to sociology, special education, rehabilitation counseling and psychology, and one year of supervised social work experience in a health care setting working directly with elderly individuals.

Other Social Services Staff - Person(s) other than the qualified social worker who are involved in providing medical social services to residents. Do not include volunteers.

Dentists - Persons licensed as dentists, according to State law where the facility is located, to provide routine and emergency dental services.

Podiatrists - Persons licensed/registered as podiatrists, according to State law where the facility is located, to provide podiatric care.

Mental Health Services - Staff (excluding those included under therapeutic services) who provide programs of services targeted to residents' mental, emotional, psychological, or psychiatric well-being and which are intended to:

- Diagnose, describe, or evaluate a resident's mental or emotional status;
- Prevent deviations from mental or emotional well-being from developing; or
- Treat the resident according to a planned regimen to assist him/her in regaining, maintaining, or increasing emotional abilities to function.

Among the specific services included are psychotherapy and counseling, and administration and monitoring of psychotropic medications targeted to a psychiatric diagnosis.

Vocational Services - Evaluation and training aimed at assisting the resident to enter, re-enter, or maintain employment in the labor force, including training for jobs in integrated settings (i.e., those which have both disabled and nondisabled workers) as well as in special settings such as sheltered workshops.

Clinical Laboratory Services - Entities that provide laboratory services and are approved by Medicare as independent laboratories or hospitals.

Diagnostic X-ray Services - Radiology services, ordered by a physician, for diagnosis of a disease or other medical condition.

Administration and Storage of Blood Services - Blood bank and transfusion services.

Housekeeping Services - Services, including those of the maintenance department, necessary to maintain the environment. Includes equipment kept in a clean, safe, functioning and sanitary condition. Includes housekeeping services supervisor and facility engineer.

Other - Record total hours worked for all personnel not already recorded, (e.g., if a librarian works 10 hours and a laundry worker works 10 hours, record 00020 in Column C).

EXHIBIT 87

DEPARTMENT OF HEALTH AND HUMAN SERVICES
CENTERS FOR MEDICARE & MEDICAID SERVICES

EXTENDED/PARTIAL EXTENDED SURVEY WORKSHEET

FACILITY	STANDARD OR ABBREVIATED SURVEY DATES
	_____ / _____ / _____ to _____ / _____ / _____ Mo Day Yr Mo Day Yr
PROVIDER NO.	EXTENDED/PARTIAL EXTENDED SURVEY DATES
	_____ / _____ / _____ to _____ / _____ / _____ Mo Day Yr Mo Day Yr

☐ Extended Survey: Substandard care determined during Standard Survey resulting in Extended Survey.
☐ Partial Extended Survey: Substandard care determined during Abbreviated Survey resulting in Partial Extended Survey.

Check all requirements not met that resulted in the Extended or Partial Extended Survey.

☐ 483.13   ☐ 483.15   ☐ 483.25

Document observations from extended/partial extended survey

Tag/Concern	

(continued on back)

Form CMS-673 (07/95)

EXHIBIT 87 *(continued)*

Document observations from extended/partial extended survey (continued)

Tag/Concern	

EXHIBIT 88

DEPARTMENT OF HEALTH AND HUMAN SERVICES
CENTERS FOR MEDICARE & MEDICAID SERVICES

MEDICATION PASS WORKSHEET

Provider Number	Surveyor Name	Date	Error Rate

Instructions: 1. Observe Pass for 20-25 opportunities for error. If one or more errors is found observe another 20-25 opportunities for error.
2. Record your observation of each opportunity for error.
3. Compare your record with physician orders.
4. Calculate and note error rate

Deficiency Formulas:

1. One or more Significant Errors = Deficiency

2. $\dfrac{\text{Significant Error} + \text{Non-Significant Error}}{\text{Doses given} + \text{Doses ordered but not given}} \times 100 \geq 5\% = \text{Deficiency}$

Identifier	Pour	Pass	Record
Resident's Full Name	Drug Prescription Name, Dose and Form	Observation of Administration	Drug Order Written As *(when different from observation)*

FORM CMS-677 (07/95)

EXHIBIT 88 *(continued)*

MEDICATION PASS WORKSHEET			
Identifier	**Pour**	**Pass**	**Record**
Resident's Full Name	Drug Prescription Name, Dose and Form	Observation of Administration	Drug Order Written As *(when different from observation)*

FORM CMS-677 (07/95)

EXHIBIT 89

DEPARTMENT OF HEALTH AND HUMAN SERVICES
CENTERS FOR MEDICARE & MEDICAID SERVICES

OFFSITE SURVEY PREPARATION WORKSHEET

Facility Name: _____   **Ombudsman Name/Number:** _____

Facility Address: _____   **Ombudsman Contact Date:** _____

Provider Number: _____   **Offsite Review Date:** _____

Total Beds: _____   **Survey Begin Date:** _____

List potential facility areas of concern and any potential residents to be reviewed during the survey. List any current complaints to be investigated onsite.

Surveyors/Discipline (list Team Coordinator first):

_____

_____

_____

_____

Form CMS-801 (07/95)

EXHIBIT 91

DEPARTMENT OF HEALTH AND HUMAN SERVICES
CENTERS FOR MEDICARE & MEDICAID SERVICES

GENERAL OBSERVATIONS OF THE FACILITY

Facility Name :_____   **Surveyor Name:**_____

Provider Number:_____   **Surveyor Number:**_____   **Discipline:**_____

Observation Dates: From _____ **To**_____

Instructions: Use the questions below to focus your observations of the facility. Include all locations used by residents (units, hallways, dining rooms, lounges, activity and therapy rooms, bathing areas, and resident smoking areas). Also check other areas that affect the residents, such as storage and utility areas. Initial that there are no concerns or note concerns and your follow-up in the space provided. Begin your observations as soon as possible after entering the facility and continue throughout the survey. Note, these tags are not all inclusive.

LIST ANY POTENTIAL CONCERNS FROM OFFSITE SURVEY PREPARATION._____

1. **HANDRAILS:** Do corridors have handrails? Are handrails affixed to walls, intact, and free of splinters? (F468)

2. **ODORS:** Is the facility free of objectionable *odors*? Are resident areas well *ventilated*? Especially observe activity areas and the dining room during activities and lunch, when the residents are using them. Are nonsmoking areas smoke free? Do smoking areas provide good quality of life for residents who smoke? (F252)

3. **CLEANLINESS:** How *clean* is the environment (walls, floors, drapes, furniture)? (F252)

4. **PESTS:** Is the facility *pest free*? (F469)

5. **LINEN:** Is the linen processed, transported, stored and handled properly to *prevent the spread of infection*? (F445)

6. **HAZARDS:** Is the facility as free of *accident hazards* as possible? Are water temperatures safe and comfortable? Are housekeeping/hazards, compounds, and other chemicals stored to prevent resident access? (F252, 323)

7. **CALL SYSTEM:** Is there a functioning *call system* in bathing areas and resident toilets in common areas? (F463)

8. **SPACE:** Do the *space and furnishings* in dining and activity areas appear sufficient to accommodate all activities? (F464)

9. **FURNISHINGS:** Are dining and activity rooms *adequately furnished*? (F464)

10. **DRUG STORAGE:** Are *drugs* and biologicals *stored properly* (locked and at appropriate temperatures)? (F432)

11. **EQUIPMENT:** Is the resident equipment in common areas *sanitary, orderly, and in good repair*? (Equipment in therapy rooms, bathing rooms, activity areas, etc.) Are equipment and supplies appropriately stored and handled in clean and dirty utility areas (sterile supplies, thermometer, etc.)? (F253)

12. **EQUIPMENT CONDITION:** [*Excluding* the kitchen] Is *essential equipment* in safe and effective operating condition (e.g. boiler room equipment, nursing unit/medication room equipment, unit refrigerators, laundry equipment, therapy equipment)? (F456)

13. **SURVEY POSTED:** Are *survey results* readily accessible to residents? Are the survey results or a notice concerning survey results posted? (F167)

14. **INFORMATION POSTED:** Is information about Medicare, Medicaid and contacting advocacy agencies posted? (Fl56)

15. **POSITIONING:** Is correct posture and comfortable positioning and assistance being provided to residents who need assistance — especially check residents who are dining or participating in activities? (F246, 311, 318)

16. **EMERGENCY:** Are staff *prepared for an emergency or disaster*? Ask two staff and a charge nurse to describe what they do in emergencies (include staff from different shifts). Evaluate the responses to determine their correctness and preparedness. (F518)

17. **EMERGENCY POWER:** Is there *emergency power*? Are staff aware of outlets, if any, powered by emergency source? (F455)

18. **WASTE:** Is waste contained in properly maintained (no breaks) cans, dumpsters or compactors with covers? (F454, 371)

THERE ARE NO IDENTIFIED CONCERNS FOR THESE REQUIREMENTS (Init.)_____

Document concerns and follow-up on back of page:_____

Form CMS-803 (7-95)

(continued)

EXHIBIT 91 *(continued)*

GENERAL OBSERVATIONS OF THE FACILITY

Tag / Concerns	Source*	Surveyor Notes (including date/time)

*Source: O = Observation, RR = Record Review, I = Interview
Form CMS-803 (7-95)

EXHIBIT 92

DEPARTMENT OF HEALTH AND HUMAN SERVICES
CENTERS FOR MEDICARE & MEDICAID SERVICES

KITCHEN/FOOD SERVICE OBSERVATION

Facility Name: _____   Surveyor Name: _____

Provider Number: _____   Surveyor Number: _____ Discipline: _____

Observation Dates/Times: _____

Instructions:

Use the questions below to focus your observations of the kitchen and the facility's storage, preparation, distribution and service of food to residents. Initial that there are no identifiable concerns or note concerns and follow-up in the space provided. All questions relate to the requirement to prevent the contamination of food and the spread of food-born illness. (F371 This tag is not all inclusive.)

LIST ANY POTENTIAL CONCERNS FROM OFFSITE SURVEY PREPARATION: _____

_____

FOOD STORAGE

1. Are the refrigerator and freezer shelves and floors clean and free of spillage, and foods free of slime and mold?

2. Is the freezer temperature 0 degrees F or below and refrigerator 41 degrees F or below (allow 2-3 degrees variance)? Do not check during meal preparation.

3. Are refrigerated foods covered, dated, labeled, and shelved to allow air circulation?

4. Are foods stored correctly (e.g., cooked foods over raw meat in refrigerator, egg and egg rich foods refrigerated)?

5. Is dry storage maintained in a manner to prevent rodent/pest infestation?

FOOD PREPARATION

6. Are cracked eggs being used only in foods that are thoroughly cooked, such as baked goods or casseroles?

7. Are frozen raw meats and poultry thawed in the refrigerator or in cold, running water? Are cooked foods cooled down safely?

8. Are food contact surfaces and utensils cleaned to prevent cross-contamination and food-borne illness?

FOOD SERVICE/SANITATION

9. Are hot foods maintained at 140 degrees F or above and cold foods maintained at 41 degrees F or below when served from tray line?

10. Are food trays, dinnerware, and utensils clean and in good condition?

11. Are the foods covered until served? Is food protected from contamination during transportation and distribution?

12. Are employees washing hands before and after handling food, using clean utensils when necessary and following infection control practices?

13. Are food preparation equipment, dishes and utensils effectively sanitized to destroy potential food borne illness? Is dishwasher's hot water wash 140 degrees F and rinse cycle 180 degrees F or chemical sanitation per manufacturer's instructions followed?

14. Is facility following correct manual dishwashing procedures (i.e., 3 compartment sink, correct water temperature, chemical concentration, and immersion time)?

NOTE: If any nutritional concerns have been identified (such as weight loss) by observation, interviews or record review, check portion sizes and how that type of food is prepared (see guidelines at 483.35). If any concerns are identified regarding meals that are not consistent in quality see guidance at Task 5B and at 483.35.

LADLES: 1/4 C = 2 oz., 1/2 C = 4 oz., 3/4 C = 6 oz., 1 C = 8 oz.

SCOOPS: #6 = 2/3 C., #8 = 1/2 C., #10 = 2/5 C., #12 = 1/3 C., #16 = 1/4 C.

THERE ARE NO IDENTIFIED CONCERNS FOR THESE REQUIREMENTS: (Init.) ____

Document concerns and follow-up on back of page.

Form CMS-804 (7-95)

(continued)

EXHIBIT 92 *(continued)*

KITCHEN/FOOD SERVICE OBSERVATION

Tag/Concerns	Source*	Surveyor Notes (including date/time)

*Source: O = Observation, RR = Record Review, I = Interview

Form CMS-804 (7-95)

EXHIBIT 93

DEPARTMENT OF HEALTH AND HUMAN SERVICES
CENTERS FOR MEDICARE & MEDICAID SERVICES

RESIDENT REVIEW WORKSHEET

Facility Name: _____   Resident Name: _____

Provider Number: _____   Resident Identifier: _____

Surveyor Name: _____   Birthdate: _____ Unit: _____ Rm #: _____

Surveyor Number: _____ Discipline: _____   Orig. Admission Date: _____ Readmission Date: _____

Survey Date: _____

Payment Source: Admission: _____

Current: _____

Diagnosis: _____

Interviewable: Yes ☐   No ☐   Type of Review: Comprehensive ☐   Focused ☐   Closed Record ☐

Selected for Individual Interview: Yes ☐   No ☐

Selected for Family Interview and Observation of Non-Interviewable Resident: Yes ☐   No ☐

Focus/Care Areas: _____

Instructions: Any regulatory areas related to the sampled resident's needs are to be included in this review.
  • Initial that each section was reviewed if there are no concerns.
  • If there are concerns, document your investigation.
  • Document all pertinent resident observations and information from resident, staff, family interviews and record
    reviews for every resident in the sample.

SECTION A: RESIDENT ROOM REVIEW: Evaluate if appropriate requirements are met in each of the following areas,
including the accommodation of needs:

• Adequate accommodations are made for resident privacy, including bed curtains.

• Call bells are functioning and accessible to residents

• Resident is able to use his/her bathroom without difficulty.

• Adequate space exists for providing care to residents.

• Resident with physical limitations (e.g., walker, wheelchair) is able to move around his/her room.

• Environment is homelike, comfortable and attractive; accommodations are made for resident personal items and his/her modifications.

• Bedding, bath linens and closet space is adequate for resident needs.

• Resident care equipment is clean and in good repair.

• Room is safe and comfortable in the following areas: temperature, water temperature, sound level and lighting.

THERE ARE NO IDENTIFIED CONCERNS FOR THESE REQUIREMENTS (Init.)_____
Document concerns and follow-up on Surveyor Notes sheet page 4.

SECTION B: RESIDENT DAILY LIFE REVIEW: Evaluate if appropriate requirements are met in each of the following areas:

• Resident appears well groomed and reasonably attractive (e.g., clean clothes, neat hair, free from facial hair).

• Staff treats residents respectfully and listens to resident requests. Note staff interaction with both communicative and non-communicative residents.

• Staff is responsive to resident requests and call bells.

• Residents are free from unexplained physical injuries and there are no signs of resident abuse. (e.g. residents do not appear frightened around certain staff members.)

• Facility activities program meets resident's individually assessed needs and preferences.

• Medically related social services are identified and provided when appropriate.

• Restraints are used only when medically necessary. *(see 483.13(a))*

• Resident is assisted with dining when necessary.

THERE ARE NO IDENTIFIED CONCERNS FOR THESE REQUIREMENTS (Init.)_____
Document concerns and follow-up on Surveyor Notes sheet page 4.

Form CMS-805(7-95)

(continued)

EXHIBIT 93 *(continued)*

Resident Review Worksheet
(continued)

SECTION C: ASSESSMENT OF DRUG THERAPIES
Review all the over-the-counter and prescribed medications taken by the resident during the last 7 days.

- Evaluate drug therapy for indications/reason, side effects, dose, review of therapy/monitoring, and evidence of unnecessary medications including antipsychotic drugs.

- Correlate drug therapy with resident's clinical condition.
- If you note concerns with drug therapy, review the pharmacist's report. See if the physician or facility has responded to recommendations or concerns.

THERE ARE NO IDENTIFIED CONCERNS FOR THESE REQUIREMENTS (Init.)_____

Medications/Dose/Schedule	Medications/Dose/Schedule	Medications/Dose/Schedule

Document concerns and follow-up on page 4.

SECTION D: RAI/CARE REVIEW SHEET *(Includes both MDS and use of RAPS):*
Reason for the most current RAI: Annual ☐   Initial ☐   Significant Change ☐
Date of Most Recent RAI _____   Date of Comparison/ Quarterly RAI _____

- For a *comprehensive review* complete a review of all care areas specific to the resident, all ADL functional areas, cognitive status, and MDS categories triggering a RAP.
- For a *focused review*:
  Phase I: Complete a review of those requirements appropriate to focus and care areas specific to the resident.
  Phase II: Complete a review of requirements appropriate to focus areas.
- For both *comprehensive* and *focused reviews* **record only the applicable sections and relevant factors about the clinical status indicating an impairment or changes between reviews.**
- If the current RAI is less than 9 months old, scan and compare with the previous RAI and most recent quarterly review.
- If the RAI is 9 months or older, compare the current RAI with the most recent quarterly review.
- Note any differences for the applicable areas being reviewed.
- Review the RAP summary and care planning.
- Look for implementation of the care plan as appropriate to the comprehensive or focused review.
- Note specifically the effects of care or lack of care.
- If the resident declined or failed to improve relative to expectations, determine if this was avoidable or unavoidable.
- For *closed records, complete a review of the* applicable areas of concern.
- Use the additional MDS item blocks on page 3 to document other sections or additional concerns.
- *Dining observation;* If there are concerns with weight loss or other nutritional issues, observe resident dining and review adequacy of meals served and menus.

THERE ARE NO IDENTIFIED CONCERNS FOR THESE REQUIREMENTS (Init.)_____
Document concerns and follow-up on page 4.

EXHIBIT 93 *(continued)*

Resident Review Worksheet
(continued)

MDS Items	RAI Status/Comparison	Care Plan Y/N	Notes/Dates/Times/Source and Tag: Observations and Interview for resident and implementation of care plan and TX, including accuracy, completeness, and how information from use of RAPs is incorporated into the resident's care. Outcome: improve/failure to improve/same/decline. If a decline or failure to improve occurred, was it avoidable or unavoidable?
Cognitive/ Decisionmaking			
Mood/Behavior/ Psychosocial			
Transfer			
Ambulation			
Dressing			
Eating			
Hygiene/ Bathing			
ROM Limits			
Bowel			
Bladder			
Activities			

Form CMS-805(7-95)   Page 3

(continued)

EXHIBIT 93 *(continued)*

Resident Review Worksheet
(continued)

Tag/Concerns	Source*	Surveyor Notes *(including date/time)*

EXHIBIT 94

DEPARTMENT OF HEALTH AND HUMAN SERVICES
CENTERS FOR MEDICARE & MEDICAID SERVICES

QUALITY OF LIFE ASSESSMENT
RESIDENT INTERVIEW

Facility Name: _____ Resident Name: _____
Provider Number: _____ Resident Identifier: _____
Surveyor Name: _____ Interview Dates/Times: _____
Surveyor Number: _____ Discipline: _____

Instructions:

For question 1, if you are meeting with the resident in a location away from the resident's room, visit the room before the interview and note anything about the room that you want to discuss. For question 7, review the RAI to determine the ADL capabilities of this resident.

Introduce yourself and explain the survey process and the purpose of the interview using the following concepts. It is not necessary to use the exact wording.

"[Name of facility] is inspected by a team from the [Name of State Survey Agency] periodically to assure that all residents receive good care. While we are here, we make a lot of observations, review the nursing home's records, and talk to residents to help us understand what it's like to live in this nursing home. We appreciate your taking the time to talk to us."

"We ask certain questions because we want to know whether you have a say in decisions affecting your nursing and medical care, your schedule and the services you receive at this facility. We want to know how you feel about your life here and whether the facility has made efforts to accommodate your preferences."

"If it is all right with you, I'd like to meet with you again later. That will give you time to think things over and to provide additional information later."

In asking the following questions, it is not necessary to use the exact wording. However, do use complete questions, not one-word probes.

Get the resident to talk about actual situations and examples by using open-ended probes, such as: "Can you tell me more about that?" or "How is that done here?" Avoid asking leading questions which suggest a certain response.

If a resident gives a response to any question that indicates there may be a concern with facility services, probe to determine if the resident has communicated the problem to facility staff and what their response was.

1. ***ROOM:*** (F177, 201, 207, 242, 250, 252, 256, 257)
   A good approach for initiating this discussion is to make a comment about something you have noticed about the resident's room, for example, "I notice that you have a lot of plants in your room."

Please tell me about your room and how you feel about it.
Do you enjoy spending time in your room?
Is there enough light for you?
Is the room temperature comfortable?
Have you lived in a different room in the facility?
   (If yes) **What was the reason for the room change?**

Did you have a choice about changing rooms?
Where was your other room? What was it like?
Is there anything you would like to change about your room?
   (If yes) **Have you talked to the facility about this?**
   How did they respond?

Form CMS-806A (07/95)   *(continued)*

EXHIBIT 94 *(continued)*

RESIDENT INTERVIEW

2. *ENVIRONMENT:* (F252, 258)

I realize that being in a nursing home is not like being in your own home, but do staff here try to make this facility seem homelike?

We've already talked about your room. How about other places you use, like the activities room and dining room? Do they seem homelike to you?

Is there anything that would make this facility more comfortable for you?

Is it generally quiet or noisy here?

What about at night?

Is the facility usually clean and free of bad smells?

3. *PRIVACY:* (F164, 174)

Are you a person who likes to have privacy sometimes?

Are you able to have privacy when you want it?

Do staff and other residents respect your privacy?

Do you have a private place to meet with visitors?

(If no phone in room) **Where do you make phone calls?**

Do you have privacy when you are on the phone? (If the resident indicates any problems with privacy, probe for specific examples. Ask if they talked to staff and what was their response.)

4. *FOOD:* (F365)

Tell me about the food here.

Do you have any restrictions on your diet?

How does your food taste?

Are you served foods that you like to eat?

Are your hot and cold foods served at a temperature you like?

Have you ever refused to eat something served to you?

(If yes) **Did the facility offer you something else to eat?**

(If the resident refused a food and did not get a substitute) **Did you ask for another food? What was the facility's response?**

5. *ACTIVITIES:* (F242, 248)

How do you find out about the activities that are going on?

Are there activities available on the weekends?

Do you participate in activities?

(If yes) What kinds of activities do you participate in?

(If resident participates) **Do you enjoy these activities?**

(If resident does not participate, probe to find out why not.)

Is there some activity that you would like to do that is not available here?

(If yes) **Which activity would you like to attend?**

Have you talked to anybody about this? What was the response?

EXHIBIT 94 *(continued)*

RESIDENT INTERVIEW

6. *STAFF:* **(F223, 241)**

Tell me how you feel about the staff members at this facility. Do they treat you with respect?

Do you feel they know something about you as a person?

Are they usually willing to take the time to listen when you want to talk about something personal or a problem you are having?

Do they make efforts to resolve your problems?

Has any resident or staff member ever physically harmed you?

Has any resident or staff member ever taken anything belonging to you without permission?

(If yes) **Can you tell me who did this?**

Has a staff member ever yelled or sworn at you?

(If yes) **Please describe what happened.**

Can you tell me who did this? Did you report this to someone?

(If yes) **How did they respond?**

7. *ADLs:* **(F216, 311, 312)**

(Tailor this question to what you have observed and what is noted in the MDS about ADL capabilities of this resident.) For example: **I see that your care plan calls for you to dress with a little help from staff. How is that working for you?**

Do you feel that you get help when you need it?

Do staff encourage you to do as much as you can for yourself?

8. *DECISIONS:* **(F154, 242, 280)**

Here at this facility, are you involved in making choices about your daily activities?

Are you involved in making decisions about your nursing care and medical treatment?

(If not, probe to determine what these choices and decisions are, and relate this information to necessary restrictions that are part of the resident's plan of care.)

Do you participate in meetings where staff plan your activities and daily medical and nursing care?

If you are unhappy with something, or if you want to change something about your care or your daily schedule, how do you let the facility know?

Do you feel the staff members listen to your requests and respond appropriately?

If the staff are unable to accommodate one of your requests, do they provide a reasonable explanation of why they cannot honor the request?

Can you choose how you spend the day?

Have you ever refused care or treatment (such as a bath or certain medication)?

(If yes) **What happened then?**

Form CMS-806A (07/95)

(continued)

EXHIBIT 94 *(continued)*

RESIDENT INTERVIEW

9. *MEDICAL SERVICES:* **(F156, 163, 164, 250, 411, 412)**

Who is your physician?

Did you choose your physician yourself?
(If no, probe for details about who selected the physician and why the resident did not do it.)

Are you satisfied with the care provided by your physician?

Can you see your doctor if you need to?

Do you see your physician here or at the office?
(If they say here) **Where in the facility does your doctor see you?**

Do you have privacy when you are examined by your physician?
(If they say they go to the office) **How do you get to the office?**

Do facility staff help you make doctor's appointments and help you obtain transportation?

Can you get to see a dentist, podiatrist, or other specialist if you need to?

10. (Write here any special items not already discussed that you have noted about this resident or about the facility that you would like to discuss with the resident.)

_____

_____

_____

_____

11. Is there anything else you would like to talk about regarding your life here?

Thank the resident. Review your notes from this interview and determine if there are any concerns you need to investigate further. Share any problems you have found with the team so they may keep them in mind during the remainder of the survey.

Form CMS-806A (07/95)

EXHIBIT 94 *(continued)*

DEPARTMENT OF HEALTH AND HUMAN SERVICES
CENTERS FOR MEDICARE & MEDICAID SERVICES

QUALITY OF LIFE ASSESSMENT
GROUP INTERVIEW

Facility Name:_____   Surveyor Name:_____
Provider Number:_____   Surveyor Number:_____
Interview Dates/Times:_____   Discipline:_____

Residents Attending: _____   _____
_____   _____
_____   _____
_____   _____
_____   _____
_____   _____

Instructions:

Introduce yourself to the group and explain the survey process and the purpose of the interview using the following
  concepts. It is not necessary to use the exact wording.

"[Name of facility] is inspected by a team from the [Name of State Survey Agency] periodically as one part of a
  process in which we evaluate the quality of life and quality of care in this facility.

While we are here, we make observations, look over the facility's records, and talk to residents about life in this
  facility.

We appreciate you taking the time to talk to us.

We would like to ask you several questions about life in the facility and the interactions of residents and staff."

1. RULES: (F151, 242, 243)

Tell me about the rules in this facility.

For instance, rules about what time residents go to bed
  at night and get up in the morning?

Are there any other facility rules you would like to
  discuss?

Do you as a group have input into the rules of this
  facility?

Does the facility listen to your suggestions?

2. PRIVACY: (F164, 174)

Can you meet privately with your visitors?

Can you make a telephone call without other people
  overhearing your conversation?

Does the facility make an effort to assure that privacy
  rights are respected for all residents?

Form CMS-806B (07/95)

(continued)

EXHIBIT 94 *(continued)*

GROUP INTERVIEW

3. *ACTIVITIES:* (F242, 248)

Activities programs are supposed to meet your interests and needs. Do you feel the activities here do that?
(If no, probe for specifics.)

Do you participate in the activities here?

Do you enjoy them?

Are there enough help and supplies available so that everyone who wants to can participate?

Do you as a group have input into the selection of the activities that are offered?

How does the facility respond to your suggestions?

Is there anything about the activities program that you would like to talk about?

Outside of the formal activity programs, are there opportunities for you to socialize with other residents?

Are there places you can go when you want to be with other residents?

(If answers are negative) Why do you think that occurs?

4. *PERSONAL PROPERTY:* (F252)

Can residents have their own belongings here if they choose to do so?

What about their own furniture?

How are your personal belongings treated here?

Does the facility make efforts to prevent loss, theft, or destruction of personal property?

Have any of your belongings ever been missing?

(If anyone answers yes) Did you talk to a staff member about this? What was their response?

5. *RIGHTS:* (F151, 153, 156, 167, 168, 170, 280)

How do residents here find out about their rights — such as voting, making a living will, getting what you need here?

Are you invited to meetings in which staff plan your nursing care, medical treatment and activities?

Do you know that you can see a copy of the facility's latest survey inspection results?

Where is that report kept here?

Do you know how to contact an advocacy agency such as the ombudsman office?

Do you know you can look at your medical record?

Have any of you asked to see your record? What was the facility's response?

Has anyone from the facility staff talked to you about these things?

Tell me about the mail delivery system here.
Is mail delivery prompt? Does your mail arrive unopened daily?

6. *DIGNITY:* (F223, 241)

How do staff members treat the residents here, not just yourselves, but others who can't speak for themselves?

Do you feel the staff here treat residents with respect and dignity?

Do they try to accommodate residents' wishes where possible?

(If answers are negative) Please describe instances in which the facility did not treat you or another resident with dignity. Did you talk to anyone on the staff about this? How did they respond?

EXHIBIT 94 *(continued)*

GROUP INTERVIEW

7. *ABUSE AND NEGLECT:* (F223)

Are you aware of any instances in which a resident was abused or neglected?

Are you aware of any instances in which a resident had property taken from them by a staff member without permission?

(If yes) **Tell me about it. How did you find out about it?**

Are there enough staff here to take care of everyone?

(If no) **Tell me more about that.**

We are willing to discuss any incidents that you know of in private if you would prefer. If so, just stop me or one of the other surveyors anytime, and we'll listen to you.

8. *COSTS:* (F156, 207)

Are residents here informed by the facility about which items and services are paid by Medicare or Medicaid and which ones you must pay for?

If there was any change in these items that you must pay for, were you informed?

Are you aware of any changes in the care any resident has received after they went from paying for their care to Medicaid paying?

(If answers suggest the possibility of Medicaid discrimination, probe for specific instances of differences in care.)

9. *BUILDING:* (F256, 257, 258,463,465,483)

I'd like to ask a few questions about the building, including both your bedroom and other rooms you use such as the dining room and activities room.

Is the air temperature comfortable for you?

Is there good air circulation or does it get stuffy in these rooms?

What do you think about the noise level here? Is it generally quiet or noisy? How about at night?

Do you have the right amount of lighting in your room to read or do whatever you want to do?

How is the lighting in the dining rooms and activity rooms?

Do you ever see insects or rodents here?

(If yes) **Tell me about it.**

10. *FOOD:* (F364, 365, 367)

The next questions are about the food here.

Is the flavor and appearance of your food satisfactory?

Outside of the dietary restrictions some of you may have, do you receive food here that you like to eat?

If you have ever refused to eat a particular food, did the facility provide you with something else to eat? (If no, probe for specifics.)

Is the temperature of your hot and cold foods appropriate?

Are the meats tender enough?

About what time do you receive your breakfast, lunch, and dinner?

Are the meals generally on time or late?

What are you offered for a bedtime snack?

If you ever had a concern about your food, did you tell the staff? What was their response?

EXHIBIT 94 *(continued)*

GROUP INTERVIEW

11. *COUNCIL:* (F243)

(If you are speaking with a resident council)

Does the facility help you with arrangements for council meetings?

Do they make sure you have space to meet?

Can you have meetings without any staff present if you wish?

How does the council communicate its concerns to the facility?

How does the administrator respond to the council's concerns?

If the facility cannot accommodate a council request, do they give you a reasonable explanation?

12. *GRIEVANCES:* (F165, 166)

Have any of you or the group as a whole ever voiced a grievance to the facility?

How did staff react to this?

Did they resolve the problem?

Do you feel free to make complaints to staff? If not, why not (probe for specific examples)**?**

13. Identify here any issues you would like to discuss with the group that have not been covered in the questions above.

_____

_____

_____

_____

14. Is there anything else about life here in the facility that you would like to discuss?

Thank the group for their time. After the interview, follow up on any concerns that need further investigation. Document your follow up on Resident Review or Supervisor Notes Worksheets. Share these concerns with the team.

EXHIBIT 94 *(continued)*

DEPARTMENT OF HEALTH AND HUMAN SERVICES
CENTERS FOR MEDICARE & MEDICAID SERVICES

**QUALITY OF LIFE ASSESSMENT
FAMILY INTERVIEW**

Facility Name: _____   **Resident Name:** _____
Provider Number: _____   **Resident Identifier:** _____
Surveyor Name: _____   **Person Interviewed:** _____
Surveyor Number: _____ **Discipline:** _____   **Relationship to Resident:** _____
Method of Contact: In person ☐ **Phone** ☐   **Interview Dates/Times:** _____

Instructions:

This interview is intended to be conducted with a person (family, friend or guardian) who is the one acting on behalf of the resident and authorizing care. Prior to the interview, complete as many questions as you can through review of the resident assessment, care plan and any activities or social service assessment.

Adapt these questions and probes as necessary to make them applicable to this resident.

Introduce yourself and explain the survey process and the purpose of the interview using the following concepts. It is not necessary to use the exact wording.

"[Name of facility] is inspected by a team from the [Name of State Survey Agency] periodically to assure that residents receive quality care. While we are here, we make observations, review the nursing home's records, and talk to residents and family members or friends who can help us understand what it's like to live in this nursing home. We appreciate your taking the time to talk to us.

"We ask these questions because we want to know about your opportunity for involvement in decision about _____ 's care and schedule, your views on services he/she receives here, and in general, what you think of the facility. We want to know if the facility has obtained information about _____'s past and current preferences in order to provide the highest quality of care. We also want to find out about the admission process and what the facility discussed with you about costs and payment for _____'s stay here.

Question 1 below screens the family member to see if she/he knows the resident well enough to complete the rest of the interview. Based on answers to question 1, decide whether you can complete the interview, complete it partially if the family member knows some things, or conclude the interview. If you decide you must conclude this interview, ask a general question that lets the family member say what they wish to say about the facility such as: "Is there anything you would like to tell me about this facility and how your relative is treated?".

---

1. (Ask about the nature and extent of the relationship between interviewee and resident both prior to and during nursing home residence):

With whom did your relative/friend live before coming to the nursing home? (If the resident did not live with this person) About how often did you see her/him?

How often do the resident and you see each other now?

Are you familiar with _____'s preferences and daily routines when he/she was more independent and more able to make choices and express preferences? (If the resident has had a lifelong disability, ask about choice and preferences prior to moving to this facility. Adapt question 2 and 3 also.)

EXHIBIT 94 *(continued)*

FAMILY INTERVIEW

To the extent that the interviewee is knowledgeable about the resident's past life, ask the following:

2. I have some questions about _____'s life-style and preferences when she/he was more independent and able to express preferences. Would you tell me about:

Did he/she enjoy any particular activities or hobbies?
Was she/he social or more solitary?
Types of social and recreational activities;

Eating habits, food likes and dislikes;
Sleeping habits, alertness at different times of the day;
Religious/spiritual activities;
Work, whether in or out of the home;
Things that gave him/her pleasure.

3. The next questions are about the resident's lifelong general personality. How would you describe:

General manner; for example, was she/he thought to be quiet, happy, argumentative, etc.?
How she/he generally adapted to change, prior to the current disability. How, for example, did the resident react to moving to a new residence, to losing a loved one, and to other changing life situations?

Characteristic ways of talking — was she/he talkative or usually quiet, likely to express herself/himself or not?

4. Have any of the preferences and personality characteristics that you told me about changed, either due to a change in her/his condition or due to relocation to this facility?

Have her/his daily routines and activities changed in a substantial way since moving here?
(If yes) Please describe these differences.

EXHIBIT 94 *(continued)*

FAMILY INTERVIEW

5. **(For all the items below: If the family member describes any problems, probe for specific information. Ask if they have talked to staff, and what was the facility's response. If the resident's payment source changed from private pay or Medicare to Medicaid, inquire if there were any changes in any of the following after the payment source changed.)**

   Please share with me your observations, either positive things or concerns, about all of the following items. If you have no information about these issues that is OK.

   Meals and snacks (F242, 310, 365, 366, 367)
   Routines and activities (F242, 245, 248)
   Visitor policies and hours, privacy for visits when desired (F164, 172)
   Care by nursing home staff (F241, 309–312)

   Noise level of the facility (F258)
   Privacy when receiving care (F164)
   Transfers (F177, 201, 203–207)
   Security and personal property (F159, 223, 252)
   Cleanliness and odor (F252–254)

6. **Did you participate in the admission process?**
   (If yes) Were you told anything about using Medicare or Medicaid to pay for _____'s stay here?
   (If yes) What did they tell you?
   (If resident's care is being paid by Medicaid) Were you asked to pay for any extras above the Medicaid rate?
   (If yes) What were these? Did you have a choice about receiving these services?
   When your relative/friend moved here, did the facility ask you to pay out of your savings or your relative's savings? (F156, 208)

7. **Are you the person who would be notified if _____'s condition changed. (If yes) Have you been notified when there have been changes in your relative's condition? Are you involved in _____'s care planning? (F157)**

8. **"Is there anything else that I have not asked that is important to understand about _____'s everyday life here?"**

   When finished: "Thank you for your help. You will be able to examine a copy of the results of this survey in about ___ days."

Form CMS-806C (07/95)

EXHIBIT 94 *(continued)*

DEPARTMENT OF HEALTH AND HUMAN SERVICES
CENTERS FOR MEDICARE & MEDICAID SERVICES

QUALITY OF LIFE ASSESSMENT
OBSERVATION OF NON- INTERVIEWABLE RESIDENT

1. **Special items to observe:** _____

_____

_____

2. *RESIDENT AND ENVIRONMENT:*

Physical condition of resident (comfort, positioning, etc.) (F246)

Appearance (grooming and attire) (F241)

Physical environment (comfort, safety, privacy, infection control, stimulation, personal belongings, homelike) (F164, 246, 252, 441, 444, 459)

Level of assistance received. Note instances of too much or too little and resulting problem (e.g., violation of dignity). (F241, 309–312)

Privacy afforded when care is given (F164)

Use of restraints and/or other restrictions on behavior (F221)

Do staff intervene to assist resident if there is a problem and the resident tries to indicate this? (F312)

3. *DAILY LIFE:*

The agreement of the daily schedule and activities with assessed interests and functional level (Note during activities if cues/prompts and adapted equipment are provided as needed and according to care plan.) (F242, 255)

Restriction of choices that the resident can make (e.g., resident reaching out for a drink or pushing away food or medication and facility response) (F155, 242)

Consistency of TV or radio being on or off with assessed interests (F242, 280)

4. *INTERACTIONS WITH OTHERS:*

Do staff individualize their interactions with this resident, based on her/his preferences, capabilities, and special needs? (F241, 246)

What is the resident's response to staff interactions (smiling, attempting to communicate, distressed, anxious, etc.)? (F241, 246)

Do staff try to communicate in a reassuring way? (Note staff tone of voice and use of speech.) While staff are giving care, do they include resident in conversation or do staff talk to each other as if resident is not there? (F241, 223)

Evidence of a roommate problem that could be addressed by the facility (F250)

Consistency of opportunities for socializing with regard to assessed interests and functional level (Note time and situations when isolated.) (F174, 242, 248, 250)

Location of resident: segregated in some way, in a special unit, or fully integrated with other residents (Note any adverse consequences for resident.) (F223)

Use the Resident Review or Surveyor Notes Worksheet to follow-up on any concerns. Share any concerns with the team.

Form CMS-806C (07/95)

EXHIBIT 95

DEPARTMENT OF HEALTH AND HUMAN SERVICES
CENTERS FOR MEDICARE & MEDICAID SERVICES

SURVEYOR NOTES WORKSHEET

Facility Name:_____   **Surveyor Name:**_____

Provider Number:_____   **Surveyor Number:**_____ **Discipline:**_____

Observation Dates: From _____ **To** _____

TAG/CONCERNS	DOCUMENTATION

Form CMS-807 (7/95)

EXHIBIT 95 *(continued)*

SURVEYOR NOTES WORKSHEET

TAG/CONCERNS	DOCUMENTATION

Form CMS-807 (7/95)

EXHIBIT 96

OSCAR REPORT 3
HISTORY FACILITY PROFILE

PAGE: 1

FACILITY

PROVIDER #:
PHONE NUMBER:
PARTICIPATION DATE: 11/28/1969

FACILITY BEDS
TOTAL: 83
CERTIFIED: 83

TYPE ACTION: RECERTIFICATION
TYPE OWNERSHIP: FOR PROFIT – CORPORATION

STATE'S REGION CODE: 001

COMPLIANCE STATUS: FACILITY MEETS REQUIREMENTS BASED ON AN ACCEPTABLE PLAN OF CORRECTION

LTC ADMISSION/SUSPENSION DATES

ADMISSION SUSPENDED:
SUSPENSION RESCINDED:

TOTAL CERTIFIED BEDS: 83

18	18/19	19	ICF/MR
-	83	-	

RESIDENT CENSUS ON 10/03/2001

	TOTAL:	73
	MEDICARE:	6
	MEDICAID:	61
	OTHER:	6

CURRENT SURVEY REVISIT DATES - 12/13/2001 11/21/2001

PRIOR 3 SURVEY 05/1998	S/S CODE	PRIOR 2 SURVEY 04/1999	S/S CODE	PRIOR 1 SURVEY 07/2000	S/S CODE	CURRENT SURVEY 10/03/2001	S/S CODE	PLAN/DATE OF CORRECT		PROGRAM REQUIREMENTS
									REQ	F0159-FACILITY MANAGEMENT OF RES FUNDS
X	D	X		X	C				REQ	F0164-PERSONAL PRIVACY/CONFIDENTIALITY OF RECORDS
						X C	C	11/21/2001	REQ	F0167-SURVEY RESULTS READILY ACCESSIBLE TO RESIDENTS
									REQ	F0221-RIGHT TO BE FREE FROM PHYSICAL RESTRAINTS NOT REQ
		X		X	D		D		REQ	F0224-FACILITY PROHIBITS ABUSE, NEGLECT
X	D	X	G			X C	D	11/21/2001	REQ	F0225-NOT EMPLOY PERSONS GUILTY OF ABUSE
				X	D				REQ	F0241-DIGNITY
				X	D				REQ	F0248-ACTIVITY PROGRAM MEETS INDIVIDUAL NEEDS
X	D	X	D	X	D				REQ	F0250-MEDICALLY RELATED SOCIAL SERVICES
X	B								REQ	F0252-SAFE/CLEAN/COMFORTABLE/HOMELIKE ENVIRONMENT
				X	C				REQ	F0253-HOUSEKEEPING & MAINTENANCE SERVICES
X	E								REQ	F0272-COMPREHENSIVE ASSESSMENTS
		X	D		D	X C	D	11/21/2001	REQ	F0274-ASSESSMENT AFTER A SIGNIFICANT CHANGE
		X	D		D				REQ	F0278-ACCURACY OF ASSESSMENTS/COORD W/PROFESSIONALS
X	D	X	H						REQ	F0279-DEVELOP COMPREHENSIVE CARE PLANS
X	E	X		X	D				REQ	F0281-SERVICES PROVIDED MEET PROFESSIONAL STANDARDS
						X C	D	12/13/2001	REQ	F0282-SERVS BY QUALIFIED PERSONS IN ACCORD W/ CARE PLAN
X	G	X	D			X C	D	11/21/2001	REQ	F0310-ADLS DO NOT DECLINE UNLESS UNAVOIDABLE
X	E	X	G			X C	D	11/21/2001	REQ	F0312-ADL CARE PROVIDED FOR DEPENDENT RESIDENTS
									REQ	F0314-PROPER TREATMENT TO PREVENT/HEAL PRESSURE SORES
X	E	X	D	X	D		D		REQ	F0316-APPROPRIATE TREATMENT FOR INCONTINENT RES
									REQ	F0318-RANGE OF MOTION TREATMENT & SERVICES
X	D	X	G	X	G	X C	D	11/21/2001	REQ	F0322-PROPER CARE & SERVICES FOR RES W/ NG TUBE
		X	D			X C	G	11/21/2001	REQ	F0324-SUPERVISION/DEVICES TO PREVENT ACCIDENTS
X	D								REQ	F0325-RES MAINTAIN NUTRITIONAL STATUS UNLESS UNAVOIDABL
									REQ	F0327-FACILITY PROVIDES SUFFICIENT FLUID INTAKE

C=DATE OF CORRECTION   N=NO DATE GIVEN   P=PLAN OF CORRECTION   R=REFUSED TO CORRECT   W=WAIVED   X=DEFICIENT
COP = CONDITION   REQ = REQUIREMENT

1RUN DATE OF REPORT: 07/03/2003

LAST FILE UPDATE: 07/02/2003

497

EXHIBIT 96 (continued)

OSCAR REPORT 3
HISTORY FACILITY PROFILE

PAGE: 2

FACILITY   PROVIDER #:

PRIOR 3 SURVEY 05/1998	S/S CODE	PRIOR 2 SURVEY 04/1999	S/S CODE	PRIOR 1 SURVEY 07/2000	S/S CODE	CURRENT SURVEY 10/03/2001	S/S CODE	PLAN/DATE OF CORRECT	PROGRAM REQUIREMENTS
X	G				F				REQ F0329-DRUG REGIMEN IS FREE FROM UNNECESSARY DRUGS
X	E				C				REQ F0332-MEDICATION ERROR RATES OF 5% OR MORE
		X	F	X	D				REQ F0353-SUFFICIENT NURSING STAFF ON A 24-HOUR BASIS
				X	F				REQ F0364-FOOD PROPERLY PREPARED, PALATABLE, ETC.
				X	D				REQ F0367-THERAPEUTIC DIET PRESCRIBED BY PHYSICIAN
X	C	X	C	X					REQ F0371-STORE/PREPARE/DISTRIB FOOD UNDER SANITARY CONDS
									REQ F0426-FACILITY PROVIDES PHARMACEUTICAL SERVICES
		X	D	X	D				REQ F0432-DRUGS STORED IN LOCKED COMPARTMENTS/UND PROP TEMP
									REQ F0441-FACILITY ESTABLISHES INFECTION CONTROL PROG
						X	C	D 11/21/2001	REQ F0444-WASH HANDS WHEN INDICATED
						X	C	C 11/21/2001	REQ F0445-HANDLE LINENS TO PREVENT SPREAD OF INFECTION
		X	F						REQ F0465-ENVIRONMENT IS SAFE/FUNCTIONAL/SANITARY/COMFORTAB
		X	C						REQ F0466-PROCEDURES TO ENSURE WATER AVAILABILITY
		X	F						REQ F0493-GOVERNING BODY APPOINTS ADMIN; MANAGES FACILITY
		X	D						REQ F0514-CLINICAL RECORDS MEET PROFESSIONAL STANDARDS

EDITION OF LSC APPLIED

85 EXIST PRIOR 3 SURVEY 05/1998	85 EXIST PRIOR 2 SURVEY 04/1999	85 EXIST PRIOR 1 SURVEY 07/2000	85 EXIST CURRENT SURVEY 10/09/2001	PLAN/DATE OF CORRECTION	LSC DEFICIENCIES - BLDG NO. 01
X					K0012-CONSTRUCTION TYPE
	X				K0017-CORRIDOR WALLS
X	X	X	X C	11/20/2001	K0025-SMOKE PARTITION CONSTRUCTION
X	X	X			K0029-HAZARDOUS AREAS - SEPARATION
X	X				K0038-EXIT ACCESS
X	X		X C	11/20/2001	K0046-EMERGENCY LIGHTING
	X				K0047-EXIT SIGNS
X					K0048-EVACUATION PLAN
X	X	X C	X C	11/20/2001	K0050-FIRE DRILLS
X	X		X C	11/20/2001	K0051-FIRE ALARM SYSTEM
	X				K0052-TESTING OF FIRE ALARM
					K0056-AUTOMATIC SPRINKLER SYSTEM
X	X				K0062-SPRINKLER SYSTEM MAINTENANCE
	X				K0066-SMOKING REGULATIONS
X	X				K0067-VENTILATING EQUIPMENT
X	X				K0069-COOKING EQUIPMENT
X	X	X C	X C	11/20/2001	K0072-FURNISHING AND DECORATIONS
X	X	X C	X C	11/20/2001	K0076-MEDICAL GAS SYSTEM
					K0130-OTHER

C=DATE OF CORRECTION   N=NO DATE GIVEN   P=PLAN OF CORRECTION   R=REFUSED TO CORRECT   W=WAIVED   F=FSES   X=DEFICIENT
COP = CONDITION   REQ = REQUIREMENT

RUN DATE OF REPORT: 07/03/2003   LAST FILE UPDATE: 07/02/2003

498

EXHIBIT 96 (continued)

OSCAR REPORT 4
FULL FACILITY PROFILE

PAGE: 1

FACILITY

PROVIDER #:	TYPE ACTION: RECERTIFICATION
PHONE NUMBER:	TYPE OWNERSHIP: FOR PROFIT - CORPORATION
PARTICIPATION DATE: 07/01/1967	

STATE'S REGION CODE: 001

FACILITY BEDS
TOTAL: 83
CERTIFIED: 83

TOTAL CERTIFIED BEDS: 83

COMPLIANCE STATUS: FACILITY MEETS REQUIREMENTS BASED ON AN ACCEPTABLE PLAN OF CORRECTION

RESIDENT CENSUS ON 10/09/2001   LTC ADMISSION/SUSPENSION DATES

TOTAL:	73	ADMISSION SUSPENDED:
MEDICARE:	6	SUSPENSION RESCINDED:
MEDICAID:	61	
OTHER:	6	

18	18/19	19	ICF/MR
—	—	83	—

PROGRAM REQUIREMENTS

SURVEY DATES FROM: 10/01/2001 TO: 10/03/2001
EXTENDED SURVEY DATES FROM: TO:
DATE PROVIDER SIGNED POC: 10/22/2001
REVISIT DATES: 12/13/2001 11/21/2001

					# AND PERCENT OF FACILITIES NOT MEETING REQUIREMENT - AFTER 09/30/1990					
					STATE		REGION		NATION	
S/S CODE	TAG #	REQUIREMENT	PLAN/DATE OF CORRECTION	STATUS OF DEFICIENCY	#	%	#	%	#	%
C	F0167	SURVEY RESULTS READILY ACCESSIBLE TO RESIDENTS	11/21/2001	DEFICIENCY CORRECTED	4	2.3	56	3.3	371	3.7
D	F0225	NOT EMPLOY PERSONS GUILTY OF ABUSE	11/21/2001	DEFICIENCY CORRECTED	22	13.0	190	11.3	1132	11.4
D	F0274	ASSESSMENT AFTER A SIGNIFICANT CHANGE	11/21/2001	DEFICIENCY CORRECTED	17	10.0	95	5.6	401	4.0
D	F0282	SERVS BY QUALIFIED PERSONS IN ACCORD W/ CARE PLA	12/13/2001	DEFICIENCY CORRECTED	67	39.6	260	15.5	1040	10.4
D	F0310	ADLS DO NOT DECLINE UNLESS UNAVOIDABLE	11/21/2001	DEFICIENCY CORRECTED	1	0.5	24	1.4	124	1.2
D	F0312	ADL CARE PROVIDED FOR DEPENDENT RESIDENTS	11/21/2001	DEFICIENCY CORRECTED	51	30.1	214	12.8	1172	11.8
G	F0322	PROPER CARE & SERVICES FOR RES W/ NG TUBE	11/21/2001	DEFICIENCY CORRECTED	18	10.6	141	8.4	564	5.6
G	F0324	SUPERVISION/DEVICES TO PREVENT ACCIDENTS	11/21/2001	DEFICIENCY CORRECTED	20	11.8	233	13.9	1896	19.1
D	F0444	WASH HANDS WHEN INDICATED	11/21/2001	DEFICIENCY CORRECTED	33	19.5	152	9.1	820	8.2
C	F0445	HANDLE LINENS TO PREVENT SPREAD OF INFECTION	11/21/2001	DEFICIENCY CORRECTED	6	3.5	55	3.2	297	2.9

BUILDING CHARACTERISTICS

BUILDING NUMBER	TYPE OF BUILDING	EDITION OF LSC APPLIED	LSC COMPLIANCE STATUS
01	BUILDING	85 EXIST	FACILITY MEETS REQUIREMENTS BASED ON AN ACCEPTABLE POC

LSC DEFICIENCIES

SURVEY DATES FROM: 10/01/2001 TO: 10/03/2001
EXTENDED SURVEY DATES FROM: TO:
DATE PROVIDER SIGNED POC: 10/29/2001
REVISIT DATES: 11/20/2001

					# AND PERCENT OF FACILITIES NOT MEETING REQUIREMENT - AFTER 09/30/1990					
					STATE		REGION		NATION	
BUILDING NUM	TAG #	REQUIREMENT	PLAN/DATE OF CORRECTION	STATUS OF DEFICIENCY	#	%	#	%	#	%

LAST FILE UPDATE: 07/02/2003

RUN DATE OF REPORT: 07/03/2003

499

EXHIBIT 96 (*continued*)

OSCAR REPORT 4
FULL FACILITY PROFILE

LSC DEFICIENCIES

FACILITY

PROVIDER #:

SURVEY DATES FROM: 10/01/2001 TO: 10/03/2001
EXTENDED SURVEY DATES FROM: TO:
DATE PROVIDER SIGNED POC: 10/29/2001
REVISIT DATES: 11/20/2001

BUILDING NUM	TAG #	REQUIREMENT	PLAN/DATE OF CORRECTION	STATUS OF DEFICIENCY	NOT MEETING REQUIREMENT - AFTER 09/30/1990 STATE		REGION		NATION	
					#	%	#	%	#	%
01	K0025	SMOKE PARTITION CONSTRUCTION	11/20/2001	DEFICIENCY CORRECTED	35	20.7	147	8.8	1057	10.6
01	K0046	EMERGENCY LIGHTING	11/20/2001	DEFICIENCY CORRECTED	10	5.9	87	5.2	589	5.9
01	K0050	FIRE DRILLS	11/20/2001	DEFICIENCY CORRECTED	56	33.1	186	11.1	764	7.6
01	K0051	FIRE ALARM SYSTEM	11/20/2001	DEFICIENCY CORRECTED	44	26.0	155	9.2	589	5.9
01	K0076	MEDICAL GAS SYSTEM	11/20/2001	DEFICIENCY CORRECTED	38	22.4	143	8.5	738	7.4
01	K0130	OTHER	11/20/2001	DEFICIENCY CORRECTED	49	28.9	230	13.7	1379	13.8

1RUN DATE OF REPORT: 07/03/2003

LAST FILE UPDATE: 07/02/2003

EXHIBIT 96 (continued)

OSCAR REPORT 4
FULL FACILITY PROFILE

FACILITY

PROVIDER #:

RESIDENT CHARACTERISTICS

		FACILITY #	FACILITY %	STATE %	REGION %	NATION %
F075	NUMBER OF RESIDENTS WHO ARE MEDICARE BENEFICIARIES.	6	8.2	10.9	12.6	11.1
F076	NUMBER OF RESIDENTS WHO ARE MEDICAID RECIPIENTS.	61	83.5	72.7	71.7	67.6
F077	NUMBER OF RESIDENTS NOT MEDICARE OR MEDICAID BENEFICIARIES.	6	8.2	16.3	15.6	21.1
F078	TOTAL NUMBER OF RESIDENTS/CLIENTS	73	100.0	100.0	100.0	100.0
F079	BATHING – NUMBER OF INDEPENDENT RESIDENTS.	2	2.7	4.0	3.8	4.3
F080	BATHING – NUMBER OF RESIDENTS ASSISTED BY STAFF.	36	49.3	52.8	51.6	56.1
F081	BATHING – NUMBER OF RESIDENTS DEPENDENT ON STAFF.	35	47.9	43.0	44.4	39.5
F082	DRESSING – NUMBER OF INDEPENDENT RESIDENTS.	8	10.9	10.8	9.6	11.2
F083	DRESSING – NUMBER OF RESIDENTS ASSISTED BY STAFF.	30	41.0	54.4	53.5	56.2
F084	DRESSING – NUMBER OF RESIDENTS DEPENDENT ON STAFF.	35	47.9	34.6	36.7	32.5
F085	TRANSFERRING – NUMBER OF INDEPENDENT RESIDENTS.	21	28.7	24.4	21.5	23.4
F086	TRANSFERRING – NUMBER OF RESIDENTS ASSISTED BY STAFF.	23	31.5	42.8	46.0	49.2
F087	TRANSFERRING – NUMBER OF RESIDENTS DEPENDENT ON STAFF.	29	39.7	32.6	32.4	27.2
F088	TOILET USE – NUMBER OF INDEPENDENT RESIDENTS.	19	26.0	20.0	16.7	18.4
F089	TOILET USE – NUMBER OF RESIDENTS ASSISTED BY STAFF.	22	30.1	39.0	41.2	46.4
F090	TOILET USE – NUMBER OF RESIDENTS DEPENDENT ON STAFF.	32	43.8	40.8	42.0	35.0
F091	EATING – NUMBER OF INDEPENDENT RESIDENTS.	21	28.7	48.9	46.1	48.3
F092	EATING – NUMBER OF RESIDENTS ASSISTED BY STAFF.	27	36.9	26.5	30.5	32.3
F093	EATING – NUMBER OF RESIDENTS DEPENDENT ON STAFF.	25	34.2	24.4	23.3	19.2
F094	CONTINENCE – NUMBER OF RESIDENTS WITH INDWELLING OR EXTERNAL CATHETER.	6	8.2	5.2	6.2	6.3
F095	NUMBER OF RESIDENTS WITH CATHETERS PRESENT ON ADMISSION	4	5.4	4.0	4.3	4.4

RUN DATE OF REPORT: 07/03/2003

LAST FILE UPDATE: 07/02/2003

EXHIBIT 96 (continued)

OSCAR REPORT 4
FULL FACILITY PROFILE

FACILITY

PROVIDER #:

RESIDENT CHARACTERISTICS

		FACILITY #	FACILITY %	STATE %	REGION %	NATION %
F096	CONTINENCE – NUMBER OF RESIDENTS OCCASIONALLY OR FREQUENTLY INCONTINENT OF BLADDER.	30	41.0	56.7	57.6	56.3
F097	CONTINENCE – NUMBER OF RESIDENTS OCCASIONALLY OR FREQUENTLY INCONTINENT OF BOWEL.	35	47.9	51.2	52.6	46.5
F098	CONTINENCE – NUMBER OF RESIDENTS ON INDIVIDUALLY WRITTEN BLADDER TRAINING PROGRAM.	4	5.4	10.0	5.8	6.0
F099	CONTINENCE – NUMBER OF RESIDENTS ON INDIVIDUALLY WRITTEN BOWEL TRAINING PROGRAM.	4	5.4	7.2	4.0	3.7
F100	MOBILITY – NUMBER OF RESIDENTS WHO ARE BEDFAST MOST OR ALL OF THE TIME.	1	1.3	8.2	6.6	4.0
F101	MOBILITY – NUMBER OF RESIDENTS IN CHAIRS MOST OR ALL OF THE TIME.	57	78.0	55.6	57.6	56.9
F102	MOBILITY – NUMBER OF INDEPENDENTLY AMBULATORY RESIDENTS	1	1.3	11.8	11.4	13.2
F103	MOBILITY – NUMBER OF RESIDENTS NEEDING ASSISTANCE OR ASSISTIVE DEVICE FOR AMBULATION.	14	19.1	27.1	27.0	30.8
F104	MOBILITY – NUMBER OF PHYSICALLY RESTRAINED RESIDENTS.	11	15.0	4.4	9.4	8.8
F105	MOBILITY – NUMBER OF RESIDENTS ADMITTED WITH ORDERS FOR RESTRAINTS.	0	0.0	0.4	1.3	2.0
F106	MOBILITY – NUMBER OF RESIDENTS WITH CONTRACTURES	19	26.0	31.3	31.5	31.1
F107	MOBILITY – NUMBER OF RESIDENTS WITH CONTRACTURES AT TIME OF ADMISSION.	17	23.2	20.1	17.8	19.3
F108	MENTAL STATUS – NUMBER OF RESIDENTS WITH MENTAL RETARDATION.	3	4.1	4.5	2.9	2.6
F109	MENTAL STATUS – NUMBER OF RESIDENTS WITH DOCUMENTED SIGNS AND SYMPTOMS OF DEPRESSION.	36	49.3	39.7	40.7	41.6
F110	MENTAL STATUS – NUMBER OF RESIDENTS WITH DOCUMENTED PSYCHIATRIC DIAGNOSIS (EXCLUDING DEMENTIAS AND DEPRESSION.)	7	9.5	18.6	18.2	17.5
F111	MENTAL STATUS – NUMBER OF RESIDENTS WITH DEMENTIA: MULTI-INFARCT, SENILE, ALZHEIMER'S TYPE, OR OTHER THAN ALZHEIMER'S TYPE	20	27.3	53.8	48.3	46.0

RUN DATE OF REPORT: 07/03/2003

OSCAR REPORT 4

EXHIBIT 96 (continued)

FULL FACILITY PROFILE

PROVIDER #:

RESIDENT CHARACTERISTICS

FACILITY

		FACILITY #	FACILITY %	STATE %	REGION %	NATION %
F112	MENTAL STATUS – NUMBER OF RESIDENTS WITH BEHAVIORAL SYMPTOMS.	2	2.7	26.0	29.0	30.5
F113	MENTAL STATUS – NUMBER OF RESIDENTS WITH BEHAVIORAL SYMPTOMS RECEIVING A BEHAVIOR MANAGEMENT PROGRAM.	1	1.3	18.0	12.3	13.6
F114	MENTAL STATUS – NUMBER OF RESIDENTS RECEIVING HEALTH REHABILITATIVE SERVICES FOR MI/MR.	0	0.0	4.3	3.0	3.1
F115	SKIN INTEGRITY – NUMBER OF RESIDENTS WITH PRESSURE SORES, EXCLUDING STAGE 1.	3	4.1	5.5	7.4	7.2
F116	SKIN INTEGRITY – NUMBER OF RESIDENTS WITH PRESSURE SORES ON ADMISSION.	0	0.0	3.3	3.9	3.7
F117	NUMBER OF RESIDENTS RECEIVING PREVENTIVE SKIN CARE.	4	5.4	77.8	74.9	69.6
F118	SKIN INTEGRITY – NUMBER OF RESIDENTS WITH SKIN RASHES.	2	2.7	3.7	4.8	5.3
F119	SPECIAL CARE – NUMBER OF RESIDENTS RECEIVING HOSPICE CARE BENEFIT.	1	1.3	2.7	2.7	2.0
F120	SPECIAL CARE – NUMBER OF RESIDENTS RECEIVING RADIATION THERAPY.	0	0.0	0.0	0.1	0.1
F121	SPECIAL CARE – NUMBER OF RESIDENTS RECEIVING CHEMOTHERAPY.	0	0.0	0.1	0.2	0.4
F122	SPECIAL CARE – NUMBER OF RESIDENTS RECEIVING DIALYSIS.	0	0.0	0.9	1.4	1.2
F123	NUMBER OF RESIDENTS RECEIVING INTRAVENOUS THERAPY, PARENTERAL NUTRITION, AND/OR BLOOD TRANSFUSIONS.	0	0.0	0.6	1.3	1.3
F124	SPECIAL CARE – NUMBER OF RESIDENTS RECEIVING RESPIRATORY TREATMENT.	4	5.4	8.4	9.7	9.7
F125	SPECIAL CARE – NUMBER OF RESIDENTS RECEIVING TRACHEOSTOMY CARE.	0	0.0	0.2	0.6	0.9
F126	SPECIAL CARE – NUMBER OF RESIDENTS RECEIVING OSTOMY CARE	6	8.2	6.5	5.4	4.3
F127	SPECIAL CARE – NUMBER OF RESIDENTS RECEIVING SUCTIONING	0	0.0	1.1	1.3	1.4
F128	SPECIAL CARE – NUMBER OF RESIDENTS RECEIVING INJECTIONS	17	23.2	14.1	15.1	13.8

RUN DATE OF REPORT: 07/03/2003

OSCAR REPORT 4

(continued)

EXHIBIT 96 (continued)

FACILITY

PROVIDER #:

FULL FACILITY PROFILE

RESIDENT CHARACTERISTICS

		FACILITY #	FACILITY %	STATE %	REGION %	NATION %
F129	SPECIAL CARE - NUMBER OF RESIDENTS RECEIVING TUBE FEEDINGS.	4	5.4	11.1	9.4	6.9
F130	SPECIAL CARE - NUMBER OF RESIDENTS RECEIVING MECHANICALLY ALTERED DIETS INCLUDING PUREED AND ALL CHOPPED FOOD.	38	52.0	39.9	39.7	35.9
F131	SPECIAL CARE - NUMBER OF RESIDENTS RECEIVING SPECIALIZED REHABILITATIVE SERVICES.	21	28.7	13.2	16.1	15.6
F132	SPECIAL CARE - NUMBER OF RESIDENTS USING ASSISTIVE DEVICES WHILE EATING.	15	20.5	5.4	5.4	8.0
F133	MEDICATIONS - NUMBER OF RESIDENTS RECEIVING PSYCHOACTIVE DRUGS.	48	65.7	60.1	60.1	58.8
F134	MEDICATIONS - NUMBER OF RESIDENTS RECEIVING ANTIPSYCHOTIC MEDICATIONS.	29	39.7	23.1	25.6	24.5
F135	MEDICATIONS - NUMBER OF RESIDENTS RECEIVING ANTIANXIETY MEDICATIONS.	5	6.8	15.8	18.6	15.3
F136	MEDICATIONS - NUMBER OF RESIDENTS RECEIVING ANTIDEPRESSANT MEDICATIONS.	34	46.5	44.5	40.9	40.6
F137	MEDICATIONS - NUMBER OF RESIDENTS RECEIVING HYPNOTIC MEDICATIONS.	0	0.0	4.1	6.6	4.8
F138	MEDICATIONS - NUMBER OF RESIDENTS RECEIVING ANTIBIOTICS.	8	10.9	7.0	8.2	7.6
F139	MEDICATIONS - NUMBER OF RESIDENTS ON PAIN MANAGEMENT PROGRAM.	12	16.4	23.1	17.9	21.9
F140	OTHER - NUMBER OF RESIDENTS WITH UNPLANNED SIGNIFICANT WEIGHT LOSS/GAIN.	1	1.3	8.5	8.3	7.6
F141	OTHER - NUMBER OF RESIDENTS WHO DO NOT COMMUNICATE IN DOMINANT LANGUAGE OF FACILITY, INCLUDING THOSE WHO USE SIGN LANGUAGE.	0	0.0	0.3	1.6	2.8
F142	OTHER - NUMBER OF RESIDENTS WHO USE NON-ORAL COMMUNICATION DEVICES.	0	0.0	2.8	3.3	3.7

RUN DATE OF REPORT: 07/03/2003

OSCAR REPORT 4

EXHIBIT 96 (continued)

FULL FACILITY PROFILE

FACILITY

PROVIDER #:

RESIDENT CHARACTERISTICS

	FACILITY #	FACILITY %	STATE %	REGION %	NATION %
F143 OTHER – NUMBER OF RESIDENTS WITH ADVANCE DIRECTIVES.	48	65.7	42.3	53.3	61.6
F144 THE NUMBER OF RESIDENTS WHO RECEIVED INFLUENZA IMMUNIZATIONS.	51	69.8	56.8	53.9	63.8
F145 THE NUMBER OF RESIDENTS WHO RECEIVED PNEUMOCOCCAL VACCINE	0	0.0	23.3	24.2	34.4

1RUN DATE OF REPORT: 07/03/2003

LAST FILE UPDATE: 07/02/2003

(continued)

505

EXHIBIT 96 (continued)

OSCAR REPORT 4
FULL FACILITY PROFILE

FACILITY

PROVIDER #:

TYPE OF DEFICIENCY	TOTAL THIS FACILITY	AVERAGE NUMBER OF DEFICIENCIES PER FACILITY		
		STATE	REGION	NATION
CONDITION/LEVEL A	0	0.00	0.00	00.00
REQUIREMENT	10	5.99	6.47	06.04
HEALTH TOTAL	10	5.99	6.47	06.04
LIFE SAFETY CODE	6	3.65	1.92	02.24
LIFE SAFETY CODE + HEALTH	16	9.65	8.39	08.28

506

EXHIBIT 259

MINIMUM DATA SET AUTOMATION CONTRACT/AGREEMENT APPROVAL RO CHECKLIST

Background: All certified nursing homes are required to encode and transmit MDS records to a repository maintained by the State in accordance with HCFA-established record specifications and time frames. Provider costs will be compensated through the Medicare and Medicaid programs according to the rules for such reimbursement effective in each State. It is expected that overall responsibility for fulfilling requirements to operate the State MDS data system will rest with the State survey agency. However, the State survey agency may enter an agreement with the State Medicaid agency, another State component or a private contractor to perform day-to-day operations of the system. **Before entering an agreement with a subcontractor, i.e., if the State MDS system is operated by an entity other than the survey agency, the survey agency must receive HCFA RO approval. Such agreements must include the following provisions:**

1. Meets confidentiality requirements: Federal Privacy Act, 5 U.S.C. Section 522a; HIPAA of 1996; other applicable Federal data acts; Section 1902 (a)(7) of the Social Security Act; applicable State standards; and industry security standards.

2. Gives State survey agency real-time access to the system to fully support all MDS-driven functions which will be required of the survey agency (e.g., quality indicator reporting, survey targeting), or if contractor is performing analysis for State agency details how.

3. Complies with need for high capacity, fault-tolerant network connections to ensure reliable support for the State survey agencies, HCFA's national database and any other daily operations (e.g., FI Medical Case Review, OIG or DOJ Fraud and Abuse activities), which will be affected by this system. Assures hardware will be properly maintained and upgraded as necessary to meet any future HCFA or State survey agency requirements. Assures adequate backup of all data.

4. Covers State survey agency responsibilities for reporting MDS data to a central repository at HCFA. Designates responsibilities for edits and "cleanness" of data. Designates responsibilities for generating and communicating facility error reports. Describes what kinds of communication will be established, e.g., a State-specific Internet and/or Intranet web pages, newsletters, their content, and who will produce/maintain/distribute these communications. If there is a separate database, designates who is responsible for operating and maintaining the HCFA-provided equipment and who will assure the viability of the HCFA database.

5. Covers responsibilities of contractor and/or State for training and support operations: Including at least who will provide facility and MDS software vendor startup training, and ongoing customer/facility support/troubleshooting; provide internal training and daily user support within the State agency; work with

(continued)

EXHIBIT 259 *(continued)*

program staff to integrate the MDS system into State survey agency functions; train State survey agency staff on aspects of analytical system (e.g., ASPEN upgrades and performance measure/"quality indicator" linked reports); handle System Operations -- functions associated with transmission logging, error tracking and resolution, system archival and process reporting; designates who is responsible for determining facility transmission schedules

6. Delineates how State will fund the monthly line charges associated with installation, maintenance, and transmission of the MDS data from the facilities to the contractor and between the contractor and State, e.g., built into contract costs or is an outside ongoing cost to the State survey agency..

7. Specifies whether it is the contractor's or the State survey agency's responsibility for systems maintenance for commercial "off-the-shelf" MDS hardware and software components. For example, are these covered under typical umbrella service agreements that the State or contractor may already have in place for maintenance of data processing equipment? If not, what is the process?

EXHIBIT 260

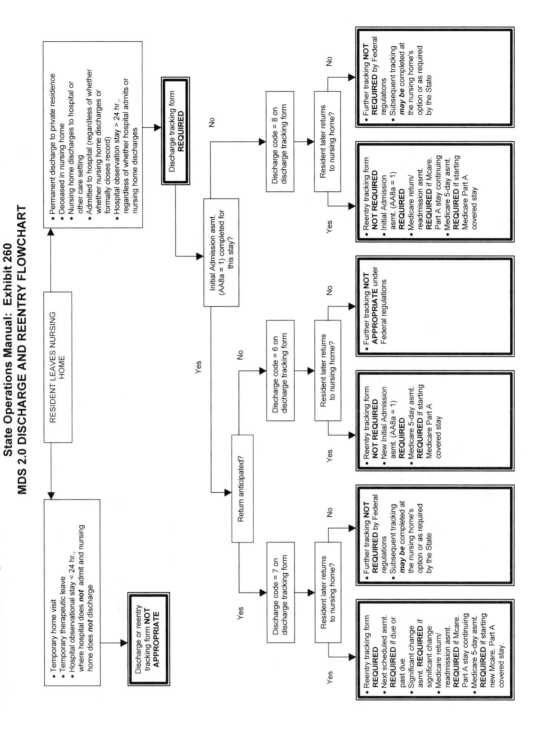

State Operations Manual: Exhibit 260
MDS 2.0 DISCHARGE AND REENTRY FLOWCHART

HCFA'S RAI Version 2.0 Q & A'S

RESIDENT LEAVES NURSING HOME

- Temporary home visit
- Temporary therapeutic leave
- Hospital observational stay < 24 hr., where hospital does **not** admit and nursing home does **not** discharge

Discharge or reentry tracking form **NOT APPROPRIATE**

- Permanent discharge to private residence
- Deceased in nursing home
- Nursing home discharges to hospital or other care setting
- Admitted to hospital (regardless of whether whether nursing home discharges or formally closes record)
- Hospital observation stay > 24 hr., regardless of whether hospital admits or nursing home discharges

Discharge tracking form **REQUIRED**

Initial Admission asmt. (AA8a = 1) completed for this stay?

Yes → Return anticipated?

No → Discharge code = 8 on discharge tracking form

Return anticipated? — Yes
Discharge code = 7 on discharge tracking form

Resident later returns to nursing home?

- **Yes:**
  - Reentry tracking form **REQUIRED**
  - Next scheduled asmt. **REQUIRED** if due or past due
  - Significant change asmt. **REQUIRED** if significant change
  - Medicare return/ readmission asmt. **REQUIRED** if Mcare. Part A stay continuing
  - Medicare 5-day asmt. **REQUIRED** if starting new Mcare. Part A covered stay.

- **No:**
  - Further tracking **NOT REQUIRED** by Federal regulations
  - Subsequent tracking **may be** completed at the nursing home's option or as required by the State

Return anticipated? — No
Discharge code = 6 on discharge tracking form

Resident later returns to nursing home?

- **Yes:**
  - Reentry tracking form **NOT REQUIRED**
  - New Initial Admission asmt. (AA8a = 1) **REQUIRED**
  - Medicare 5-day asmt. **REQUIRED** if starting Medicare Part A covered stay

- **No:**
  - Further tracking **NOT APPRIATE** under Federal regulations

Initial Admission asmt. — No
Discharge code = 8 on discharge tracking form

Resident later returns to nursing home?

- **Yes:**
  - Reentry tracking form **NOT REQUIRED**
  - Initial Admission asmt. (AA8a = 1) **REQUIRED**
  - Medicare return/ readmission asmt. **REQUIRED** if Mcare. Part A stay continuing
  - Medicare 5-day asmt. **REQUIRED** if starting Medicare Part A covered stay

- **No:**
  - Further tracking **NOT REQUIRED** by Federal regulations
  - Subsequent tracking **may be** completed at the nursing home's option or as required by the State

509

EXHIBIT 261

PRIVACY ACT STATEMENT - HEALTH CARE RECORDS

THIS STATEMENT GIVES YOU ADVICE REQUIRED BY LAW (the Privacy Act of 1974).
THIS STATEMENT IS NOT A CONSENT FORM. IT WILL NOT BE USED TO RELEASE OR TO USE YOUR HEALTH CARE INFORMATION.

I. AUTHORITY FOR COLLECTION OF YOUR INFORMATION, INCLUDING YOUR SOCIAL SECURITY NUMBER, AND WHETHER OR NOT YOU ARE REQUIRED TO PROVIDE INFORMATION FOR THIS ASSESSMENT.
Sections 1102(a), 1154, 1861(o), 1861(z), 1863, 1864, 1865, 1866, 1871, 1891(b) of the Social Security Act.

Medicare and Medicaid participating home health agencies must do a complete assessment that accurately reflects your current health and includes information that can be used to show your progress toward your health goals. The home health agency must use the "Outcome and Assessment Information Set" (OASIS) when evaluating your health. To do this, the agency must get information from every patient. This information is used by the Centers for Medicare & Medicaid Services (CMS, the federal Medicare & Medicaid agency) to be sure that the home health agency meets quality standards and gives appropriate health care to its patients. You have the right to refuse to provide information for the assessment to the home health agency. If your information is included in an assessment, it is protected under the federal Privacy Act of 1974 and the "Home Health Agency Outcome and Assessment Information Set" (HHA OASIS) System of Records. You have the right to see, copy, review, and request correction of your information in the HHA OASIS System of Records.

II. PRINCIPAL PURPOSES FOR WHICH YOUR INFORMATION IS INTENDED TO BE USED

The information collected will be entered into the Home Health Agency Outcome and Assessment Information Set (HHA OASIS) System No. 09-70-9002. Your health care information in the HHA OASIS System of Records will be used for the following purposes:
- support litigation involving the Centers for Medicare & Medicaid Services;
- support regulatory, reimbursement, and policy functions performed within the Centers for Medicare & Medicaid Services or by a contractor or consultant;
- study the effectiveness and quality of care provided by those home health agencies;
- survey and certification of Medicare and Medicaid home health agencies;
- provide for development, validation, and refinement of a Medicare prospective payment system;
- enable regulators to provide home health agencies with data for their internal quality improvement activities;
- support research, evaluation, or epidemiological projects related to the prevention of disease or disability, or the restoration or maintenance of health, and for health care payment related projects; and
- support constituent requests made to a Congressional representative.

III. ROUTINE USES

These "routine uses" specify the circumstances when the Centers for Medicare & Medicaid Services may release your information from the HHA OASIS System of Records without your consent. Each prospective recipient must agree in writing to ensure the continuing confidentiality and security of your information. Disclosures of the information may be to:
1. the federal Department of Justice for litigation involving the Centers for Medicare & Medicaid Services;
2. contractors or consultants working for the Centers for Medicare & Medicaid Services to assist in the performance of a service related to this system of records and who need to access these records to perform the activity;
3. an agency of a State government for purposes of determining, evaluating, and/or assessing cost, effectiveness, and/or quality of health care services provided in the State; for developing and operating Medicaid reimbursement systems; or for the administration of Federal/State home health agency programs within the State;
4. another Federal or State agency to contribute to the accuracy of the Centers for Medicare & Medicaid Services' health insurance operations (payment, treatment and coverage) and/or to support State agencies in the evaluations and monitoring of care provided by HHAs;
5. Quality Improvement Organizations, to perform Title XI or Title XVIII functions relating to assessing and improving home health agency quality of care;
6. an individual or organization for a research, evaluation, or epidemiological project related to the prevention of disease or disability, the restoration or maintenance of health, or payment related projects;
7. a congressional office in response to a constituent inquiry made at the written request of the constituent about whom the record is maintained.

IV. EFFECT ON YOU, IF YOU DO NOT PROVIDE INFORMATION

The home health agency needs the information contained in the Outcome and Assessment Information Set in order to give you quality care. It is important that the information be correct. Incorrect information could result in payment errors. Incorrect information also could make it hard to be sure that the agency is giving you quality services. If you choose not to provide information, there is no federal requirement for the home health agency to refuse you services.

NOTE: This statement may be included in the admission packet for all new home health agency admissions. Home health agencies may **request** you or your representative to sign this statement to document that this statement was given to you. **Your signature is NOT required.** If you or your representative sign the statement, the signature merely indicates that you received this statement. You or your representative must be supplied with a copy of this statement.

CONTACT INFORMATION

If you want to ask the Centers for Medicare & Medicaid Services to see, review, copy, or correct your personal health information that the Federal agency maintains in its HHA OASIS System of Records:

Call 1-800-MEDICARE, toll free, for assistance in contacting the HHA OASIS System Manager.
TTY for the hearing and speech impaired: 1-877-486-2048.

EXHIBIT 262

CMS's RAI Version 2.0 Manual   **CH 5: Submission and Correction**

CORRECTION POLICY FLOWCHART

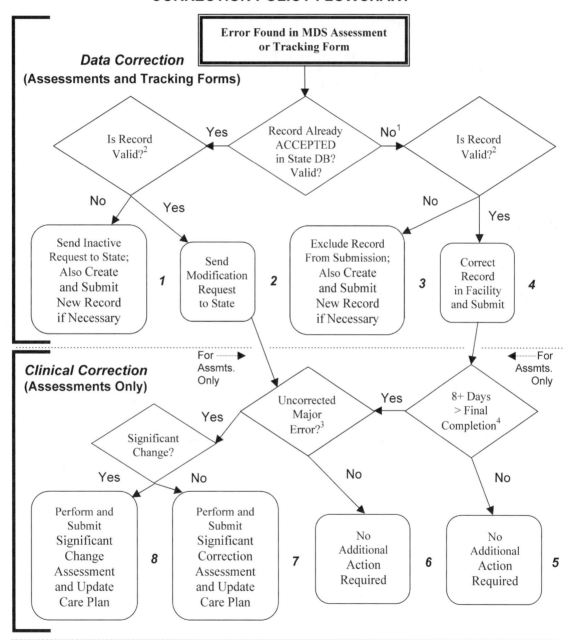

---

[1]Record has not been data entered, has not been submitted, or has been submitted and rejected.

[2]The record is **valid** if **event occurred**, **resident** and **reasons for assessment are correct**, and **submission is required**.

[3]The assessment in error contains a Major error that has not been corrected by a subsequent assessment.

[4]Final completion is Item VB4 for a comprehensive and R2b for all other assessments.

EXHIBIT 263

CMS's RAI Version 2.0 Manual   **CH 5: Submission and Correction**

- **Assessment Transmission:** Comprehensive assessments must be transmitted electronically within 31 days of the Care Plan Completion Date (VB4). All other MDS or MPAF assessments must be submitted within 31 days of the MDS Completion Date (R2b).
- **Tracking Form Transmission:** Tracking forms must be transmitted within 31 days of the Event Date (R4 for Discharge records; A4 for Reentry records).
- **Monthly Transmission Requirements:** A facility must, at least on a monthly basis, electronically transmit to the State MDS database encoded, accurate and complete MDS assessments conducted during the previous month.

SUBMISSION TIME FRAME FOR MDS RECORDS

Type of Record	Primary Reason (AA8a)	Secondary Reason (AA8b)	Final Completion or Event Date	Submit By
Admission Assmt.	01	All values	VB4	VB4 + 31
Annual Assmt.	02	All values	VB4	VB4 + 31
Sign. Change Assmt.	03	All values	VB4	VB4 + 31
Sign. Correction Full Assmt.	04	All values	VB4	VB4 + 31
Quarterly Assmt.	05	All values	R2b	R2b + 31
Sign. Correction Quarterly Assmt.	10	All values	R2b	R2b + 31
Assmt. for Medicare (with AA8a = 00)	00	1, 2, 3, 4, 5, 7 or 8	R2b	R2b + 31
Discharge Tracking	06, 07, 08	Blank	R4	R4 + 31
Reentry Tracking	09	Blank	A4a	A4a + 31
Correction Request	All values	All values	AT6	AT6 + 31

Table Legend:

ITEM   DESCRIPTION

VB4 .... Date of the signature of the person completing the care planning decision on the RAP Summary sheet (Section V), indicating which RAPs are addressed in the care plan (Care Plan Completion Date).

R2b .... Date of the RN assessment coordinator's signature, indicating that the MDS is complete (MDS Completion Date).

R4 .... Date of death or discharge

A4a .... Date of reentry

AT6 .... Date of the RN coordinator's signature on the Correction Request form certifying completion of the correction request information and the corrected assessment or tracking form information.

EXHIBIT 264

DEPARTMENT OF HEALTH AND HUMAN SERVICES
CENTERS FOR MEDICARE & MEDICAID SERVICES

RESIDENT CENSUS AND CONDITIONS OF RESIDENTS

Provider No.	Medicare	Medicaid	Other	Total Residents
	F75	F76	F77	F78

ADL	Independent	Assist of One or Two Staff	Dependent
Bathing	F79	F80	F81
Dressing	F82	F83	F84
Transferring	F85	F86	F87
Toilet Use	F88	F89	F90
Eating	F91	F92	F93

A. Bowel/Bladder Status

F94____ With indwelling or external catheter

F95 Of total number of residents with catheters, ____ were present on admission.

F96____ Occasionally or frequently incontinent of bladder

F97____ Occasionally or frequently incontinent of bowel

F98____ On individually written bladder training program

F99____ On individually written bowel training program

B. Mobility

F100____ Bedfast all or most of time

F101____ In chair all or most of time

F102____ Independently ambulatory

F103____ Ambulation with assistance or assistive device

F104____ Physically restrained

F105 Of total number of residents restrained,____ were admitted with orders for restraints.

F106____ With contractures

F107 Of total number of residents with contractures, ____ had contractures on admission.

C. Mental Status

F108____ With mental retardation

F109____ With documented signs and symptoms of depression

F110____ With documented psychiatric diagnosis (exclude dementias and depression)

F111____ Dementia: multi-infarct, senile, Alzheimer's type, or other than Alzheimer's type

F112____ With behavioral symptoms

F113 Of the total number of residents with behavioral symptoms, the total number receiving a behavior management program ____.

F114____ Receiving health rehabilitative services for MI/MR

D. Skin Integrity

F115____ With pressure sores (exclude Stage I)

F116 Of the total number of residents with pressure sores excluding Stage I, how many residents had pressure sores on admission?____.

F117____ Receiving preventive skin care

F118____ With rashes

(continued)

EXHIBIT 264 *(continued)*

RESIDENT CENSUS AND CONDITIONS OF RESIDENTS

E. Special Care

F119____ Receiving hospice care benefit

F120____ Receiving radiation therapy

F121____ Receiving chemotherapy

F122____ Receiving dialysis

F123____ Receiving intravenous therapy, parenteral nutrition, and/or blood transfusion

F124____ Receiving respiratory treatment

F125____ Receiving tracheostomy care

F126____ Receiving ostomy care

F127____ Receiving suctioning

F128____ Receiving injections (exclude vitamin B12 injections)

F129____ Receiving tube feedings

Fl30____ Receiving mechanically altered diets including pureed and all chopped food (not only meat)

F131____ Receiving specialized rehabilitative services (Physical therapy, speech-language therapy, occupational therapy)

F132____ Assistive devices while eating

F. Medications

F133____ Receiving any psychoactive medication

    F134____ Receiving antipsychotic medications

    F135____ Receiving antianxiety medications

    F136____ Receiving antidepressant medications

    F137____ Receiving hypnotic medications

F138____ Receiving antibiotics

F139____ On pain management program

G. Other

F140____ With unplanned significant weight loss/gain

F141____ Who do not communicate in the dominant language of the facility (include those who use sign language)

F142____ Who use non-oral communication devices

F143____ With advance directives

F144____ Received influenza immunization

F145____ Received pneumococcal vaccine

I certify that this information is accurate to the best of my knowledge.

Signature of Person Completing the Form	Title	Date

TO BE COMPLETED BY SURVEY TEAM

F146   Was ombudsman office notified prior to survey?   Yes ☐   No ☐

F147   Was ombudsman present during any portion of the survey?   Yes ☐   No ☐

F148   Medication error rate ____%

EXHIBIT 264 *(continued)*

RESIDENT CENSUS AND CONDITIONS OF RESIDENTS
(use with Form CMS-672)

GENERAL INSTRUCTIONS
THIS FORM IS TO BE COMPLETED BY THE FACILITY AND REPRESENTS THE
CURRENT CONDITION OF RESIDENTS AT THE TIME OF COMPLETION

There is not a federal requirement for automation of the 672 form. The facility may continue to complete the 672 with manual methods. The facility may use the MDS data to start the 672 form, but must verify all information, and in some cases, re-code the item responses to meet the intent of the 672 to represent current resident status according to the definitions of the 672. Since the census is designed to be a representation of the facility during the survey, it does not directly correspond to the MDS in every item.

For the purpose of this form "the facility" equals certified beds (i.e., Medicare and/or Medicaid certified beds). For the purpose of this form "residents" means residents in certified beds regardless of payor source.

Following the definition of each field, the related MDS 2.0 codes and instructions will be noted within square brackets ([ ]).

Where coding refers to the admission assessment, use the first assessment done after the most recent admission or readmission event.

Complete each item by specifying the number of residents characterized by each category. If no residents fall into a category enter a "0".

INSTRUCTIONS AND DEFINITIONS

Provider No. - Enter the facility's assigned provider number. Leave blank for initial certifications.

Block F75 - Enter the number of facility residents, whose primary payer is Medicare. [code manually]

Block F76 - Enter the number of facility residents, whose primary payer is Medicaid. [code manually]

Block F77 - Enter the number of facility residents, whose primary payer is neither Medicare nor Medicaid. [code manually]

Block F78 - Enter the number of total residents for whom a bed is maintained, on the day the survey begins, including those temporarily away in a hospital or on leave. [Total residents in nursing facility or on bedhold]

ADLS (F79 – F93)
To determine resident status, unless otherwise noted, consider the resident's condition for the 7 days prior to the survey. [Horizontal totals must equal the number in F78; Manually re-code all "8" responses.]

Bathing (F79 – F81)
The process of bathing the body (excluding back and shampooing hair). This includes a full-body bath/shower, sponge bath, and transfer into and out of tub or shower. [F79: G2A = 0; F80: G2A = 1, 2, 3; F81: G2A = 4]

Many facilities routinely provide "setup" assistance to all residents such as drawing water for a tub bath or laying out bathing materials. If this is the case and the resident requires no other assistance, count the resident as independent.

Dressing (F82 – F84)
How the resident puts on, fastens, and takes off all items of street clothing, including donning or removing prostheses (e.g., braces and artificial limbs). [F82: G1Ag = 0; F83: G1Ag = 1, 2, 3; F84: G1Ag = 4]

Many facilities routinely set out clothes for all residents. If this is the case and this is the only assistance the resident receives, count the resident as independent. However, if a resident receives assistance with donning a brace, elastic stocking, a prosthesis and so on, securing fasteners, or putting a garment on, count the resident as needing the assistance of 1 or 2 staff.

(continued)

EXHIBIT 264 *(continued)*

RESIDENT CENSUS AND CONDITIONS OF RESIDENTS
(use with Form CMS-672)

Transferring (F85 – F87)
How the resident moves between surfaces, such as to and from the bed, chair, wheelchair or to and from a standing position. (EXCLUDE transfers to and from the bath or toilet). [F85: G1Ab = 0; F86: GlAb = 1, 2, 3; F87: GlAb = 4]

Many facilities routinely provide "setup" assistance to all residents, such as handing the equipment (e.g., sliding board) to the resident. If this is the case and is the only assistance required, count the resident as independent.

Toilet Use (F88 – F90)
How the resident uses the toilet room (or bedpan, bedside commode, or urinal). How resident transfers on and off toilet, cleans self after elimination, changes sanitary napkins, ostomy, external catheters, and adjusts clothing prior to and after using toilet. If all that is done for the resident is to open a package (e.g., a clean sanitary pad), count the resident as independent. [F88: GlAi = 0; F89: G1Ai = 1, 2, 3; F90: G1Ai = 4]

Eating (F91 – F93)
How resident eats and drinks regardless of skill. Many facilities routinely provide "setup" activities, such as opening containers, buttering bread, and organizing the tray; if this is the case and is the extent of assistance, count this resident as independent. [F91: G1Ah = 0; F92: G1Ah = 1, 2, 3; F93: G1Ah = 4]

A. BOWEL/BLADDER STATUS (F94 – F99)

F94 - With an indwelling or an external catheter
The number of residents whose urinary bladder is constantly drained by a catheter (e.g., a Foley catheter, a suprapubic catheter) or who wears an appliance that is applied over the penis and connected to a drainage bag to collect urine from the bladder (e.g., a Texas catheter). [H3c or d = check]

F95 - Of the total number of residents with catheters
The number of residents who had a catheter present on admission. For a resident readmitted from a hospital with a catheter, count this resident as admitted with a catheter. [H3c or d = check and A8a = 1 or A8b = 1 or 5]

F96 - Occasionally or frequently incontinent of bladder
The number of residents who have an incontinent episode two or more times per week. Do not include residents with an indwelling or external catheter. [Hlb = 2, 3 or 4 and H3c and d are not = check]

F97 - Occasionally or frequently incontinent of bowel
The number of residents who have a loss of bowel control two or more times per week. [H1a = 2, 3 or 4]

F98 - On individually written bladder training program
The number of residents with a detailed plan of care to assist the resident to gain and maintain bladder control (e.g., pelvic floor exercises). Count all residents on training programs including those who are incontinent. [H3b = check]

F99 - On individually written bowel training program
The number of residents with a detailed plan of care to assist the resident to gain and maintain bowel control (e.g., use of diet, fluids, and regular schedule for bowel movements). Count all residents on training programs including those who are incontinent. [code manually]

B. MOBILITY (F100 – F107)

[Total for Fl00 – F103 should = F78; Algorithm to force mutual exclusivity: Test for each resident. If F100 = 1 then add 1 to F100, and go to the next resident; If F101 = 1 then add 1 to F101 and go to the next resident; If F103 = 1 then add 1 to F103 and go to the next resident; If F102 = 1 then add 1 and go to the next resident.]

F100 - Bedfast all or most of time The number of residents who were in bed or recliner 22 hours or more per day in the past 7 days. Includes bedfast with bathroom privileges. [G6a = check and G5d is not = check]

F101 - In chair all or most of time The number of residents who depend on a chair for mobility. Includes those residents who can stand with assistance to pivot from bed to wheelchair or to otherwise transfer. The resident cannot take steps without extensive or constant weight-bearing support from others and is not bedfast all or most of the time. [G5d = check]

F102 - Independently ambulatory The number of residents who require no help or oversight; or help or oversight was provided only 1 or 2 times during the past 7 days. Do not include residents who use a cane, walker or crutch. [G1Ac = 0 and GlAd = 0 and G5a is not = check]

EXHIBIT 264 *(continued)*

RESIDENT CENSUS AND CONDITIONS OF RESIDENTS
(use with Form CMS-672)

F103 - Ambulation with assistance or assistive devices
The number of residents who required oversight, cueing, physical assistance or who used a cane, walker, crutch. Count the use of lower leg splints, orthotics, and braces as assistive devices. [G1Ac or d = 1, 2 or 3 or G5a = check]

F104 - Physically restrained The number of residents whose freedom of movement and/or normal access to his/her body is restricted by any manual method or physical or mechanical device, material or equipment that is attached or adjacent to his/her body and cannot be easily removed by the resident. [Any P4c, d or e = 1 or 2]

F105 - Of total number of restrained residents, number admitted or readmitted with an order for restraint. [Code manually when criteria for F104 is met and P4c, d or e = 1 or 2 and A8a = 1 or A8b = 1 or 5]

F106 - With contractures The number of residents that have a restriction of full passive range of motion of any joint due to deformity, disuse, pain, etc. Includes loss of range of motion in fingers, wrists, elbows, shoulders, hips, knees and ankles. [Any G4Aa, b, c, d, e or f = 1 or 2]

F107 - Of total of residents with contractures, the number who had a contracture(s) on admission. [Code when criteria for F106 is met on admission or readmission assessment and A8a = 1 or A8b = 1 or 5.]

C. MENTAL STATUS (F108 – F114)

F108 - With mental retardation Identify the total number of residents in all of the categories of developmental disability regardless of severity, as determined by the State Mental Health or State Mental Retardation Authorities. [Any AB10b, c, e or f = check]

F109 - With documented signs and symptoms of depression The total number of residents with documented signs and symptoms of depression as defined by MDS (Mood and Behavior Section). [I1ee = check or E1a, e, l or m > 0]

F110 - With documented psychiatric diagnosis (exclude dementias and depression) The number of residents with primary or secondary psychiatric diagnosis including:
• Schizophrenia
• Schizo-affective disorder
• Schizophreniform disorder
• Delusional disorder
• Psychotic mood disorders (including mania and depression with psychotic features, acute psychotic episodes, brief reactive psychosis, and atypical psychosis). [I1dd, ff, or gg = check. Code manually for other psychiatric diagnoses listed here]

F111 - Dementia: Multi-infarct, senile, Alzheimer's type, or other than Alzheimer's type The number of residents with a primary or secondary diagnosis of dementia or organic mental syndrome including multi-infarct, senile type, Alzheimer's type, or other than Alzheimer's type. [I1q or u = check]

F112 - With behavioral symptoms The number of residents with one or more of the following symptoms: wandering, verbally abusive, physically abusive, socially inappropriate/disruptive, resistive to care. (See MDS Section (Mood and Behavioral Patterns)). [Any E4Aa, b, c, d or e = 1, 2 or 3]

F113 - Of the total number with behavioral symptoms, the number receiving a behavior management program. The number of residents with behavior symptoms who are receiving an individualized care plan/program designed to address behavioral symptoms (as listed above). [Manually code when criteria for F112 is met and P2a = check and P2c or d = check]

F114 - Receiving health rehabilitative services for MI/MR The number of residents for whom the facility is providing health rehabilitative services for MI/MR as defined at 483.45(a). [Use item for Residents who meet F108 or F110, then code manually]

D. SKIN INTEGRITY (F115 – F118)

Fl15 - With pressure sores The number of residents with ischemic ulcerations and/or necrosis of tissues overlying a bony prominence (exclude Stage I). [Any M1b, c or d > 0 or M2a > 1 Code for first assessment after latest admission or re-admission]

F116 - Of the total number of residents with pressure sores excluding Stage I, the number who had pressure sores on admission or who were readmitted with a new pressure sore (exclude Stage I). [Code when criteria for field 115 are met and A8a = 1 or A8b = 1 or 5.]

(continued)

EXHIBIT 264 *(continued)*

RESIDENT CENSUS AND CONDITIONS OF RESIDENTS
(use with Form CMS-672)

F117 - Receiving preventive skin care The number of residents receiving non-routine skin care provided according to a physician's order, and/or included in the resident's comprehensive plan of care (e.g., hydrocortisone ointment to areas of dermatitis three times a day, granulex sprays, etc.) [Any M5a, b, c, d, e, f, g, h, or i = check]

Fl18 - With rashes Enter the number of residents who have rashes which may or may not be treated with any medication or special baths, etc. (e.g., but not limited to antifungals, cortisteroids, emollients, dipherydramines or scabiciduls, etc.) [M4d = check]

E. SPECIAL CARE (F119 – F132)

F119 - Receiving hospice care Number of residents who have elected or are currently receiving the hospice benefit. [P1ao = check]

F120 - Receiving radiation therapy The number of residents who are under a treatment plan involving radiation therapy. [P1ah = check]

F121 - Receiving chemotherapy The number of residents under a specific treatment plan involving chemotherapy. [P1aa = check]

F122 - Receiving dialysis The number of residents receiving hemodialysis or peritoneal dialysis either within the facility or offsite. [P1ab = check]

F123 - Receiving intravenous therapy, IV nutritional feedings and/or blood transfusion The number of residents receiving fluids, medications, all or most of their nutritional requirements and/or blood and blood products administered intravenously. [K5a = check or P1ac = check or P1ak check]

F124 - Receiving respiratory treatment The number of residents receiving treatment by the use of respirators/ventilators, oxygen, IPPB or other inhalation therapy, pulmonary toilet, humidifiers, and other methods to treat conditions of the respiratory tract. This does not include residents receiving tracheotomy care or respiratory suctioning. [P1ag = check or P1al = check or P1bdA > 0]

F125 - Receiving tracheotomy care The number of residents receiving care involved in maintenance of the airway, the stoma and surrounding skin, and dressings/ coverings for the stoma. [P1aj = check]

F126 - Receiving ostomy care The number of residents receiving care for a colostomy, ileostomy, uretrostomy, or other ostomy of the intestinal and/or urinary tract. DO NOT include tracheotomy. [P1af– check]

F127 - Receiving suctioning The number of residents that require use of a mechanical device which provides suction to remove secretions from the respiratory tract via the mouth, nasal passage, or tracheotomy stoma. [P1ai = check]

F128 - Receiving injections The number of residents that have received one or more injections within the past 7 days. (Exclude injections of Vitamin B 12.) [Review residents for whom 03 = 1, 2, 3, 4, 5, 6 or 7. Omit from count any resident whose only injection currently is B12.]

F129 - Receiving tube feeding The number of residents who receive all or most of their nutritional requirements via a feeding tube that delivers food/nutritional substances directly into the GI system (e.g., nasogastric tube, gastrostomy tube). [K5b = check]

F130 - Receiving mechanically altered diets The number of residents receiving a mechanically altered diet including pureed and/or chopped foods (not only meat). [K5c = check]

F131 - Receiving rehabilitative services The number of residents receiving care designed to improve functional ability provided by, or under the direction of a rehabilitation professional (physical therapist, occupational therapist, speech-language pathologist. (Exclude health rehab. for MI/MR.) [P1baA or P1bbA or P1bcA > 0]

F132 - Assistive devices with eating The number of residents who are using devices to maintain independence and to provide comfort when eating (i.e., plates with guards, large handled flatware, large handle mugs, extend hand flatware, etc.). [K5g = check]

EXHIBIT 264 *(continued)*

RESIDENT CENSUS AND CONDITIONS OF RESIDENTS
(use with Form CMS-672)

F. MEDICATIONS (F133 – F139)

F133 - Receiving psychoactive drugs The number of residents that receive drugs classified as antidepressants, antianxiety, sedative and hypnotics, and antipsychotics. [Any O4a, b, c or d = 1, 2, 3, 4, 5, 6 or 7].

Use the following lists to assist you in determining the number of residents receiving psychoactive drugs. These lists are not meant to be all inclusive; therefore, a resident receiving a psychoactive drug not on this list, should be counted under F133 and any other drug category that applies - F134, F135, F136, and/or F137.

F134 - Receiving antipsychotic medications
[O4a = 1, 2, 3, 4, 5, 6 or 7]
Clorazil (Clozapine)
Haldol (Haloperidol)
Haldol Deconate (Haloperiodal Deconate)
Inapsine (Droperidol)
Loxitane (Loxapine)
Mellaril (Thioridazine)
Moban (Molindone)
Navane (Theothixene)
Olazapine (Zyprexa)
Orap (Pimozide)
Prolixin, Deconoate (Fluphenazine Deconate)
Prolixin, Permitil (Fluphenazine)
Quetiapine (Seroquel)
Risperdal (Risperidone)
Serentil (Mesoridazine)
Sparine (Promazine)
Stelazine (Trifluoperazine)
Taractan (Chlorprothixene)
Thorazine (Chlorpromazine)
Tindel (Acetophenazine)
Trilafon (Perphenazine)

F135 - Receiving antianxiety medications
[O4b = 1, 2, 3, 4, 5, 6 or 7]
Ativan (Lorazepam)   Serax (Oxazepam)
Centrax (Prazepam)   Valium (Diazepam)
Klonopin (Clonazepam)   Vistaril, Atarax (Hydrox-
Librium (Chlordiazepoxide) yzine)
Paxipam (Halazepam)   Xanax (Alprazolam)

F136 - Receiving antidepressant medications
[O4c = 1, 2, 3, 4, 5, 6, 7]
Asendin (Amoxapine)
Aventlyl, Pamelor (Nortriptyline)
Bupropion (Wellbutrin)
Desyrel (Trazodone)
Effexor (Venlafaxine)

Elavil (Amtriptyline)
Lithonate, Lithane (Lithium)
Ludiomil (Maprotiline)
Marplan (Isocarboxazid)
Nardil (Phenelzine)
Nefazodone (Serzone)
Norpramin (Desipramine)
Parnate (Tranylcypromine)
Paroxetine (Paxil)
Prozac (Fluoxetine)
Sertraline (Zoloft)
Sinequan (Doxepin)
Tofranil (Imipramine)
Vivactil (Protriptyline)

F137 - Receiving hypnotic medications
[O4d = 1, 2, 3, 4, 5, 6 or 7]
Dalmane (Flurazepam)   Quazepam (Doral)
Estazolam (ProSom)   Restoril (Temazepam)
Halcion (Triazolam)   Zolpidem (Ambien)

F138 - Receiving antibiotics The number of residents receiving sulfonamides, antibiotics, etc., either for prophylaxis or treatment. [Code manually]

F139 - On a pain management program The number of residents with a specific plan for control of difficult to manage or intractable pain, which may include self medication pumps or regularly scheduled administration of medication alone or in combination with alternative approaches (e.g., massages, heat, etc.). [Code manually when any J3a, b, c, d, e, f, g, h, i or j = check]

G. OTHER RESIDENT CHARACTERISTICS (F140 – F146)

F140 - With unplanned or significant weight loss/gain The number of residents who have experienced gain or loss of 5% in one month or 10% over six months. [K3a or K3b = 1 and K5h is not = check]

F141 - Who do not communicate in the dominant language at the facility The number of residents who only express themselves in a language not dominant at the facility (e.g., this would include residents who speak only Spanish, but the majority of staff that care for the residents speak only English). [code manually]

(continued)

EXHIBIT 264 *(continued)*

RESIDENT CENSUS AND CONDITIONS OF RESIDENTS
(use with Form CMS-672)

F142 - Who use non-oral communication devices
(e.g., picture board, computers, sign-language). [Any
C3b, c, d, e,or f = check]

F143 - Who have advanced directives (living will/
durable power of attorney) The number of residents
who have advanced directives, such as a living will or
durable power of attorney for health care, recognized
under state law and relating to the provisions of care
when the individual is incapacitated.
[Any Al0a, b, c, f, g, or h = check]

F144 - Received influenza immunization The
number of residents known to have received the
influenza immunization within the last 12 months.
[code manually]

F145 - Received pneumococcal vaccine   The number
of residents known to have received the pneumococcal
vaccine. [code manually]

F146 - Ombudsman notice - LEAVE BLANK
This will be completed by survey team. Indicate yes or
no whether Ombudsman office was notified prior to
survey.

F147 - LEAVE BLANK This will be completed by
the survey team. Indicate whether Ombudsman was
present at any time during the survey, 1 (yes) or 2 (no).

F148 - Medication error rate - LEAVE BLANK
This will be completed by the survey team.

EXHIBIT 265

Roster/Sample Matrix

DEPARTMENT OF HEALTH AND HUMAN SERVICES
CENTERS FOR MEDICARE & MEDICAID SERVICES

Offsite   Phase I   Phase 2   Prov. #

Total Sample:
Phase 1
Phase 2
Individual Interview (I)
Family Interview (F)
Closed Record (CL)
Comprehensive (C)
Focused Review (F)

Resident Characteristics

Review — Interview: Indiv/Fam; Closed Rec/Compr/Focus

For Surveyor Use

Column	Label	Group
1	Privacy/Dignity Issues	
2	Social Services	
3	Choices	
4	Abuse/Neglect	
5	Clean/Comfort/Homelike	
6	Falls/Fx/Abras/Bruise	
7	Behavior Symp/Depression	
8	9 or more Meds	
9	Cognitive Impairment	
10	Incont/Toilet Program	Elimination
11	Catheter	Elimination
12	Fecal Impaction	Elimination
13	UTI/Inf Control/Antibio	
14	Wt/Nutr/Swallow/Denture	Nutrition
15	Tube Feeding	Nutrition
16	Dehydration	Nutrition
17	Bedfast Residents	Phys. Funct
18	ADL Decline/Concern	Phys. Funct
19	ROM/Contract/Position	Phys. Funct
20	Psychoactive Meds	
21	Physical Restraints	
22	Activities	Q of Life
23	Pressure Sores/Ulcers	
24	Pain/Comfort	
25	Language/Communication	
26	Vision/Hearing/Devices	
27	Specialized Rehab	
28	Assistive Devices	
29	Hospice	
30	Dialysis	
31	O$_2$/Respiratory	
32	Admit/Trans/Disch	
33	MR/MI (Non-Dementia)	
34		
35		

Resident Number
Resident Room
Surveyor Assigned
Resident Name

Form CMS-802 (7/99)

EXHIBIT 266

DEPARTMENT OF HEALTH AND HUMAN SERVICES
CENTERS FOR MEDICARE & MEDICAID SERVICES

ROSTER/SAMPLE MATRIX PROVIDER INSTRUCTIONS
(use with FORM CMS-802)

The Roster/Sample Matrix form (CMS-802) is used by the facility to list all current residents (including residents on bedhold) and to note pertinent care categories. **The facility completes the following: resident name, resident room, and columns 6–33, which are described below.** All remaining columns are for Surveyor Use Only.

There is not a federal requirement for automation of Form CMS-802. The facility may continue manual coding of Form CMS-802. The facility may use MDS data to provide a "worksheet" of the form, but must amend item responses as necessary to represent current resident status on the first day of the survey. The MDS crosswalk items below are provided as a reference point, but the form is to be completed using the time frames and other specific instructions below. The information required on the Provider Instructions is not based on the Quality Measures/Indicators.

For each resident mark all columns that are pertinent.

6. **Falls/Fx/Abrasions/Bruises –** If the resident currently has abrasions, bruises, skin tears; has fallen within the past 30 days; or has had a fracture within the last 180 days.
   - Mark A if the resident has abrasions, skin tears or bruises, Fx for fractures and F for fallen.
   Crosswalk:
   If M4a checked or M4f checked, then 802 - 6 = A.
   If I1m checked or I1p checked or J4c checked or J4d checked, then 802 - 6 = Fx.
   If J4a checked, then 802 - 6 F.

7. **Behavioral Symptoms/Depression –** If the resident has behavioral symptoms or symptoms of depression, as listed in the MDS, mark this column.
   - Mark B for behavior and D for depression.
   Crosswalk:
   If E4A a, b, c, d or e are greater than 0, then 802 - 7 = B.
   If E5 = 2, then 802 - 7 = B.
   If E1a,b, c, d, e, f, g, h, i, j, k, l, m, n, o, p are greater than 0, then 802 - 7 = D.
   If E2 = 2,then 802 - 7 = D.
   If E3 = 2, then 802 - 7 = D.
   If I1ee checked, then 802 - 7 = D.

8. **9 or More Medications –** If the resident is using 9 or more medications, check this column.
   Crosswalk:
   If O1 is greater than 8, then 802 - 8 = checked.

9. **Cognitive Impairment –** If the resident is cognitively impaired, check this column.
   Crosswalk:
   If B5a, b, c, d, e or f are greater than 0, then 802 - 9 = checked.
   If B2a or b = 1, then 802 - 9 = checked.
   If B4 is greater than 1, then 802 - 9 = checked.

10. **Incontinence/Toileting Programs –** If the resident is incontinent of bladder, mark I. If the resident is on a bladder training program, mark T.

Crosswalk:
If H1b = 3 or 4, then 802 - 10 = I.
If H4 = 2 then 802 - 10 = I.
If H3b checked, then 802 - 10 = T.

11. **Catheter –** If the resident has an indwelling urinary catheter, check this column.
   Crosswalk:
   If H3d checked, then 802 - 11 = checked.

12. **Fecal Impaction –** If the resident has had fecal impaction within the last 90 days, check this column. Note: MDS item H2d only includes the past 14 days.
   Crosswalk:
   If H2d checked, then 802 - 12 = checked.

13. **UTI/Infection Control/Antibiotics –** If the resident has an infection or is on antibiotics, check this column.
   Crosswalk:
   Consider I2a, b, c, d, e, f, g, h, i, j, k, l checked or M6b checked, then 802 - 13 = checked, but amend this information to show the resident's condition on the day of the survey.

14. **Weight Change/Nutrition/Swallowing/Dentures –** If the resident has had an unintended weight loss/gain of 5% in one month or 10% in six months, has had chronic insidious weight loss or is at nutritional risk, mark this column. If the resident is in a restorative dining program, has chewing or swallowing problems that may affect dietary intake, or has dentures, mark this column.
   - Mark W for weight change, S for chewing or swallowing problems, D for dentures, and R for restorative dining program.
   Crosswalk:
   If J1a checked, then 802 - 14 = W.
   If K3a = 1, then 802 - 14 = W.
   If K3b = 1, then 802- 14 = W.
   If K1b checked, then 802 - 14 = S.

EXHIBIT 266 *(continued)*

ROSTER/SAMPLE MATRIX PROVIDER INSTRUCTIONS
(use with FORM CMS-802)

If K1a checked, then 802 - 14 = S.

If L1b = check, then 802 - 14 = D.

If P3h is greater than 0, then 802 - 14 = R.

Note: MDS items for weight change do not differentiate between planned and unintended changes. Code only unintended changes.

No crosswalk is available for chronic insidious weight loss or nutritional risk. Insidious weight loss is a slow, steady, and persistent weight loss over time that when reviewed in the aggregate is clinically significant. Code manually with a W for either.

15. **Tube Feedings** – If the resident has a feeding tube, check this column.
   Crosswalk:
   If K5b checked, then 802 - 15 = checked.

16. **Dehydration** – If the resident has problems with dehydration, check this column.
   Crosswalk:
   If J1c or d checked, then 802 - 16 = checked.
   Also consider I3 = 276.5.

17. **Bedfast Residents** – If the resident is bedfast, check this column.
   Crosswalk:
   If G6a checked then, 802 - 17 = checked.

18. **ADL Decline/Concern** – If the resident has shown a decline in ADL areas check this column.
   Crosswalk:
   If G9 = 2, then 802 - 18 = checked.

19. **ROM/Contractures/Positioning** – If the resident has functional limitations in range of motion, check this column.
   Crosswalk:
   Use codes below as reference, then determine if functional limitation in range of motion is present.
   If G4Aa, b, c, d, e or f are greater than 0, then 802 - 19 = checked.

20. **Psychoactive Meds** – If the resident receives any psychoactive medications, mark this column.
   • Mark P for antipsychotic, A for antianxiety, D for antidepressant, and H for hypnotic.
   Crosswalk:
   If O4a is greater than 0, then 802 - 20 = P.
   If O4b is greater than 0, then 802 - 20 = A.
   If O4c is greater than 0, then 802 - 20 = D.
   If O4d is greater than 0, then 802 - 20 = H.

21. **Physical Restraints** – If the resident has a physical restraint, check this column.
   • Mark N for non-siderail devices and S for siderails.
   Crosswalk:
   If P4 c, d, or e are greater than 0, then 802 - 21 = N.
   If P4a or b are greater than 0 and G6b not checked, then 802 - 21 = S.

22. **Activities** – If the resident has little or no activity or has indicated a desire for change in type or extent of activity, check this column.
   Crosswalk:
   If N2 is greater than 1, then 802 - 22 = checked.
   If N5a or b are greater than 1, then 802 - 22 = checked.

23. **Pressure Sores/Ulcers** – If the resident has a stage 2, 3 or 4 pressure sore(s), check this column.
   Crosswalk:
   If M2a is greater than 1, then 802 - 23 = checked.

24. **Pain/Comfort** – If the resident needs pain or comfort measures or is on a pain management program check this column.
   Crosswalk:
   If J2a = 2, then 802 - 24 = checked.
   If J2b = 3, then 802 - 24 = checked.
   No crosswalk is available for pain management program. Code manually.

25. **Language/Communication** – Enter a code in this item if the resident uses a language other than the dominant language of the facility or exhibits difficulty communicating his/her needs. This must be individually determined. In some facilities the predominant language is other than English, such as Spanish, Navajo, or French.
   • Mark L if resident uses a language other than the dominant language of the facility. (If a resident uses American Sign Language, consider this a different language and mark L.) Mark C if the resident has communication difficulties.
   Crosswalk:
   For Dominant Language, AB8a must be individually determined, based on the predominant language spoken within the facility. If the resident's primary language is different, then 802 - 25 = L.
   If C3d, e or f checked, then 802 - 25 = C.
   If C4 = 2 or 3, then 802 - 25 = C.
   If C5 = 1 or 2, then 802 - 25 = C.
   If I1r checked, then 802 - 25 = C.

(continued)

EXHIBIT 266 *(continued)*

ROSTER/SAMPLE MATRIX PROVIDER INSTRUCTIONS
(use with FORM CMS-802)

---

26. Vision/Hearing/Devices – If the resident has significant impairment of vision or hearing, or uses devices to aid vision or hearing, mark this column.
  • Mark V for visual impairment, H for hearing impairment, and D for use of devices (glasses or hearing aids).
Crosswalk:
If D1 is greater than 1, then 802 - 26 = V.
If D2a or b checked, then 802 - 26 = V.
If C1 = 2 or 3, then 802 - 26 = H.
If D3 = 1, then 802 - 26 = D.
If C2 a or b is checked, then 802 - 26 = D.

27. Specialized Rehab – If the resident is receiving specialized rehabilitative services, mark the following:
  S   for speech/language therapy
  O   for occupational therapy
  P   for physical therapy
  H   for health rehabilitative services for MI/MR
Crosswalk:
If P1bAa is greater than 0, then 802 - 27 = S.
If P1bAb is greater than 0, then 802 - 27 = O.
If P1bAc is greater than 0, then 802 - 27 = P.
If P1bAe is greater than 0, then 802 - 27 = H.
There is no code for services for mental retardation.
Code manually as H.

28. Assistive Devices – If the resident uses special devices to assist with eating or mobility (e.g., tables, utensils, hand splints, canes, crutches, etc.) and other assistive devices, check this column.
Crosswalk:
If K5g checked, then 802 - 28 = checked.
If G5a checked, then 802 - 28 = checked.
If G6e checked, then 802 - 28 = checked.
If P3c is greater than 0, then 802 - 28 = checked.

29. Hospice – If the resident is receiving Hospice Care, check this column.
Crosswalk:
If P1ao checked, then 802 - 29 = checked.

30. Dialysis – If the resident is receiving dialysis, check this column.
Crosswalk:
If P1 ab checked, then 802 - 30 = checked.

31. Oxygen/Respiratory Care – If the resident has a tracheotomy, ventilator, resident needs suctioning, or is receiving oxygen therapy, etc., check this column.
Crosswalk:
At item P1a, if g, i, j or l checked, then 802 - 31 = checked.
If P1bAd is greater than 0, then 802 - 31 = checked.

32. Adm./Transfer/Discharge – Enter a code in this column if the resident was admitted within the past 30 days or is scheduled to be transferred or discharged within the next 30 days.
  • Mark A for an admission. Code for first assessment after initial admission or readmission after discharge without expectation of return. Mark T for a transfer and D for a discharge.
Crosswalk:
If today's date minus AB1 is less than or equal to 30 days, then 802 - 32 = A.
No codes are available for transfer and discharge anticipated. Code manually.

33. MR/MI (Non Dementia) – Enter a code in this column if the resident has a diagnosis of mental retardation or mental illness.
  • Mark MR for mental retardation or MI for mental illness not classified as dementia.
Crosswalk:
If AB10 b, e or f checked, then 802 - 33 = MR.
If I1 dd ee, ff or gg checked, then 802 - 33 = MI.

EXHIBIT 267

DEPARTMENT OF HEALTH AND HUMAN SERVICES
CENTERS FOR MEDICARE & MEDICAID SERVICES

ROSTER/SAMPLE MATRIX INSTRUCTIONS FOR SURVEYORS
(use with FORM CMS-802)

The Roster/Sample Matrix (CMS-802) is a tool for selecting the resident sample and may be used for recording information from the tour. When using the form to identify the resident sample, indicate by a check whether this CMS-802 is being used for the sample from Offsite, Phase 1 or Phase 2. The horizontal rows list residents chosen for review (or residents encountered during the tour) and indicate the characteristics/concerns identified for each resident.

Use the resident sample selection table to identify the number of residents required in the sample.

In the vertical columns under the heading **Review,** code the Interview: Individual /Family column with '**I**' for each resident receiving a Resident Interview or with '**F**' for any non-interviewable resident receiving a Family Interview/Observation. **Code** the Closed Record/Comprehensive/Focused Review column with '**CL**' for a closed record review, '**C**' for a resident chosen for a comprehensive review or '**F**' for a resident chosen for a focused review.

Use the vertical columns numbered 1 through 35 to check the characteristics for each resident, as appropriate. The bolded language in columns 6 through 23 corresponds to fields in the Facility Quality Measure/Indicator (QM/QI) Report. Some columns capture language from more than one QM/QI, as well as non-indicator characteristics; e.g., QM/QI's 1.1 and 1.2 and residents with abrasions and bruises in column 6; QM/QI's 2.1, 2.2 and 2.3 in column 7; QM/QI's 5.1 and 5.3 in column 10 and QM/QI's 10.1, 10.2, and 10.3 in column 20.

During each portion of the survey (Offsite, Phase I, Phase 2) highlight the vertical columns for each characteristic identified as a potential facility concern.

Resident Number – Number each line sequentially down the rows continuing the numbering sequence for any additional pages needed. These numbers may be used as resident identifiers for the sample.

Resident Room – Identify room no. for the resident listed.

Surveyor Assigned – List initials or surveyor number of surveyor assigned to review each resident.

Resident Name – List the name of the resident.

COLUMNS 6–35: Highlight each column that is an area of concern. For each resident entered on the roster/sample matrix, check all columns that pertain to the resident according to the Offsite and Sample Selection Tasks of the Survey. The term QM/QI Report refers to the Resident Level/Quality Measure/Indicator Reports.

1. **Privacy/Dignity** – Concerns about residents' right to privacy (accommodations, written and telephone communication, visitation, personal care) or concerns that the facility does not maintain or enhance residents' dignity.

2. **Social Services** – Concerns about medically related social services; e.g., interpersonal relationships, grief, clothing.

3. **Choices** – Concerns about residents' ability to exercise their rights as citizens; freedom from coercion, discrimination or reprisal; self determination and participation; choice of care and schedule, etc.

4. **Abuse/Neglect** – Concerns about resident abuse, neglect or misappropriation of resident property, or how the facility responds to allegations of abuse, neglect or misappropriation of resident property.

5. **Clean/Comfortable/Homelike** – Concerns about the facility environment including cleanliness, lighting levels, temperature, comfortable sound levels, or homelike environment and the residents ability to use their personal belongings and individualize their room to the extent possible.

6. **Falls/Fractures/Abrasions/Bruises** (QM/QI 1.1, 1.2) – Concerns about residents with bruises, skin tear, abrasions, history of accidents or incidence of a new fracture or a fall or QM/QI Report indicates accidents or falls.

7. **Behavioral Symptoms/Depression** (QM/QI 2.1, 2.2, and 2.3) – Concerns about incidence or prevalence of resident behaviors that need to be addressed by the facility (e.g., verbal or physical outbursts, withdrawing/isolation) or residents indicated on the QM/QI Report as having behavioral symptoms affecting others or symptoms of depression with or without antidepressant therapy.

8. **9 or more Medications** (QM/QI 3.1) – Residents identified during the tour or on the QM/QI Report as using 9 or more medications.

9. **Cognitive Impairment** (QM/QI 4.1) – Concerns for residents with cognitive impairment or residents identified as becoming cognitively impaired on the QM/QI Report.

10. **Incontinence/Toiling Programs** (QM/QI 5.1 and 5.3) – Concerns related to resident incontinence and facility toileting programs including residents identified as such on the QM/QI Report.

11. **Catheter** (QM/QI 5.2) – Concerns related to catheter use in the facility or residents identified on the QM/QI Report.

12. **Fecal Impaction** (QM/QI 5.4) – Concerns related to management of constipation or residents having a fecal impaction as identified on the QM/QI Report. *This condition is considered a sentinel event.*

(continued)

EXHIBIT 267 *(continued)*

ROSTER/SAMPLE MATRIX INSTRUCTIONS FOR SURVEYORS

13. **UTI/Infection Control/Antibiotics** (QM/QI 6.1) – Concerns about presence or prevalence of resident infections, facility infection control practices, residents receiving antibiotics, or residents identified as having a UTI on the QM/QI Report.

14. **Weight Change/Nutrition/Swallowing/Dentures** (QM/QI 7.1) – Concerns about residents with nutritional needs, chewing or swallowing problems that may affect intake (including the use of dentures), experiencing significant or chronic insidious unintended weight change, being on a restorative dining program or residents identified on the QM/QI Report as having a weight loss.

15. **Tube Feedings** (QM/QI 7.2) – Concerns related to residents having a feeding tube or identified on the QM/QI Report as having a feeding tube.

16. **Dehydration** (QM/QI 7.3) – Concerns about residents who show signs or symptoms or have risk factors for dehydration or who are identified on the QM/QI Report as having dehydration. *This condition is considered a sentinel event.*

17. **Bedfast Residents** (QM/QI 9.2) – Concerns about residents identified on the QM/QI Report or observed to be spend most time in bed or chair.

18. **ADL Decline/Concern** (QM/QI 9.1 and 9.3) – Concern that resident receives appropriate treatment and services to maintain or improve ability or concerns about residents identified on the QM/QI Report as having an ADL decline.

19. **ROM/Contractures/Positioning** (QM/QI 9.4) – Concerns about the occurrence, prevention or treatment of contractures. Concerns with staff provision or lack of provision of splints, ROM, the appropriate positioning of residents or residents identified on the QM/QI Report as having a decline in ROM.

20. **Psychoactive Meds** (QM/QI 10.1, 10.2 and 10.3) – Concerns about the use of psychoactive medications or residents identified on QM/QI Report with antipsychotic use in the absence of psychotic or related conditions or use of antianxiety or hypnotic medications.

21. **Physical Restraints** (QM/QI 11.1) – Concerns about the use of physical restraints or residents identified on the QM/QI Report as physically restrained daily (excluding side rails).

22. **Activities** (QM/QI 11.2) – Concerns about activities meeting cultural needs, interests, preferences, etc. of residents or residents identified on the QM/QI Report as having little or no activity.

23. **Pressure Sores/Ulcers** (QM/QI 12.1 and 12.2) (QM/QI 13.3 for PAC residents) – Concerns about the occurrence, assessment, prevention or treatment of pressure ulcers or other necessary skin care or residents identified on the QI Report as having stage 1–4 pressure ulcers. *Residents who flag at low risk for this QM/QI are considered to have a sentinel event.*

24. **Pain/Comfort** (QM/QI 8.1 and for PAC residents 13.2) – Concerns about timely assessment and intervention with residents needing pain or comfort measures or who are on a pain management program.

25. **Language/Communication** – Concerns about the facility assisting those residents with communication difficulties to communicate at their highest practicable level or residents identified as speaking other than the dominant language of the facility.

26. **Vision/Hearing/Devices** – Concerns about the facility assisting those residents with visual or hearing impairments to function at their highest practicable level including those residents who have glasses or hearing aids.

27. **Specialized Rehab** – Concerns about the facility's provision or lack of provision of Specialized Rehabilitative Services including:
    • Physical therapy
    • Speech/language pathology
    • Occupational therapy
    • Health rehabilitative services for MI/MR

28. **Assistive Devices** – Concerns about the need for, absence of or use of special devices to assist residents in eating (e.g., tables, utensils, hand splints, etc.) or concerns about any other assistive devices (e.g., canes, crutches, etc.).

29. **Hospice** – Concerns for residents who have elected the hospice benefit, whether the resident lives in the facility or is temporarily receiving inpatient services or respite care.

30. **Dialysis** – Concern about care and coordination of services for residents receiving hemo or peritoneal dialysis either in the facility or at another site.

31. **Oxygen/Respiratory Care** – Concerns about care provided to residents with tracheotomies or ventilators, residents needing suctioning, and residents receiving oxygen, etc.

32. **Adm./Transfer/Discharge** – Concerns about care/tx for residents recently admitted. Concerns about resident preparation and procedures for transfer or discharge.

33. **MR/MI(NonDementia)** – Concerns related to the care and treatment of residents with mental retardation or mental illness.

34–35. Note any other concerns; e.g., residents who are comatose or have special care areas (e.g., prosthesis, side rails, ostomy, injection, special foot care and IV's, including total parenteral nutrition) that may be of concern in the column. If during the Offsite prep, concerns arise about the accuracy of the MDS, enter MDS accuracy as a concern. Also add concerns with delirium (QM/QI 13.1) in these fields.

EXHIBIT 268
Rev. 9, 08/05/2005

Facility Characteristics Report

Facility Name	LISA01	
City/State	SACRAMENTO,CA	
Provider Number	855134	
Login/Internal ID	LISA01/1234	

Run Date	04/21/05 09:55:36
Report Period	09/01/04 - 02/28/05
Comparison Group	07/01/04 - 12/31/04
Report Version Number	1.07

	Facility			Comparison Group	
	Num	**Denom**	**Observed Percent**	**State Average**	**National Average**
Gender					
Male	9	46	19.6%	33.0%	31.3%
Female	37	46	80.4%	67.0%	68.7%
Age					
<25 years old	0	46	0.0%	0.3%	0.5%
25-54 years old	0	46	0.0%	9.0%	5.8%
55-64 years old	0	46	0.0%	7.4%	6.7%
65-74 years old	4	46	8.7%	12.6%	13.3%
75-84 years old	24	46	52.2%	30.6%	32.7%
85+ years old	18	46	39.1%	40.0%	40.9%
Payment Source (all that apply)					
Medicaid per diem	0	46	0.0%	45.0%	44.7%
Medicare per diem	0	46	0.0%	28.4%	30.3%
Medicare ancillary Part A	37	46	80.4%	15.1%	18.2%
Medicare ancillary Part B	0	46	0.0%	6.0%	8.4%
Self or family pays for full per diem	9	46	19.6%	20.0%	15.1%
Medicaid resident liability or Medicare co-payment	0	46	0.0%	5.4%	10.6%
Private insurance per diem (including co-payment)	1	46	2.2%	10.7%	10.4%
All other per diem	0	46	0.0%	2.1%	3.2%
Diagnostic Characteristics					
Psychiatric diagnosis	0	46	0.0%	18.1%	13.1%
Mental retardation	0	46	0.0%	2.0%	2.7%
Hospice	0	46	0.0%	2.7%	3.2%
Type of Assessment					
Admission assessment	37	46	80.4%	30.7%	31.2%
Annual assessment	1	46	2.2%	11.6%	10.9%
Significant change in status assessment	0	46	0.0%	7.5%	8.4%
Significant correction of prior full assessment	0	46	0.0%	0.0%	0.0%
Quarterly assessment	8	46	17.4%	50.2%	49.4%
Significant correction of prior quarterly assessment	0	46	0.0%	0.0%	0.0%
All other assessment types	0	46	0.0%	0.0%	0.0%
Stability of Conditions					
Conditions/disease make resident unstable	8	46	17.4%	42.5%	41.8%
Acute episode or chronic flareup	36	46	78.3%	17.3%	17.1%
End-stage disease, 6 or fewer months to live	0	46	0.0%	2.0%	2.8%
Discharge Potential					
No discharge potential	8	46	17.4%	66.6%	65.7%
Discharge potential within 30 days	32	46	69.6%	9.5%	10.6%
Discharge potential 30-90 days	2	46	4.3%	5.1%	5.5%
Uncertain discharge potential	4	46	8.7%	17.9%	17.4%

EXHIBIT 269
Rev. 9, 08/05/2005

Facility Quality Measure/Indicator Report

Page 1 of 2

Facility Name	LISA01		**Run Date**	05/20/05 16:01:28
City/State	SACRAMENTO,CA		**Report Period**	09/01/04 - 02/28/05
Provider Number	855134		**Comparison Group**	07/01/04 - 12/31/04
Login/Internal ID	LISA01/1234		**Report Version Number**	1.07

Measure ID	Domain/Measure Description	Num	Denom	Facility Observed Percent	Adjusted Percent	Comparison Group State Average	National Average	State Percentile
Chronic Care Measures								
	Accidents							
1.1	Incidence of new fractures	1	109	0.9%	-	1.9%	2.1%	29
1.2	Prevalence of falls	5	109	4.6%	-	12.3%	12.9%	8
	Behavior/Emotional Patterns							
2.1	Residents who have become more depressed or anxious	9	109	8.3%	-	16.1%	15.7%	23
2.2	Prevalence of behavior symptoms affecting others: Overall	16	106	15.1%	-	23.3%	18.9%	26
2.2-HI	Prevalence of behavior symptoms affecting others: High risk	15	86	17.4%	-	26.1%	22.1%	29
2.2-LO	Prevalence of behavior symptoms affecting others: Low risk	1	20	5.0%	-	8.7%	8.1%	49
2.3	Prevalence of symptoms of depression without antidepressant therapy	0	106	0.0%	-	6.7%	5.3%	0
	Clinical Management							
3.1	Use of 9 or more different medications	76	109	69.7%	-	56.2%	60.2%	84
	Cognitive Patterns							
4.1	Incidence of cognitive impairment	1	22	4.5%	-	15.0%	12.3%	23
	Elimination/Incontinence							
5.1	Low-risk residents who lost control of their bowels or bladder	42	67	62.7%	-	47.1%	46.8%	88
5.2	Residents who have/had a catheter inserted and left in their bladder	7	109	6.4%	5.8%	5.2%	7.7%	62
5.3	Prevalence of occasional or frequent bladder or bowel incontinence without a toileting plan	32	33	97.0%	-	54.9%	44.2%	85
5.4	Prevalence of fecal impaction	0	109	0.0%	-	0.2%	0.1%	0
	Infection Control							
6.1	Residents with a urinary tract infection	8	109	7.3%	-	8.5%	9.5%	44
	Nutrition/Eating							
7.1	Residents who lose too much weight	6	90	6.7%	-	10.9%	10.0%	21
7.2	Prevalence of tube feeding	24	109	22.0%	-	9.0%	7.2%	96 *
7.3	Prevalence of dehydration	2	109	1.8%	-	0.5%	0.4%	93 *
	Pain Management							
8.1	Residents who have moderate to severe pain	13	109	11.9%	9.4%	9.8%	7.8%	61
	Physical Functioning							
9.1	Residents whose need for help with daily activities has increased	6	77	7.8%	-	15.6%	17.5%	16
9.2	Residents who spend most of their time in bed or in a chair	29	106	27.4%	-	8.1%	5.5%	98 *
9.3	Residents whose ability to move in and around their room got worse	6	52	11.5%	10.1%	14.0%	15.7%	33
9.4	Incidence of decline in ROM	4	105	3.8%	-	8.1%	8.5%	27

Note: Dashes represent a value that could not be computed

EXHIBIT 269 (Cont.)

Facility Quality Measure/Indicator Report

Facility Name	LISA01	
City/State	SACRAMENTO,CA	
Provider Number	855134	
Login/Internal ID	LISA01/1234	

Run Date	05/20/05 16:01:28
Report Period	09/01/04 - 02/28/05
Comparison Group	07/01/04 - 12/31/04
Report Version Number	1.07

				Facility		Comparison Group		
Measure ID	**Domain/Measure Description**	**Num**	**Denom**	**Observed Percent**	**Adjusted Percent**	**State Average**	**National Average**	**State Percentile**
Chronic Care Measures								
	Psychotropic Drug Use							
10.1	Prevalence of antipsychotic use, in the absence of psychotic or related conditions: Overall	18	100	18.0%	-	26.7%	22.0%	20
10.1-HI	Prevalence of antipsychotic use, in the absence of psychotic or related conditions: High risk	7	11	63.6%	-	47.7%	46.0%	83
10.1-LO	Prevalence of antipsychotic use, in the absence of psychotic or related conditions: Low risk	11	86	12.8%	-	22.2%	18.1%	18
10.2	Prevalence of antianxiety/hypnotic use	20	100	20.0%	-	18.6%	18.8%	58
10.3	Prevalence of hypnotic use more than two times in last week	3	109	2.8%	-	3.8%	4.1%	47
	Quality of Life							
11.1	Residents who were physically restrained	8	109	7.3%	-	9.8%	7.1%	40
11.2	Prevalence of little or no activity	65	106	61.3%	-	10.5%	9.2%	99 *
	Skin Care							
12.1	High-risk residents with pressure ulcers	13	75	17.3%	-	17.1%	15.2%	58
12.2	Low-risk residents with pressure ulcers	1	34	2.9%	-	2.9%	3.4%	64 *
Post-Acute Care(PAC) Measures								
13.1	Short-stay residents with delirium	5	86	5.8%	5.2%	4.8%	3.4%	69
13.2	Short-stay residents who had moderate to severe pain	44	86	51.2%	-	23.5%	23.7%	92 *
13.3	Short-stay residents with pressure ulcers	20	83	24.1%	23.4%	19.7%	18.8%	67

Note: Dashes represent a value that could not be computed

EXHIBIT 270
Rev. 9, 08/05/2005

Resident Level Quality Measure/Indicator Report: Chronic Care Sample

Facility Name LISA01
City/State SACRAMENTO, CA
Provider Number 855134
Login/Internal ID LISA01/1234

Run Date 05/21/05 10:06:04
Report Period 09/01/04 - 02/28/05
Report Version Number 1.07

Resident Int Id	Resident Name	A/Ba	NewFract	Falls	Depression	Problem Behavior Hi	Problem Behavior Lo	Dprs No Tx	9+ Meds	Cog Impair	Bwl/Blad Incnt Lo	Cath Insert	Incnt No TP	Fecal Impct	UTIs	WtLoss	Tube Feed	Dhyd	Mod/Sevr Pain	ADL Help Incrs	Most Time Chair	Move Ability Wrse	Decln ROM	Antipsy w/o Psychotic Condition Hi	Antipsy w/o Psychotic Condition Lo	Anti-anx/Hpnot	Hpnot 2x Week	Phys Rstrn	Little Activ	Pressure Ulcers Hi	Pressure Ulcers Lo	Count
																																Count
Active Residents																																
999999	DOE, JANE	05							X		X				X														X			5
999999	DOE, JANE	01		X					X		X		X			X			X													4
999999	DOE, JOHN	05									X																					X	1
999999	DOE, JANE	05		X					X								X		X										X	X		4
999999	DOE, JOHN	01		X					X				X						X							X						6
999999	DOE, JANE	01				X			X			X	X			X			X		X					X			X	X		4
999999	DOE, JANE	01				X			X			X	X						X											X		5
999999	DOE, JOHN	05		X					X										X									X				4
999999	DOE, JANE	05							X			X	X						X					X		X	X	X	X	X		5
999999	DOE, JOHN	05							X		X					X	X				X				X	X			X	X		6
999999	DOE, JOHN	01							X		X		X								X	X			X				X		X	9
999999	DOE, JANE	05									X				X						X	X			X				X		X	3
999999	DOE, JANE	01							X			X					X		X		X											5
999999	DOE, JOHN	02										X														X			X			6
999999	DOE, JANE	01		X		X			X				X						X									X				3
999999	DOE, JOHN	01									X	X													X	X	X					7
999999	DOE, JANE	02																															0
999999	DOE, JOHN	05															X		X		X				X	X			X		X	3
999999	DOE, JANE	05																			X								X	X		5
999999	DOE, JOHN	05																			X				X	X			X	X		5
999999	DOE, JANE	05							X								X				X								X	X		3
999999	DOE, JOHN	05															X								X				X	X	X	5
999999	DOE, JOHN	05																X								X			X		X	3

Note: X=triggered, blank=not triggered or excluded.

EXHIBIT 270 (Cont.)

Resident Level Quality Measure/Indicator Report: Post Acute Care Sample Page 1 of 1

Facility Name	LISA01
City/State	SACRAMENTO,CA
Provider Number	855134
Login/Internal ID	LISA01/1234

Run Date	05/09/05 16:18:49
Report Period	09/01/04 - 02/28/05
Report Version Number	1.07

Resident Int Id	Resident Name	Delrm	Mod/Sevr Pain	Press Ulcer	Count
Active Residents					
999999	DOE, JANE				0
999999	DOE, JANE				0
999999	DOE, JANE				0
999999	DOE, JOHN				0
Discharged Residents					
999999	DOE, JANE				0
999999	DOE, JANE				0
999999	DOE, JOHN	X			1
999999	DOE, JANE			X	1
999999	DOE, JOHN				0
999999	DOE, JOHN				0
999999	DOE, JOHN				0
999999	DOE, JANE				0
999999	DOE, JANE				0
999999	DOE, JANE		X		1
999999	DOE, JANE				0
999999	DOE, JANE				0
999999	DOE, JOHN				0
999999	DOE, JANE	X			1
999999	DOE, JANE		X		1
999999	DOE, JOHN		X		1

Note: X=triggered, blank=not triggered or excluded.

EXHIBIT 271
Rev. 9, 08/05/2005

QM/QI Reports Technical Specifications: Version 1.0

Introduction

The measures contained on the Quality Measure/Indicator (QM/QI) Reports are calculated in two major steps. In the first step, two samples of assessments are selected: a chronic care sample and a post-acute care (PAC) sample. In the second step, logic is applied to the two samples of assessments to produce the chronic care and PAC measures. The purpose of this document is to describe the technical details that are involved in these two steps.

This document is divided into three major sections. The first section describes the logic that is used to calculate each of the measures on the QM/QI Reports. The second and third sections describe the criteria that are used to select the assessment records for the chronic care and post-acute care resident samples.

Calculation Logic

The table below[1] lists all of the measures that are on the QM/QI Reports and describes the logic that is used to calculate each measure. The table contains three columns:

- Measure description
- Measure specifications
- Covariates/Risk adjustment

The contents of these columns are described below.

Measure Description Column

- **Measure number.** Each measure is assigned a number that corresponds to the numbering in the QM/QI Reports.
- **Measure description.** This is a brief description of the measure.
- **Source.** The QM/QI Reports combine the publicly reported Quality Measures (QMs) and the CHSRA Quality Indicator (QI) measures. For QM measures, the "source" indicates "QM" and lists the abbreviation that has been assigned to the measure. For the QI measures, the "source" says QInn where "nn" is a number that corresponds to the measure's number on the prior CHSRA QI reports. For example, "QI01" refers to QI #1.

---

[1] This table is based upon information presented in two documents: (1) *National Nursing Home Quality Measures User's Manual, November, 2004 (v1.2)*, and (2) *Facility Guide for the Nursing Home Quality Indicators, September 28, 1999*.

EXHIBIT 271 (Cont.)
QM/QI Reports Technical Specifications: Version 1.0

- **QI Replaced.** Several CHSRA QI measures were replaced by corresponding QM measures. For these measures, a "QI Replaced" entry indicates the number for the QI measure that has been replaced.

Measure Specifications Column

- **Numerator.** The numerator entry gives the logic used to determine whether a resident triggers the QM (if the resident is included in the numerator for the QM rate in the facility).
- **Denominator.** The denominator entry defines whether a resident has the necessary records available to be a candidate for the QM (inclusion of the resident in the denominator for the QM rate for the facility).
- **Exclusions.** The exclusions entry provides clinical conditions and missing data conditions that preclude a resident from consideration for the QM. An excluded resident is excluded from both the numerator and denominator of the QM rate for the facility.
- **Technical comments.** These comments provide additional technical details pertaining to the QM numerator, denominator, and exclusions. Examples of the type of information provided include specific details for calculating scale scores, definition of missing data values for an MDS item, and selection of the value for an MDS item that may come from different assessments for a resident.

Covariates/Risk Adjustment Column

- **Covariates.** The "Covariates" entry defines the calculation logic for covariates. Covariates are always prevalence indicators with a value of 1 if the condition is present and a value of 0 if the condition is not present.
- **High Risk/Low Risk.** A "High Risk" entry defines the calculation logic for a resident who is high risk for the measure. A "Low Risk" entry defines a resident who is low risk.
- **Technical comments.** In some cases, technical comments are provided to define measures or scales that are used to calculate covariates or risk groups.

Notes regarding interpreting the specifications table

- The symbol [t] indicates a target assessment, and [t-1] indicates a prior assessment.
- An MDS item has missing data if that item has an "unable to determine" response (dash in the MDS record), if that item has been skipped (blank), or if that item is not active on the assessment.
- In lists of ICD-9 codes, an asterisk (*) indicates that any value meets the requirements. For example, a code listed as 295.** indicates that any code starting with "295." meets the requirements. In this case the last 2 digits are ignored.

(continued)

EXHIBIT 271 (Cont.)
QM/QI Reports Technical Specifications: Version 1.0

Measure Description	Measure Specifications	Covariates/Risk Adjustment
	Chronic Care Measures	
Accidents		
1.1 Incidence of new fractures Source: QI01	**Numerator:** Residents with new fractures on target assessment. New fracture defined as: 1. New hip fracture (J4c[t] is checked on target assessment and J4c[t-1] is not checked on prior assessment) *OR* 2. Other new fractures (J4d[t] is checked on target assessment and J4d[t-1] is not checked on prior assessment) **Denominator:** All residents with a valid target assessment and a valid prior assessment who did not have fractures on the prior assessment (J4c[t-1] is not checked and J4d[t-1] is not checked). **Exclusions:** Residents satisfying any of the following conditions: 1. The measure did not trigger (resident not included in the numerator) and there is missing data on J4c or J4d on either the target or prior assessment (J4c[t], J4d[t], J4c[t-1], or J4d[t-1] is missing).	
1.2 Prevalence of falls Source: QI02	**Numerator:** Residents who had falls within the past 30 days (J4a is checked on the target assessment). **Denominator:** All residents with a valid target assessment. **Exclusions:** Residents satisfying any of the following conditions: 1. The target assessment is an admission (AA8a = 01) assessment. 2. J4a has missing data on the target assessment.	

EXHIBIT 271 (Cont.)
QM/QI Reports Technical Specifications: Version 1.0

Measure Description	Measure Specifications	Covariates/Risk Adjustment
Behavior/Emotional Patterns		
2.1 Residents who have become more depressed or anxious Source: QM CMOD03	**Numerator:** Residents whose Mood Scale scores are greater on target assessment relative to prior assessment (Mood Scale [t] > Mood Scale [t-1]). [The Mood Scale is defined in the Technical Comments.] **Denominator:** All residents with a valid target assessment and a valid prior assessment. **Exclusions:** Residents satisfying any of the following conditions: 1. The Mood Scale score is missing on the target assessment [t]. 2. The Mood Scale score is missing on the prior assessment [t-1] and the Mood Scale score indicates symptoms present on the target assessment (Mood Scale [t] >0). 3. The Mood Scale score is at a maximum (value 8) on the prior assessment. 4. The resident is comatose (B1 = 1) or comatose status is unknown (B1 = missing) on the target assessment. **Technical Comments** **Mood Scale Definition:** Mood Scale score is defined as the count of the number of the following eight conditions that are satisfied (range 0 through 8) on the target assessment. The mood scale has a missing value if any of the MDS items in the following eight conditions has missing data. 1. Any verbal expression of distress (E1a>0, E1c>0, E1e>0, E1f>0, E1g>0, or E1h>0). 2. Shows signs of crying, tearfulness (E1m>0). 3. Motor agitation (E1n>0). 4. Leaves food uneaten (K4c=checked) on target or last full assessment. The K4c value from the last full assessment is only considered if the target assessment is a quarterly assessment and the state quarterly assessment does not include K4c. 5. Repetitive health complaints (E1h>0).	

(continued)

EXHIBIT 271 (Cont.)
QM/QI Reports Technical Specifications: Version 1.0

Measure Description	Measure Specifications	Covariates/Risk Adjustment
2.2 Prevalence of behavior symptoms affecting others **2.2-HI High risk** **2.2-LO Low risk** **Source:** QI03	6. Repetitive/recurrent verbalizations (E1a>0, E1c>0, or E1g>0). 7. Negative statements (E1a>0, E1e>0, or E1f>0). 8. Mood symptoms not easily altered (E2=2). *Numerator:* Residents with behavioral symptoms affecting others on target assessment. Behavioral symptoms affecting others: Verbally abusive (E4bA >0); OR physically abusive (E4cA > 0); OR socially inappropriate /disruptive behavior (E4dA > 0). *Denominator:* All residents with a valid target assessment. *Exclusions:* Residents satisfying any of the following conditions: 1. The target assessment is an admission (AA8a = 01) assessment. 2. The measure did not trigger (resident not included in the numerator) and there is missing data on E4bA, E4cA, or E4dA. 3. The resident does not qualify as high risk and B2a, B4, I1ff or I1gg has missing data—i.e., the risk group is unknown. *Note:* Three separate measures are defined: (1) for all residents (overall), (2) for residents defined as high risk, and (3) for residents defined as low risk. The only difference between the three measures is the denominator definition and use of exclusions as follows: *Denominator for overall:* All residents with a valid target assessment with only the first 2 exclusions applied. *Denominator for high risk:* All residents with a valid target assessment who are defined as high risk, with all 3 exclusions applied. *Denominator for low risk:* All residents with a valid target assessment who are defined as low risk, with all 3 exclusions applied.	*High Risk:* Presence of Cognitive Impairment (see technical note, below) on the target assessment. OR Psychotic disorders (I3a-I3e = ICD-9 295.**-295.**; 297.**-298.** or I1gg schizophrenia is checked) on the target assessment or on the most recent full assessment. The I3a-I3e values from both the target assessment and the last full assessment are always considered. The I1gg value from the last full assessment is only considered if the target assessment is a quarterly assessment and the state quarterly assessment does not include I1gg. OR Manic-depressive (I3 a-I3e =ICD-9 296.**-296.** or I1ff is checked) on the target assessment or on the most recent full assessment. The I3a-I3e values from both the target assessment and the last full assessment are always considered. The I1ff value from the last full assessment is only considered if the target assessment is a quarterly assessment and the state quarterly assessment does not include I1ff. *Low Risk:* All other residents that are not high risk.

EXHIBIT 271 (Cont.)
QM/QI Reports Technical Specifications: Version 1.0

Measure Description	Measure Specifications	Covariates/Risk Adjustment
		Technical Comments
		Cognitive Impairment Definition. Resident has impairment in daily decision making ability (B4 >0) and has short term memory problems (B2a=1).
2.3 Prevalence of symptoms of depression without antidepressant therapy Source: QI05	**Numerator:** Residents with symptoms of depression (see technical comments, below) and no antidepressant therapy (O4c=0) on the target assessment. **Denominator:** All residents with a valid target assessment. **Exclusions:** Residents satisfying any of the following conditions: 1. The target assessment is an admission (AA8a = 01) assessment. 2. The measure did not trigger (resident not included in the numerator) and the following 2 conditions are both satisfied: (a) there is missing data on any of the following items: B1, E1a, E1g, E1j, E1n, E1o, E1p, E2, E4eA, K3a, N1a, N1b, N1c, N1d, or O4c and (b) the measure could have triggered if there had been no missing data. **Technical Comments** **Symptoms of Depression Definition.** Sad mood (E2 = 1 or 2) and at least 2 of the following other symptoms of functional depression: 1. **Symptom 1 distress** (E1a = 1 or 2: resident made negative statements); 2. **Symptom 2 agitation or withdrawal** (E1n = 1 or 2: repetitive physical movements, or E4eA = 1, 2, or 3: resists care, or E1o = 1 or 2: withdrawal from activity, or E1p = 1 or 2: reduced social activity); 3. **Symptom 3 wake with unpleasant mood** (E1j = 1 or 2), **or not awake most of the day** (N1d is checked), **or awake 1 period of the day or less and not comatose** (N1a+N1b +N1c <= 1 and B1 = 0);	

(continued)

EXHIBIT 271 (Cont.)
QM/QI Reports Technical Specifications: Version 1.0

Measure Description	Measure Specifications	Covariates/Risk Adjustment
	4. Symptom 4 suicidal or has recurrent thoughts of death (E1g = 1 or 2); 5. Symptom 5 weight loss (K3a = 1).	
Clinical Management		
3.1 Use of 9 or more different medications Source: QI06	*Numerator:* Residents who received 9 or more different medications on target assessment: O1 (number of medications) >= 9. *Denominator:* All residents with a valid target assessment. *Exclusions:* Residents satisfying any of the following conditions: 1. The target assessment is an admission (AA8a = 01) assessment. 2. O1 has missing data on the target assessment.	
Cognitive Patterns		
4.1 Incidence of cognitive impairment Source: QI07	*Numerator:* Residents who were cognitively impaired on the target assessment and who were not cognitively impaired on the prior assessment (see technical comment below for definition of cognitive impairment). *Denominator:* Residents with a valid target assessment and a valid prior assessment who were not cognitively impaired on the prior assessment. *Exclusions:* Residents satisfying the following condition: 1. The measure did not trigger (resident not included in the numerator) and there is missing data on B4 or B2a on target or prior assessment (B4[t], B2a[t], B4[t-1], or B2a[t-1] is missing). *Technical Comments* *Cognitive Impairment Definition.* Resident has any impairment in daily decision making ability (B4 >0) and has short term memory problems (B2a=1).	

EXHIBIT 271 (Cont.)
QM/QI Reports Technical Specifications: Version 1.0

Measure Description	Measure Specifications	Covariates/Risk Adjustment
Elimination/Incontinence		

5.1 Low-risk residents who lost control of their bowels or bladder
 	
Source: QM CCNT06
 	
QI Replaced: QI08 Low Risk
	Numerator: Residents who were frequently incontinent or fully incontinent on the target assessment (H1a = 3 or 4, or H1b = 3 or 4).
	
	Denominator: All residents with a valid target assessment and not qualifying as high risk.
	
	Exclusions:
	
	1. Residents who qualify as high risk are excluded from the denominator:
	
	  a. Severe cognitive impairment on the target assessment as indicated by B4 = 3 AND B2a = 1; OR
	
	  b. Totally dependent in mobility ADLs on the target assessment: G1aA = 4 or 8 AND G1bA = 4 or 8 AND G1eA = 4 or 8.
	
	2. Residents satisfying any of the following conditions are also excluded from the risk group:
	
	  a. The target assessment is an admission (AA8a = 01) assessment.
	
	  b. The QM did not trigger (resident is not included in the QM numerator) AND the value of H1a or H1b is missing on the target assessment.
	
	  c. The resident is comatose (B1 = 1) or comatose status is unknown (B1 = missing) on the target assessment.
	
	  d. The resident has an indwelling catheter (H3d = checked) or indwelling catheter status is unknown (H3d = missing) on the target assessment.
	
	  e. The resident has an ostomy (H3i = checked) or ostomy status is unknown (H3i = missing) on the target assessment.
	
	  f. The resident does not qualify as high risk and either of the cognitive impairment items (B2a or B4) are missing on the target assessment.	

(continued)

EXHIBIT 271 (Cont.)
QM/QI Reports Technical Specifications: Version 1.0

Measure Description	Measure Specifications	Covariates/Risk Adjustment
	g. The resident does not qualify as high risk and any of the mobility ADLs (G1aA, G1bA and G1eA) is missing on the target assessment.	
5.2 Residents who have/had a catheter inserted and left in their bladder Source: QM CCAT02 QI Replaced: QI10	*Numerator:* Residents with indwelling catheters on target assessment (H3d = checked). *Denominator:* All residents with a valid target assessment. *Exclusions:* Residents satisfying any of the following conditions: 1. The target assessment is an admission (AA8a = 01) assessment. 2. H3d is missing on the target assessment.	*Covariates:* 1. Indicator of bowel incontinence on the prior assessment: Covariate = 1 if H1a = 4 Covariate = 0 if H1a = 0,1,2, or 3 2. Indicator of pressure sores on the prior assessment: Covariate = 1 if M2a = 3 or 4 Covariate = 0 if M2a = 0, 1 or 2
5.3 Prevalence of occasional or frequent bladder or bowel incontinence without a toileting plan Source: QI09	*Numerator:* Residents with no scheduled toileting program (neither H3a nor H3b is checked) on the target assessment and either or both of the following conditions on the target assessment: 1. Occasional or frequent bladder incontinence (H1b = 2 or 3), OR 2. Bowel incontinence (H1a = 2 or 3). *Denominator:* Residents with frequent incontinence or occasionally incontinent in either bladder (H1b = 2 or 3) or bowel (H1a = 2 or 3) on target assessment. *Exclusions:* Residents satisfying any of the following conditions: 1. The target assessment is an admission (AA8a = 01) assessment. 2. The measure did not trigger (resident not included in the numerator) and there is missing data on any of the following: H3a, H3b, H1a, H1b.	

EXHIBIT 271 (Cont.)
QM/QI Reports Technical Specifications: Version 1.0

Measure Description	Measure Specifications	Covariates/Risk Adjustment
5.4 Prevalence of fecal impaction Source: QI11	**Numerator:** Residents with fecal impaction (H2d is checked) on the most recent assessment. **Denominator:** All residents with a valid target assessment. **Exclusions:** Residents satisfying any of the following conditions: 1. The target assessment is an admission (AA8a = 01) assessment. 2. H2d is missing on the target assessment.	
Infection Control		
6.1 Residents with a urinary tract infection Source: QM CCNT04 QI Replaced: QI12	**Numerator:** Residents with urinary tract infection on target assessment (I2j = checked). **Denominator:** All residents with a valid target assessment. **Exclusions:** Residents satisfying any of the following conditions: 1. The target assessment is an admission (AA8a = 01) assessment. 2. I2j is missing on the target assessment.	
Nutrition/Eating		
7.1 Residents who lose too much weight Source: QM CWLS01 QI Replaced: QI13	**Numerator:** Residents who have experienced weight loss (K3a=1) of 5 percent of more in the last 30 days or 10 percent or more in the last 6 months. **Denominator:** All residents with a valid target assessment. **Exclusions:** Residents satisfying any of the following conditions: 1. The target assessment is an admission (AA8a = 01) assessment. 2. K3a is missing on the target assessment. 3. The resident is receiving hospice care (P1ao = checked) or hospice status is unknown (P1ao = missing) on the target assessment or the most recent full assessment. The P1ao value from the last full assessment is only considered if the target assessment is a quarterly assessment and the state quarterly assessment does not include P1ao.	

(continued)

EXHIBIT 271 (Cont.)
QM/QI Reports Technical Specifications: Version 1.0

Measure Description	Measure Specifications	Covariates/Risk Adjustment
7.2 Prevalence of tube feeding Source: QI14	**Numerator:** Residents with tube feeding (K5b is checked) on target assessment. **Denominator:** All residents with a valid target assessment. **Exclusions:** Residents satisfying any of the following conditions: 1. The target assessment is an admission (AA8a = 01) assessment. 2. K5b is missing on the target assessment.	
7.3 Prevalence of dehydration Source: QI15	**Numerator:** Residents with dehydration: output exceeds input (J1c is checked) on the target assessment or I3a-I3e = ICD-9 276.5 on the target assessment. **Denominator:** All residents with a valid target assessment. **Exclusions:** Residents satisfying any of the following conditions: 1. The target assessment is an admission (AA8a = 01) assessment. 2. J1c is missing on the target assessment.	
Pain Management		
8.1 Residents who have moderate to severe pain Source: QM CPAI0X	**Numerator:** Residents with moderate pain at least daily (J2a=2 AND J2b=2) OR horrible/excruciating pain at any frequency (J2b=3) on the target assessment. **Denominator:** All residents with a valid target assessment. **Exclusions:** Residents satisfying any of the following conditions: 1. The target assessment is an admission (AA8a = 01) assessment. 2. Either J2a or J2b is missing on the target assessment. 3. The values of J2a and J2b are inconsistent on the target assessment. J2a and J2b are inconsistent if either (a) J2a = 0 and J2b is not blank, or (b) J2a >0 and J2b = blank.	**Covariates:** 1. Indicator of independence or modified independence in daily decision making on the prior assessment: Covariate = 1 if B4 = 0 or 1. Covariate = 0 if B4 = 2 or 3.

EXHIBIT 271 (Cont.)
QM/QI Reports Technical Specifications: Version 1.0

Measure Description	Measure Specifications	Covariates/Risk Adjustment
Physical Functioning		
9.1 Residents whose need for help with daily activities has increased Source: QM CADL01 QI Replaced: QI17	**Numerator:** Residents with worsening (increasing MDS item score) in Late-Loss ADL self performance at target relative to prior assessment. Residents meet the definition of Late-Loss ADL worsening when at least two of the following are true: 1. Bed mobility – [Level at target assessment (G1aA[t]] – [Level at previous assessment (G1aA[t-1]))] > 0, or 2. Transfer - [Level at target assessment (G1bA[t]] – [Level at previous assessment (G1bA[t-1])] > 0, or 3. Eating - [Level at target assessment (G1hA[t]] – [Level at previous assessment (G1hA[t-1])] > 0, or 4. Toileting - [Level at target assessment (G1iA[t]] – [Level at previous assessment (G1iA[t-1])] > 0, OR at least one of the following is true: 1. Bed mobility – [Level at target assessment (G1aA[t]] – [Level at previous assessment (G1aA[t-1])] > 1, or 2. Transfer - [Level at target assessment (G1bA[t]] – [Level at previous assessment (G1bA[t-1])] > 1, or 3. Eating - [Level at target assessment (G1hA[t]] – [Level at previous assessment (G1hA[t-1])] > 1, or 4. Toileting - [Level at target assessment (G1iA[t]] – [Level at previous assessment (G1iA[t-1])] > 1. **Denominator:** All residents with a valid target and a valid prior assessment. **Exclusions:** Residents meeting any of the following conditions: 1. None of the four Late-Loss ADLs (G1aA, G1bA, G1hA, and G1iA) can show decline because each of the four have a value of 4 (total dependence) or a value of 8 (activity did not occur) on the prior assessment [t-1]. 2. The QM did not trigger (resident not included in the numerator) AND there is missing data on any one of the four Late-Loss ADLs	

(continued)

EXHIBIT 271 (Cont.)
QM/QI Reports Technical Specifications: Version 1.0

Measure Description	Measure Specifications	Covariates/Risk Adjustment
	(G1aA), G1bA, G1hA, or G1iA) on the target assessment [t] or prior assessment [t-1]. 3. The resident is comatose (B1 = 1) or comatose status is unknown (B1 = missing) on the target assessment. 4. The resident has end-stage disease (J5c = checked) or end-stage disease status unknown (J5c = missing) on the target assessment. 5. The resident is receiving hospice care (P1ao = checked) or hospice status is unknown (P1ao = missing) on the target assessment or the most recent full assessment. The P1ao value from the last full assessment is only considered if the target assessment is a quarterly assessment and the state quarterly assessment does not include P1ao.	
9.2 Residents who spend most of their time in a bed or in a chair Source: QM CBFT01 QI Replaced: QI16	*Numerator:* Residents who are bedfast (G6a is checked) on target assessment. *Denominator:* All residents with a valid target assessment. *Exclusions:* Residents meeting any of the following conditions: 1. The target assessment is an admission (AA8a = 01) assessment. 2. G6a is missing on the target assessment. 3. The resident is comatose (B1=1), or comatose status is unknown (B1= missing) on the target assessment.	
9.3 Residents whose ability to move in and around their room got worse Source: QM CMOB01	*Numerator:* Residents whose value for locomotion self performance is greater at target relative to prior assessment (G1eA[t]>G1eA[t- 1]). *Denominator:* All residents with a valid target assessment and a valid prior assessment. *Exclusions:* Residents satisfying any of the following conditions: 1. The G1eA value is missing on the target assessment [t]. 2. The G1eA value is missing on the prior assessment [t-1] and the G1eA value shows some dependence on the target assessment (G1eA[t]>0). 3. The G1eA value on the prior assessment is 4 (total dependence)	*Covariates:* 1. Indicator of recent falls on the prior assessment: Covariate = 1 if J4a checked or J4b checked Covariate = 0 if J4a not checked AND J4b not checked 2. Indicator of extensive support or more dependence in eating on the prior assessment:

EXHIBIT 271 (Cont.)
QM/QI Reports Technical Specifications: Version 1.0

Measure Description	Measure Specifications	Covariates/Risk Adjustment
	or 8 (activity did not occur). 4. The resident is comatose (B1 = 1) or comatose status is unknown (B1 = missing) on the target assessment. 5. The resident has end-stage disease (J5c = checked) or end-stage disease status is unknown (J5c = missing) on the target assessment. 6. The resident is receiving hospice care (P1ao = checked) or hospice status is unknown(P1ao = missing) on the target assessment or the most recent full assessment. The P1ao value from the last full assessment is only considered if the target assessment is a quarterly assessment and the state quarterly assessment does not include P1ao.	Covariate = 1 if G1hA = 3,4, or 8 Covariate = 0 if G1hA = 0,1, or 2 3. Indicator of extensive support or more dependence in toileting on the prior assessment: Covariate = 1 if G1iA = 3,4, or 8 Covariate = 0 if G1iA = 0,1, or 2
9.4 Incidence of decline in ROM **Source: QI18**	*Numerator:* Residents with increases in functional limitation in ROM between prior and target assessments. Functional limitation in ROM is defined as the sum of items G4aA through G4f A: G4aA + G4bA + G4cA + G4dA + G4eA + G4fA, as follows: SUM(G4aA..G4fA)[t] = functional limitation in ROM on target assessment, and SUM(G4aA..G4fA)[t-1] = functional limitation in ROM on prior assessment. Resident triggers if: SUM(G4aA..G4fA)[t] > SUM(G4aA..G4fA)[t-1] *Denominator:* All residents with a valid target assessment and a valid prior assessment. *Exclusions:* Residents satisfying any of the following conditions: 1. Residents with maximal loss of ROM on prior assessment: SUM(G4aA..G4fA)[t-1]=12. 2. Residents with missing data on either the target or prior assessment on any of the following items: G4aA, G4bA, G4cA, G4dA, G4eA, or G4fA.	

(continued)

EXHIBIT 271 (Cont.)
QM/QI Reports Technical Specifications: Version 1.0

Measure Description	Measure Specifications	Covariates/Risk Adjustment
Psychotropic Drug Use		

10.1 Prevalence of antipsychotic use, in the absence of psychotic or related conditions
 	
10.1-HI High risk
10.1-LO Low risk
 	
Source: QI19
	Numerator: Residents receiving anti-psychotics (O4a >= 1) on target assessment
	
	Denominator: All residents on target assessment, except those with psychotic or related conditions (see exclusion).
	
	Exclusions: Residents satisfying any of the following conditions:
	
	1. The target assessment is an admission (AA8a = 01) assessment.
	2. Residents with one or more of the following psychotic or related conditions on the target assessment or on the most recent full assessment. The I3a-I3e values from both the target assessment and the last full assessment are always considered. The I1gg value from the last full assessment is only considered if the target assessment is a quarterly assessment and the state quarterly assessment does not include I1gg.
	   a. I3a-I3e ICD-9 = 295.** - 295.**, 297.** - 298.**, or I1gg ICD-9 = 295.** - 295.**, 297.** - 298.**, or
	   b. I1gg schizophrenia is checked, or
	   c. Tourette's (I3a-I3e ICD-9 =307.23), or
	   d. Huntington's (I3a-I3e ICD-9 =333.4 or 333.40).
	3. Residents with hallucinations (J1i is checked) on the target assessment.
	4. Residents who do not trigger the measure (are not included in the numerator) and who have missing data on any of the following items: O4a, I1gg, or J1i.
	5. Residents who are not high risk and the following 2 conditions are both satisfied: (a) there is missing data on any of the following items: B2a, B4, E4bA, E4cA, or E4dA and (b) high risk could have resulted if there had been no missing data.
	
	Note: Three separate measures are defined, one for all residents (overall), one for residents defined as high risk, and one for residents defined as low risk. The only difference between the two measures is the denominator definition and use of exclusions as follows:
	
	Denominator for overall: All residents with a valid target
		High risk: Cognitive Impairment AND Behavior Problems on target assessment (see technical comments below for definitions).
		
		Low Risk: All other residents that are not high risk.
		
		Technical Comments
		
		Cognitive impairment definition. Any impairment in daily decision making ability (B4 >0) AND has short term memory problems (B2a=1).
		
		Behavior problems definition. Behavior problems. defined as one or more of the following less than daily or daily: verbally abusive (E4bA > 0), physically abusive (E4cA > 0), or socially inappropriate/disruptive behavior (E4dA > 0).

EXHIBIT 271 (Cont.)
QM/QI Reports Technical Specifications: Version 1.0

Measure Description	Measure Specifications	Covariates/Risk Adjustment
	assessment except those with psychotic or related conditions, with only the first 4 exclusions applied. **Denominator for high risk:** All residents with a valid target assessment who are defined as high risk except those with psychotic or related conditions, with all 5 exclusions applied. **Denominator for low risk:** All residents with a valid target assessment who are defined as low risk except those with psychotic or related conditions, with all 5 exclusions applied.	

10.2 Prevalence of antianxiety/hypnotic use
 	
Source: QI20
	Numerator: Residents who received antianxiety or hypnotics (O4b or O4d >= 1) on target assessment.
	
	Denominator: All residents on target assessment, except those with psychotic or related conditions (see exclusion).
	
	Exclusions: Residents satisfying any of the following conditions:
	
	1. The target assessment is an admission (AA8a = 01) assessment.
	2. Residents with one or more of the following psychotic disorders on the target assessment or on the most recent full assessment The I3a-I3e values from both the target assessment and the last full assessment are always considered. The I1gg value from the last full assessment is only considered if the target assessment is a quarterly assessment and the state quarterly assessment does not include I1gg.
	    a. I3a-I3e ICD-9 = 295.** - 295.**, 297.** - 298.**, or
	    b. I1gg schizophrenia is checked, or
	    c. Tourette's (I3a-I3e ICD-9 =307.23), or
	    d. Huntington's (I3a-I3e ICD-9 =333.4 or 333.40)
	3. Residents with hallucinations (J1i is checked) on the target assessment.
	4. Residents who do not trigger the measure (are not included in the numerator) and who have missing data on any of the following items: O4b, O4d, I1gg, or J1i.	

(continued)

EXHIBIT 271 (Cont.)
QM/QI Reports Technical Specifications: Version 1.0

Measure Description	Measure Specifications	Covariates/Risk Adjustment
10.3 Prevalence of hypnotic use more than two times in last week Source: QI21	*Numerator:* Residents who received hypnotics more than 2 times in last week (O4d > 2) on the target assessment. *Denominator:* All residents with a valid target assessment. *Exclusions:* Residents satisfying any of the following conditions: 1. The target assessment is an admission (AA8a = 01) assessment. 2. O4d is missing on the target assessment.	
Quality of Life		
11.1 Residents who were physically restrained Source: QM CRES01 QI Replaced: QI22	*Numerator:* Residents who were physically restrained daily (P4c or P4d or P4e = 2) on target assessment. *Denominator:* All residents with a valid target assessment. *Exclusions:* Residents satisfying any of the following conditions: 1. The target assessment is an admission (AA8a = 01) assessment. 2. The QM did not trigger (resident is not included in the QM numerator) AND the value of P4c or P4d or P4e is missing on the target assessment.	
11.2 Prevalence of little or no activity Source: QI23	*Numerator:* Residents with little or no activity (N2 = 2 or 3) on the target assessment. *Denominator:* All residents with a valid target assessment. *Exclusions:* Residents satisfying any of the following conditions: 1. The target assessment is an admission (AA8a = 01) assessment. 2. The resident is comatose (B1=1). 3. N2 or B1 is missing on the target assessment.	

EXHIBIT 271 (Cont.)
QM/QI Reports Technical Specifications: Version 1.0

Measure Description	Measure Specifications	Covariates/Risk Adjustment
Skin Care		
12.1 High-risk residents with pressure ulcers Source: QM CPRU02 QI Replaced: QI24 High Risk	***Numerator:*** Residents with pressure sores (Stage 1-4) on target assessment (M2a >0 OR I3a-I3e = ICD-9 707.0*) who are defined as high risk (see denominator definition). ***Denominator:*** All residents with a valid target assessment and any one of the following high-risk criteria: 1. Impaired in bed mobility or transfer on the target assessment as indicated by G1aA = 3, 4, or 8 OR G1bA = 3, 4, or 8. 2. Comatose on the target assessment as indicated by B1 = 1. 3. Suffer malnutrition on the target assessment as indicated by I3a through I3e = 260, 261, 262, 263.0, 263.1, 263.2, 263.8, or 263.9. ***Exclusions:*** Residents satisfying any of the following conditions are excluded: 1. The target assessment is an admission (AA8a = 01) assessment. 2. The QM did not trigger (resident is not included in the QM numerator) AND the value of M2a is missing on the target assessment.	
12.2 Low-risk residents with pressure ulcers Source: QM CPRU03 QI Replaced: QI24 Low Risk	***Numerator:*** Residents with pressure sores (Stage 1-4) on target assessment (M2a >0 OR I3a-I3e = ICD-9 707.0*) who are defined as low risk (see denominator definition). ***Denominator:*** All residents with a valid target assessment who are defined as low risk. "Low risk" residents are those who do not qualify as high risk as defined in denominator definition for measure 12.1 above. ***Exclusions:*** Residents satisfying any of the following conditions are excluded from all risk groups (high and low): 1. The target assessment is an admission (AA8a = 01) assessment. 2. The QM did not trigger (resident is not included in the QM numerator) AND the value of M2a is missing on the target assessment.	

(continued)

EXHIBIT 271 (Cont.)
QM/QI Reports Technical Specifications: Version 1.0

Measure Description	Measure Specifications	Covariates/Risk Adjustment
	3. The resident does not qualify as high-risk AND the value of G1aA or G1bA is missing on the target assessment. 4. The resident does not qualify as high-risk AND the value of B1 is missing on the target assessment.	
	Post-Acute Care (PAC) Measures	
13.1 Short-stay residents with delirium Source: QM PAC-DEL0X	**Numerator:** Short-stay residents at SNF PPS 14-day assessment with at least one symptom of delirium that represents a departure from usual functioning (at least one B5a through B5f = 2). **Denominator:** All patients with a valid SNF PPS 14-day assessment (AA8b = 7). **Exclusions:** Patients satisfying any of the following conditions: 1. Patients who are comatose (B1 = 1) or comatose status is unknown (B1 = missing) on the SNF PPS 14-day assessment. 2. Patients with end-stage disease (J5c = checked) or end-stage disease status is unknown (J5c = missing) on the SNF PPS 14-day assessment. 3. Patients who are receiving hospice care (P1ao = checked) or hospice status is unknown (P1ao = missing) on the SNF PPS 14-day assessment. 4. The QM did not trigger (patient not included in the numerator) AND there is a missing value on any of the items B5a through B5f on the SNF PPS 14-day assessment.	**Covariates:** 1. Indicator of NO prior residential history preceding the current SNF stay for the patient: Covariate = 1 if there is NO prior residential history indicated by the following condition being satisfied: a. There is a recent admission assessment (AA8a = 01) AND AB5a through AB5e are not checked (value 0) and AB5f is checked (value 1). Covariate = 0 if there is prior residential history indicated by either of the following conditions being satisfied: a. There is a recent admission assessment (AA8a = 01) AND any of the items AB5a through AB5e are checked (value 1) OR AB5f is not checked (value 0). b. There is no recent admission assessment (AA8a = 01).
13.2 Short-stay residents who had moderate to severe pain Source: QM PAC-PAI0X	**Numerator:** Short-stay residents at SNF PPS 14-day assessment with moderate pain at least daily (J2a = 2 and J2b = 2) OR horrible/excruciating pain at any frequency (J2b = 3). **Denominator:** All patients with valid SNF PPS 14-day assessment (AA8b	

EXHIBIT 271 (Cont.)
QM/QI Reports Technical Specifications: Version 1.0

Measure Description	Measure Specifications	Covariates/Risk Adjustment
	= 7).	
	Exclusions: Patients satisfying any of the following conditions:	
	1. Either J2a or J2b is missing on the 14-day assessment.	
	2. The values of J2a and J2b are inconsistent on the 14-day assessment. J2a and J2b are inconsistent if either (a) J2a = 0 and J2b is not blank, or (b) J2a >0 and J2b = blank.	

13.3 Short-stay residents with pressure ulcers
 	
Source: QM PAC-PRU0X
	Numerator: Short-stay residents at SNF PPS 14-day assessment who satisfy either of the following conditions:
	
	1. On the SNF PPS 5-day assessment, the patient had no pressure sores (M2a[t-1] = 0) AND, on the SNF PPS 14-day assessment, the patient has at least a Stage 1 pressure sore (M2a[t] = 1,2,3, or 4).
	
	2. On the SNF PPS 5-day assessment, the patient had a pressure sore (M2a[t-1] = 1,2,3, or 4) AND on the SNF PPS 14-day assessment, pressure sores worsened or failed to improve (M2a[t]>= M2a[t-1]).
	
	Denominator: All patients with a valid SNF PPS 14-day assessment (AA8b = 7) AND a valid preceding SNF PPS 5-day assessment (AA8b = 1).
	
	Exclusions: Patients satisfying any of the following conditions:
	
	1. M2a is missing on the 14-day assessment [t].
	
	2. M2a is missing on the 5-day assessment [t-1] and M2a shows presence of pressure sores on the 14-day assessment (M2a = 1,2,3, or 4).
		Covariates:
		
		1. Indicator of history of resolved pressure sore on the SNF PPS 5-day assessment:
		
		    Covariate = 1 if M3 = 1
		    Covariate = 0 if M3 = 0
		
		2. Indicator of requiring limited or more assistance in bed mobility on the SNF PPS 5-day assessment:
		
		    Covariate = 1 if G1aA = 2,3,4, or 8
		    Covariate = 0 if G1aA =0 or 1
		
		3. Indicator of bowel incontinence at least one/week on the SNF PPS 5-day assessment:
		
		    Covariate = 1 if H1a = 2,3, or 4
		    Covariate = 0 if H1a = 0 or 1
		
		4. Indicator of diabetes or peripheral vascular disease on the SNF PPS 5-day assessment:
		
		    Covariate = 1 if I1a checked (value 1) OR I1j checked (value 1)

(continued)

EXHIBIT 271 (Cont.)
QM/QI Reports Technical Specifications: Version 1.0

Measure Description	Measure Specifications	Covariates/Risk Adjustment
		Covariate = 0 if I1a not checked (value 0) AND I1j not checked (value 0).
		5. Indicator of Low Body Mass Index (BMI) on the SNF PPS 5- day assessment:
		Covariate = 1 if BMI >= 12 AND <= 19 Covariate = 0 if BMI > 19 AND <= 40
		Where: BMI = weight (kg)/height^2 (m^2) = ((K2b*0.45)/(K2a)*.0254)^2)
		(Note: An implausible BMI value <12 or >40 will be treated as a missing value on this covariate.)

EXHIBIT 271 (Cont.)
QM/QI Reports Technical Specifications: Version 1.0
Selection of the Chronic Care Sample

The chronic care measure calculation sample involves selection of residents with a target assessment in the target period. For a selected resident, three different assessment records are then selected: target assessment, prior assessment and most recent full assessment.

Assessment Selected		Chronic Care Measure Selection Specifications
Target Assessment	**Selection period**	The QM/QI reports use a default 6 month target period, however the user can change this period if desired.
	Qualifying Reasons for Assessment (AA8a/AA8b)	01/*, 02/*, 03/*, 04/*, 05/*, 10/* (* indicates any value accepted)
	Selection Logic	Latest assessment with qualifying reasons for assessment and assessment reference date (A3a) within selection period.
	Rationale	Select a normal (OBRA) assessment from the target quarter. Normal OBRA assessments that are coupled with a PPS assessment (item AA8b = 1,2,3,4,5,7, or 8) are still selected. Selection ignores whether an assessment is also a PPS assessment or not.
Prior Assessment	**Selection period**	46 to 165 days before the target assessment
	Qualifying Reasons for Assessment (AA8a/AA8b)	01/*, 02/*, 03/*, 04/*, 05/*, 10/* (* indicates any value accepted)
	Selection Logic	Latest assessment with qualifying reasons for assessment and assessment reference date (A3a) in the window of 46 days to 165 days preceding the target assessment reference date (A3a).
	Rationale	Select a normal (OBRA) assessment in the 4-month window ending 46 days before the target assessment. This window insures that the gap between the prior and target assessment will not be small (gaps of 45 days or less are excluded). A 4-month window is employed to allow sufficient time to find an OBRA assessment. OBRA assessments are required every 3 months. A grace month has been added to yield a window of 4 months to account for late assessments. In the last half of 2000, scheduled OBRA assessments were late about 8 percent of the time. A relative window based on the assessment reference date (A3a) of the target assessment is used to accommodate cases in which scheduled assessments are performed early or a significant change occurs. Normal OBRA assessments that are coupled with a PPS assessment (item AA8b = 1,2,3,4,5,7, or 8) are still selected. Selection ignores whether an assessment is also a PPS assessment or not.

(continued)

EXHIBIT 271 (Cont.)
QM/QI Reports Technical Specifications: Version 1.0

Assessment Selected		Chronic Care Measure Selection Specifications
Most Recent Full Assessment	**Selection period**	Most recent 18.5 months preceding target assessment
	Qualifying Reasons for Assessment (AA8a/AA8b)	01/*, 02/*, 03/*, 04/* (* indicates any value accepted)
	Selection Logic	Latest assessment with qualifying reasons for assessment and assessment reference date (A3a) in the 18.5-month (or 562- day) period preceding the target assessment reference date (A3a).
	Rationale	Select a normal (OBRA) full assessment. Normal OBRA full assessments that are coupled with a PPS assessment (item AA8b = 1,2,3,4,5,7, or 8) are still selected. Selection ignores whether a full assessment is also a PPS assessment or not. If the target assessment is a quarterly assessment, it will at times be necessary to carry -forward items (not available on the quarterly assessment) from the most recent full assessment to that target assessment. The most recent full assessment will be used to carry forward values to a target quarterly assessment, but only if the most recent full assessment is in the 395 day period (approximately 13 months) preceding the target assessment reference date (A3a). A 13-month look-back period is employed to allow sufficient time to find an earlier OBRA full assessment. OBRA full assessments are required every 12 months. A grace month has been added to yield a look-back period of 13 months to account for late full assessments. If the prior assessment is a quarterly assessment, it will at times be necessary to carry -forward items (not available on the quarterly assessment) from the most recent full assessment to that prior assessment. The most recent full assessment will be used to carry forward values to a prior quarterly assessment, but only if the most recent full assessment is in the 395 day period (approximately 13 months) preceding the prior assessment reference date (A3a). A 13-month look-back period is employed to allow sufficient time to find an earlier OBRA full assessment. OBRA full assessments are required every 12 months. A grace month has been added to yield a look-back period of 13 months to account for late full assessments.

EXHIBIT 271 (Cont.)
QM/QI Reports Technical Specifications: Version 1.0
Selection of the Post-acute Care Sample

The post-acute measure calculation sample involves selection of residents with a 14-day SNF PPS assessment in the target period. If a resident has more than one 14-day assessment in the target period, then the latest 14-day assessment is selected. The appropriate 5-day assessment preceding the 14-day assessment is also selected, if available. One additional record is also selected, that record being the most recent admission assessment on the same date or before the selected 14-day assessment.

Assessment Selected		Post-acute Care Measure Selection Specifications
14-Day PPS Assessment	**Selection period**	The QM/QI reports use a default 6 month target period, however the user can change this period if desired.
	Qualifying Reasons for Assessment (AA8a/AA8b)	*/7 (*indicates any value accepted)
	Selection Logic	Select the latest 14-day assessment (*/7) with assessment reference date (A3a) in the selection period
	Rationale	If there are multiple qualifying assessments, the latest assessment is selected.
5-Day PPS Assessment	**Selection period**	The interval from 3 to 18 days before the selected 14-day assessment.
	Qualifying Reasons for Assessment (AA8a/AA8b)	*/1 (* indicates any value accepted)
	Selection Logic	Latest 5-day assessment with assessment reference date A3a) in the selection period for the same resident and facility.
	Rationale	Select a 5-day assessment (AA8b = 1) in the selection window preceding the selected 14-day assessment. The selection window (3 to 18 days prior to the 14-day assessment) allows for the 5-day to be completed on day 1 through day 8 of the stay and the 14-day to be completed on day 11 through day 19 of the stay, according to the SNF PPS assessment requirements. These requirements indicate that the gap between the 2 assessments should have a minimum of 3 and a maximum of 18 days. If there is more than one qualifying 5-day assessment in the selection window, then select the latest one.
Recent MDS Admission Assessment	**Selection period**	50-day period ending with the date of the selected 14-day assessment.
	Qualifying Reasons for Assessment (AA8a/AA8b)	01/* (* indicates any value accepted)
	Selection Logic	Select the latest admission assessment with assessment reference date (A3a) in the selection period.

(continued)

EXHIBIT 271 (Cont.)
QM/QI Reports Technical Specifications: Version 1.0

Assessment Selected		Post-acute Care Measure Selection Specifications
	Rationale	This admission assessment is needed to capture the facesheet item AB5 (prior institutional history). The facesheet must be completed on an admission assessment. If no facesheet record is found in the selection period, then assume that AB5a = 1, indicating residence in this facility prior to the SNF stay. The selection period allows sufficient look back to encounter a new resident's admission associated with the SNF covered stay. A SNF covered stay must begin within 30 days of the end of a qualifying hospitalization and the 14-day assessment must be performed by day 19 of the stay. This yields a look back period of 30 days plus 19 days, and this was rounded up 1 day to 50.

EXHIBIT 272

OVERVIEW OF MDS SUBMISSION RECORD
(Version 1.10 of the MDS Data Specifications)

With the new MDS 2.0 Correction Policy, previously unused space in the submission record has been assigned to accommodate information on the Correction Request Form. A submission record now consists of areas devoted to MDS Assessment or Tracking Form items **and** areas devoted to Correction Request Form information as follows:

Submission
Record

Correction Request Items	MDS Assessment or Tracking Form Items

The contents of a submission record vary depending upon whether the record is an original submission, a modification request, or an inactivation request, as displayed below:

Original
Submission
Record

BLANK	INCLUDED
Correction Request Items	MDS Assessment or Tracking Form Items

Modification
Request
Record

INCLUDED	INCLUDED
Correction Request Items	MDS Assessment or Tracking Form Items

Inactivation
Request
Record

INCLUDED	BLANK
Correction Request Items	MDS Assessment or Tracking Form Items

Exhibit 273
Correction Policy Summary Matrix

ACTIONS BY FACILITY

SCENARIO	1 Inactivate Record in State Database	2 Modify Record in State Database	3 Exclude Record from Submission	4 Correct Orig. Record In-House and Submit	5 Revise Care Plan if Necessary	6 No Sign. Change or Correct. Required	7 Perform and Submit Sign. Correction Assessment and Update Care Plan	8 Perform and Submit Sign. Change Assessment and Update Care Plan
1 Invalid asmt. (assessment) or tracking form record at State	✓							
2 Tracking form or non-OBRA asmt. error at State		✓						
2/6 Minor OBRA asmt. error at State		✓				✓		
2/7 Uncorr. Major OBRA asmt. error at State, no sign. change		✓					✓	
2/8 Uncorr. Major OBRA asmt. error at State, sign. change		✓						✓
3 Invalid assessment or tracking form record in-house			✓					
4 Tracking form or non-OBRA asmt. error in-house				✓				
4/5 Major/minor error in OBRA asmt. in edit phase in-house				✓	✓			
4/6 Minor error in OBRA asmt. in-house				✓		✓		
4/7 Uncorr. Major OBRA asmt. error in-house, no sign. change				✓			✓	
4/8 Uncorr. Major OBRA asmt. error in-house, sign. change				✓				✓

Exhibit 274

DEFINITION OF SELECTED DATES IN THE RAI PROCESS

TYPE OF RECORD	TARGET (OR EVENT) DATE	FINAL COMPLETION DATE
Assessment not Comprehensive (quarterly or full assessment without Section V)	A3a	R2b (all required assessment items complete)
Comprehensive Asmt. (includes Section V)	A3a	VB4 (final completion of comprehensive assessment and care plan)
Discharge Tracking Form	R4	R4
Reentry Tracking Form	A4a	A4a
Correction Request Form	----	AT6

Index